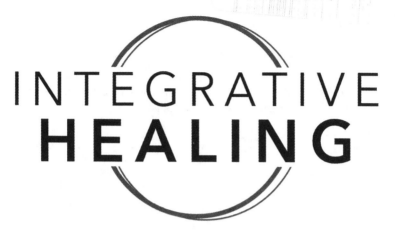

INTEGRATIVE
HEALING

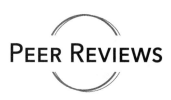

PEER REVIEWS

"This is one of the most comprehensive books I have read that integrates many aspects of mind and body medicine. Every person can find his/her own program to suit their lifestyle and needs. As a physical therapist, I recommend this book for every clinic as a reference source for patients and clinicians."

Avi Amit, PT, DPT
Director of Rehab Services
Olympia Medical Center
Los Angeles, California

"Everyone hopes to stay active and engaged throughout life. To do this you need a plan to guide you to manage stress and maintain mobility. *Integrative Healing: Developing Wellness in the Mind and Body* is this guide. Presented in an easy-to-follow format this book includes all of the pieces you need to stay active and well. You will find yourself flagging pages for reference again and again. The sources for these recommendations are noted and you can rely on this guide to supply you with a snapshot of the most valid and useful tools to help you get and stay healthy."

Tracy Gensler, MS, RD
Author of *Probiotic and Prebiotic Recipes for Health*
Coauthor of *The Anti-Aging Fitness Prescription*

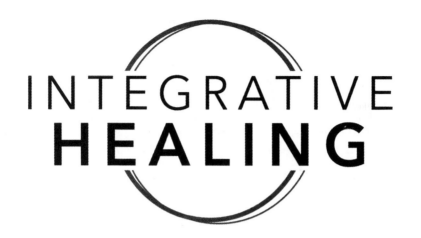

INTEGRATIVE HEALING

Developing
Wellness in the
Mind and Body

Z ALTUG PT, DPT, MS, CSCS

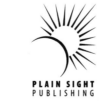

PLAIN SIGHT
PUBLISHING
An imprint of Cedar Fort, Inc.
Springville, Utah

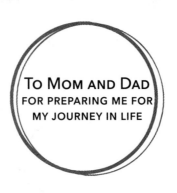

TO MOM AND DAD
FOR PREPARING ME FOR
MY JOURNEY IN LIFE

ISBN 13: 978-1-4621-2204-2

Published by Plain Sight Publishing, an imprint of Cedar Fort, Inc.
2373 W. 700 S., Springville, UT 84663
Distributed by Cedar Fort, Inc., www.cedarfort.com

LIBRARY OF CONGRESS CATALOGING-IN-PUBLICATION DATA

Names: Altug, Ziya, author.
Title: Integrative healing : developing wellness in the mind and body / Ziya Altug.
Description: Springville, Utah : Plain Sight Publishing, An imprint of Cedar Fort, Inc., [2018] | Includes bibliographical references and index.
Identifiers: LCCN 2018003807 (print) | LCCN 2018010526 (ebook) | ISBN 9781462128990 (epub, pdf, mobi) | ISBN 9781462122042 (perfect bound : alk. paper)
Subjects: LCSH: Integrative medicine. | Exercise. | Health.
Classification: LCC R733 (ebook) | LCC R733 .A528 2018 (print) | DDC 613.7--dc23
LC record available at https://lccn.loc.gov/2018003807

Cover design by Shawnda T. Craig
Cover design © 2018 Cedar Fort, Inc.
Edited by Erin Tanner, Erica Myers, and Allie Bowen
Typeset by Kaitlin Barwick

Printed in the United States of America

10 9 8 7 6 5 4 3 2 1

Printed on acid-free paper

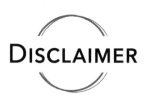

DISCLAIMER

This book is for educational purposes and is not a substitute for medical advice, diagnosis, or treatment. All reasonable effort has been made to ensure the accuracy of the information in this book. However, due to ongoing research and discoveries, the information in this book may not reflect the latest standards, developments, or treatments.

Readers who have questions about a particular condition or treatment should consult with a physician or healthcare provider. The publisher and author shall not be liable for any damages allegedly arising from the information in this book. The publisher and author are also not responsible for errors or omissions or for any consequences from the application of the information in this book and makes no warranty, expressed or implied, with respect to the currency, completeness, or accuracy of the contents of the publication. This work is merely a reference tool.

As with all health and fitness programs, the reader should get a physician's approval before beginning an exercise, nutrition, or any other self-help routine. Any practice or guideline described in this book should be applied by the reader in conjunction with the advice of his or her healthcare provider and/or fitness professional.

Remember to follow these four golden rules: 1) Do no harm. 2) If you are in doubt about something in this book, check it out with your healthcare provider and/or fitness professional. 3) Start slowly and progress gradually. 4) And, finally, listen to your mind and body and do not exceed your physical and mental abilities.

All trademarks, trade names, model names and numbers, and any other designations referred to herein are the property of their respective owners and are used solely for identification purposes.

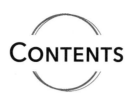

CONTENTS

Holistic Healing Box Index

Exercise Index

Warm-Up Exercises

Aerobic Exercises

Strength Exercises

Flexibility Exercises

Balance Exercises

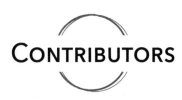

CONTRIBUTORS

JUAN CIFUENTES
Photographer
Los Angeles, California

Chapters 2, 6–11, and 13
www.juancifuentes.com

LILIAN CIFUENTES
Graphic Designer

Los Angeles, California

ROMY PHILLIPS, MFA, E-RYT 500, C-IAYT
Certified Yoga Therapist / Yoga
Practitioner

Yogathology

Los Angeles, California

www.yogathology.com

Author of *Yoga Forma: A Visual
Resource Guide for the Spine
and Lower Back* (Cedar Fort
Publishing, 2018)

Contributor to Chapter 6: Yoga
for Health

DEREK PLONKA, DPT, MTOM, L.AC, CSCS
Doctor of Physical Therapy /
Licensed Acupuncturist

Insight Wellness Clinic

Santa Monica, California

www.insightwellnessclinic.com

Contributor to portions of
Chapter 2: Managing Your Stress

Contributor to Chapter 7: Tai Chi
for Health

Contributor to Chapter 8: Qigong
for Health

MAVIS RODE, PT, DPT, CSCS
Doctor of Physical Therapy /
Pilates Practitioner

Mavis Rode Physical Therapy

Los Angeles, California

www.mrodept.com

Contributor to Chapter 9: Pilates
for Health

BRIDGET QUEBODEAUX, GCFP, LMFT
Guild Certified Feldenkrais
Practitioner^cm and Licensed
Marriage and Family Therapist

Center for Physical Health

Los Angeles, CA

www.feldenkraiswestla.com

www.emotion-focused.com

Contributor to Chapter 10:
Feldenkrais Method® for Health

LEAH ZHANG, MFA, AmSAT, CEAS II
Alexander Technique Teacher /
Certified Ergonomics Specialist

Leah Zhang Alexander Technique
Studio

Los Angeles, CA

www.leahteachesalexander.com

Contributor to Chapter 11:
Alexander Technique for Health

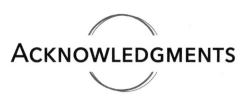

ACKNOWLEDGMENTS

First, I thank my family for their support and encouragement in all my creative pursuits. I also thank my brother, Aykut Altug, for his meticulous editing of the manuscript.

I would like to thank Debbie Cheung at the Institute for Natural Resources for introducing me to Cedar Fort Publishing.

I thank the entire team at Cedar Fort Publishing for their effort and enthusiasm, with special thanks to Bryce Mortimer, Jessica Pettit, Kaitlin Barwick, Vikki Downs, Shawnda Craig, Erin Tanner, Erica Myers, and Allie Bowen.

I thank Lilian Cifuentes for being the model in the chapter 13 exercise photographs.

I thank photographer Juan Cifuentes for all the exercise photographs in chapters 2, 6 through 11, and 13.

I thank physical therapist Marc A. Pierre, MS, PT for letting us use his clinic, The Center for Physical Health in Los Angeles, for the Feldenkrais Method photo shoot.

I thank Allen Au for being the model for the Alexander Technique photographs in chapter 11.

I thank all my contributors for providing amazing content.

Finally, I thank my physical therapy patients and clients for asking great questions and helping me to keep my knowledge current.

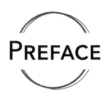

PREFACE

Dear Reader,

The purpose of *Integrative Healing: Developing Wellness in the Mind and Body* is to provide an evidence-based practical, foundation which bridges the gap between Eastern and Western movement systems and practices. The book is written in a format that largely uses bullet points, checklists, tables, charts, and boxes to help readers easily extract and use the information.

Integrative Healing can be used by a wide range of people, including the following:

- **Individual consumers** looking for simple tips and guidelines to supplement the advice provided by their healthcare professionals. As a reader, you will work with your healthcare provider to decide which strategies in this reference book will best serve your needs. There is no substitute for proper medical care.
- **Healthcare professionals** (such as physicians, physical therapists, occupational therapists, speech therapists, respiratory therapists, athletic trainers, nurses, pharmacists, registered dietitians, psychologists, psychiatrists, addiction counselors, marriage and family therapists, chiropractors, osteopathic physicians, naturopathic physicians, homeopaths, and acupuncturists), **Fitness professionals** (such as personal trainers, conditioning coaches, and exercise physiologists), **Practitioners** (such as massage therapists, bodyworkers, art therapists, music therapists, and recreational therapists and also practitioners of yoga, tai chi, qigong, Pilates, the Feldenkrais Method, and the Alexander Technique) to educate their patients or clients on evidence-based self-management strategies for holistic health, healing, and wellness.
- **Coaches** to discuss various performance-enhancing and healing strategies with their athletes.
- **Parents** to discuss various healthy lifestyle behaviors with their children to take advantage of the prime growing and learning years.

I look forward to serving as your guide as you embark on your mind body journey for improving your health.

Z Altug, PT, DPT, MS, CSCS
Los Angeles, CA

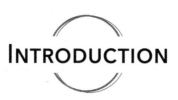

INTRODUCTION

Integrative Healing is about including advice and recommendations from your doctor and healthcare provider in your health and wellness program. However, it is also about incorporating lifestyle changes such as managing stress, getting adequate sleep, eating nourishing foods, meditating, and performing fun and meaningful exercises. As my dad, a physician specializing in internal medicine for 46 years, would say, "Feeling well is rarely a random event." In other words, many aspects of our health are not random. Our health is mainly a result of our habits (such as to smoke or not smoke), choices (such as our choice to eat healthy foods or going for the quick and unhealthy fast food), and the environments (such as work and relationships) we put ourselves in.

This book is not obsessed with or focused on a particular philosophy, such as being on Paleo (Paleolithic), Keto (Ketogenic), vegan (vegetarian), or IF (intermittent fasting) diets, or a type of exercise such as HIIT (high intensity interval training), functional training, or body weight training. The focus of this book is to help you explore and discover which nutrition, exercise, sleep, mindfulness, and stress management approaches work best for your mind and body. Mind and body practices can allow your mind and body to slow down from overthinking things (mental stress) and overdoing things (physical stress). This book is written through my personal experiences, my clinical practice, and from the evidence provided in research.

WHAT DOES "INTEGRATIVE, ALTERNATIVE, AND COMPLEMENTARY MEDICINE" MEAN?

The National Center for Complementary and Integrative Health (nccih.nih.gov) defines the terms as follows:

- "If a non-mainstream practice is used **together with** conventional medicine, it's considered 'complementary.'"
- "If a non-mainstream practice is used **in place of** conventional medicine, it's considered 'alternative.'"
- Integrative health care involves "bringing conventional and complementary **approaches together** in a coordinated way." The integrative approach typically involves pain management, relief of symptoms, and promoting healthy behaviors.

The integrative health care movement has expanded so much is recent years that mainstream medical facilities are now offering nontraditional strategies to help patients and families manage their health. For a list of some of the current medical institutions participating in integrative medicine, refer to the Academic Consortium for Integrative Medicine & Health (www.imconsortium.org).

WHAT IS MIND BODY MEDICINE?

The mind body medicine model includes self-care and self-awareness as a key component of care, treats the person in a holistic manner, aims to get at the root cause of an illness or disease, and encourages adopting a healthy lifestyle, which includes wholesome nutrition, meaningful exercise, restorative sleep, stress management strategies, meditation, mindfulness, balance between work and rest, and finally, involvement in healthy relationships. Some of the basic foundations of mind body medicine are that the program accounts for differences in each individual (not everyone gets the same program), the program is sustainable (the program is not a one-month- and-done routine), and the program is meaningful to the person. Some of the clinical uses of mind body medicine (or integrative healing) include treatment and care for anxiety, attention-deficit/hyperactivity disorder (ADHD), central sensitization (or heightened sensitivity to pain), depression, fibromyalgia, headache or migraines, pain, pain catastrophizing, post-traumatic stress disorder, sleep disorders, and chronic stress.

MY PERSONAL HEALING JOURNEY

In a viewpoint published in the JAMA Network in 2017 (Ioannidis 2017), the authors conclude that "As a general rule, if an author's living example could be reasonably expected to influence how some readers perceive an article, disclosure should be encouraged. Authors who have strong beliefs and make highly committed choices for diet or other behaviors should not hesitate to disclose them. Doing so may help everyone understand who is promoting what and why." I agree! For this reason, I am disclosing some of my ongoing personal experiences in improving my health in this section.

I was diagnosed with Hashimoto's thyroiditis in 2004 by my family physician. My symptoms at the time included severe fatigue, anxiety, mental fogginess, and periodic panic attacks. I was also about 25 pounds overweight even though I exercised every day, which included some high-intensity workouts. Even my job as a physical therapist was very active, so it wasn't like I was sitting at a desk all day. Something was just not right in my body.

I followed the advice of my doctors (family physician and *endocrinologist*), but I also took charge of my health by improving many aspects of my life. Those changes had a positive effect on my personal health and my medical condition. Some of you may be curious about the changes I made. I know many of my patients in physical therapy routinely ask me what I did to make improvements in my health and how I maintain these changes. Well, here is what I did to improve my health:

1. **Physical Examination:** I get a yearly medical checkup from my family physician at UCLA and undergo any needed tests (such as blood tests and urinalysis). It was my family physician who discovered my Hashimoto's thyroiditis and then referred me to an amazing endocrinologist at UCLA. I receive great care and I am very grateful for their knowledge and compassion. A simple, yearly medical exam saved me from suffering for many years with the symptoms I mentioned above. I firmly believe everyone should get a yearly medical exam just to monitor things and catch any potential problems early on. A yearly physical exam is something I have been getting since I was around 10 years old, since my father was a physician specializing in internal medicine. Thanks Dad!

2. **More Knowledge:** In addition to the information and guidance my physicians have provided (and continue to provide), I also needed to do my part by taking charge of my health. I have never smoked, do not drink alcohol, do not consume caffeine or soft drinks, eat a healthy diet, usually get enough sleep and stay physically active, but I still needed some changes in my lifestyle. I needed better strategies to control my fast-paced, Type A personality, fine-tune my diet, and change my constant high-intensity approach to exercise. First, I read the book *Hashimotos's Thyroiditis: Lifestyle Interventions for Finding and Treating the Root Cause* (2013) by pharmacist Izabella Wentz. Now she has the new book *Hashimoto's Protocol* (2017). I also learned many things from the *Thyroid Healthy* (2014) book by pharmacist Suzy Cohen. Both authors deliver amazing practical content. Thank you both for helping make improvements in my life! You never know what kind of amazing life-changing gems you are going to find in any book you read. See Box 6: Hashimoto's Thyroiditis in chapter 4 if you are interested in this topic.

3. **Diet Change:** After reading the books by both pharmacists, I modified my diet so it agrees with my body physiology. Even though I use the "food first" approach to nutrition, I do take some low-dose supplements for my needs. Through some trial and error, I found this approach works for me. However, I am always open-minded enough to allow for future changes.

4. **Modified Exercises:** I now exercise at lower intensities (yes, my Type A personality is now under control) and do movements and activities for fun. I engage in some weight training, walking, yoga, tai chi, qigong, and basketball. I guess I finally realized I am not an elite athlete and do

not need to train like one! I also tell my patients that I was apparently born to be a rabbit (fast and swift) but I aspire to be like a turtle (slow and calm).

5. **Quality Sleep:** I make sure that every night I get 8 to 9 hours of restful sleep.

6. **Meditate:** I meditate and do self-hypnosis every morning right after my calisthenics and qigong routine. This sets up my day by getting my body moving in a relaxed manner.

7. **Manage Stress:** My stress management strategies include playing with my cats, listening to music, watching comedy shows, learning about astronomy, and writing. Yes, writing this book has been a very pleasant experience!

8. **Limit Media Exposure:** I minimize my exposure to bad news since the news is now a 24-hour cycle. Yes, the news keeps us informed, but I don't think the human mind and body were meant to be exposed to a continuous cycle of bad news coming at us from every angle. I also limit my time on social media since I want time to be in nature, and talk to my friends and family in person. My mother also taught me to always save time to explore my world through travel, books, music, and art. And I do. Thanks Mom!

9. **Enjoy Family, Friends, and Job:** I am very grateful that I enjoy my job as a physical therapist and I get along very well with my coworkers, family, and friends. I did not need to makes changes in this area.

10. **Minimize Potentially Harmful Chemicals**: Finally, I have minimized the use of unnecessary chemicals in my personal care products and during household cleaning. I try to use simple and natural alternatives when I can. For example, I use baking soda mixed with some water as my deodorant (warning: baking soda like Arm & Hammer may irritate some skin types and it does not function as an antiperspirant—which is fine by me since I do not want to block things in this sensitive area). It works for me!

11. **Daily Journal**: I have kept a daily journal / diary for many years (more on that later in the book) to help me monitor and modify my diet, exercise, and other lifestyle habits as needed. The journal and my morning 20-minute exercise and meditation routine, followed by a nice breakfast, helps to kick off my day on a positive note.

So, that's my story in case you are wondering how I made lifestyle changes to improve my health. Please note that I am not trying to encourage anyone to do things the way I do. I follow a Paleo diet, but you may be best suited to follow a vegetarian diet. No problem. I do qigong and yoga, but you may do Pilates and play softball. Awesome! I routinely tell my patients in physical therapy that what I am showing them is "a way" and not "the way." Use what you wish from my personal stories and interpretations in this book, but by all means, please find "your way." So yes, I have to work at my lifestyle changes every day but in the long run, it's all worth it. Staying healthy allows me to continue doing the job I love. I am grateful I am able to help others and along the way I hope I am able to make a small but positive difference in the world. It is my sincere wish that each of you discover something in this book to help you improve your health and overall well-being so you have a pleasant journey in life.

What Is Unique about This Book?

You may ask how this health and wellness book is so different than the others on the market. Let me count the ways. My book is:

- **A Hybrid:** The book is part reference and resource manual and also part workbook to help you find relevant topics for your needs and apply that information in an easy-to-use manner.
- **Clinically Relevant:** I bring my 28 years of practical experiences and scientific inquiries as a licensed physical therapist and make them available in this book. If you wish to know more about my background than what is written in the book bio, please see my LinkedIn page for my full professional resume.
- **Evidence-Based:** The book uses mainly evidence-based research to explain the facts and benefits of the recommend strategies. The book has over 750 scientific references.
- **Reviewed:** The book is peer-reviewed by professionals in the field to ensure quality.
- **Practical:** The book outlines many easy-to-use training programs that may be performed in the comfort of your home.
- **Mindful:** The book includes many strategies to help you stay relaxed and focused on what is important to you.
- **Integrative:** The book draws information from Eastern and Western approaches to wellness.
- **Holistic:** The book has contributors from a variety of disciplines who are experienced professionals in their respective fields.
- **User-friendly:** The book is written in an easy-to-read format with lists, tables, and boxes and uses just enough prose to provide practical examples.
- **Full of Practical Lessons:** The Mind Body Health section outlines ready-to-use introductory lessons for yoga, tai chi, qigong, Pilates, Feldenkrais Method, and the Alexander Technique.

Your Holistic Health Team

Be sure to check out Appendix A: Medical and Wellness Associations for further information regarding your holistic care.

Icons Used In the Book

There are several icons used in this book. They are there to give you visual cues about the practical mental and physical training programs throughout the book. Here are the icons I will use:

 This icon lets you know that there is a practical mental training or relaxation program you may use.

 This icon lets you know that there is a practical physical training or activity program you may use.

 This icon lets you know that there is a healthy choice you can make.

How to Proceed from Here

You can read the book from the beginning or jump around to chapters which interest you most. I will also post lots of free bonus materials to this book on my website and other social media. So stay tuned! You already know that I don't have all the answers to health and wellness, but *your* mind and body does. This book is a tool to help you search for the answers for your optimal health and well-being. Okay, let's dive into the book and begin your journey.

Reference

Ioannidis JPA, Trepanowski JF. (2017). Disclosures in nutrition research: Why it is different. *JAMA*. Electronic publication ahead of print.

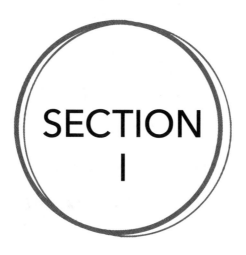

SECTION I

LIFESTYLE MEDICINE

This section introduces you to some key concepts you can use to make lifestyle changes for improving your health and well-being.

Many of the leading causes of death in the United States are related to lifestyle factors such as lack of exercise and sleep, poor diet, uncontrolled stress, obesity, tobacco use, and overconsumption of alcohol. Lifestyle medicine helps in the treatment and prevention of many medical conditions such as anxiety, cancer, cardiovascular disease, dementia, depression, hypertension, obesity, osteoarthritis, sarcopenia, stroke, and type-2 diabetes. The four primary pillars of lifestyle medicine include nutrition, stress management, adequate sleep, and exercise.

CHAPTER 1

MINDFULNESS AND
RELAXATION TRAINING

"Wherever you go, there you are."

—Jon Kabat-Zinn, PhD

I routinely tell my patients that "your body believes what your brain tells it." Of course this is an oversimplification, but there is a purpose to the statement. In athletic competition, if our brain is thinking I can't do something or is focused on negative thoughts, there is a good chance the body won't be able to perform the way we want it to (Josefsson et al. 2017). The same holds true for my patients trying to accomplish a task, such as going down stairs or crossing a city street without fear. Once the person has the necessary strength, balance, and stamina, they ultimately need to believe and be confident that they can do the task.

So what does this have to do with mindfulness and relaxation? First, a person needs to be connected to the moment or a task at hand before they can be highly successful at it. Then they need to be relaxed and calm enough to perform the task. This isn't always true but highly desirable. For example, even a sprinter trying to run at full speed needs to have a certain amount of focus and relaxation while running in order to allow for fluid motion and prevent unnecessary tension. Another way to think of it is that you can't step on the gas pedal and the brake at the same time if you want to accomplish certain tasks. So in my clinical world, I have found that being mindful can help unlock the mind and the body.

WHAT IS MINDFULNESS?

There are several interpretations as to what mindfulness means. One definition is that mindfulness-based stress reduction is "the use of meditation and self-awareness to enhance one's ability to cope with challenging circumstances and psychological tensions" (Venes 2017). Another way to look at it is that "Mindfulness meditation is a technique to help us quiet the mind" (Savel et al. 2017). You will read about more interpretations in this chapter and throughout the book. The main purpose of this chapter is to share my collection of practical mindfulness routines for you to try. This way, you can see which one(s) works best for your needs. However, I do want to point to one of my clinical observations about being mindful and relaxed. Simply doing mindfulness exercises may not be enough to "quiet the mind." The person may have to dig deeper to find the root cause of their anxiety or mental unrest. Perhaps the root cause is eating trigger foods or nutrient deficiencies, lack of quality sleep, or not engaging in a fun or meaningful exercise program. It could also be that a person may need counseling and the expert guidance of a psychologist or psychiatrist. However, using the techniques outlined in this chapter and book can serve as good adjuncts to other medical care.

WHAT ARE THE BENEFITS OF MINDFULNESS TRAINING?

According to the UCLA Mindful Awareness Research Center, the benefits of mindfulness training may impact your health in the following ways (UCLA Mindful Awareness Research Center 2017):

- Help you to reduce stress
- Help to reduce chronic physical pain
- Serve as a boost to the immune system
- Help reduce emotional reactivity
- Help increase self-awareness
- Help improve attention and concentration
- Help you enhance positive emotions
- Help you cultivate well-being and happiness
- Impact the brain in a positive manner

DIAPHRAGMATIC BREATHING AND SPINE DECOMPRESSION

Purpose: To relax the mind and body, and decompress the spine. Diaphragmatic breathing (or belly breathing or abdominal breathing) may be helpful for stress reduction, relaxation, pain control, lymphedema, and thoracic outlet syndrome (Kisner et al. 2018).

Positions: Supine position (lying down on your back, face-up) for relaxation and decompression, or a seated position for relaxation only.

Technique and Design:

- Start by lying on your back with knees bent to approximately 90 degrees, feet shoulder-width apart.

- Breathe in through your nose as if trying to draw in a pleasant aroma. Then, breathe out as if you want to make the flame of a candle in front of your mouth start to flicker without blowing it out (Eherer et al. 2012).
- Once you are good at this exercise in a lying position, try it when sitting, standing, or doing gentle stretches.
- Do one set of 10 to 20 slow breaths for a brief relaxation period. For a more extended relaxation period and also to decompress the spine, try lying on your back with your legs either straight or elevated (supported on pillows, a bolster or cushion, or placed on a sofa or chair) for 5 to 15 minutes. May be performed daily.

Precaution: If your chest rises more than your abdomen, you might be performing the exercise incorrectly. Try again, and be patient. It takes practice and a little coordination to master this exercise.

Alternate Spine Decompression Strategies:

- Try a sidelying position with the knees bent, while hugging a pillow with your arms, and placing a separate pillow between your knees (do for 5 to 15 minutes)
- Try assuming a hands-and-knees position (do for one minute)
- Try partially hanging from a pull-up bar or a doorframe, with your feet still touching the ground (do three sets for 10 to 15 seconds)
- Try relaxing in a pool (do for 5 to 15 minutes)
- Try reclining in a good reclining chair (do for 5 to 15 minutes)
- Try a rocking chair (do for 5 to 15 minutes)
- Speak with a medical professional about using a spine belt or brace
- Speak with a medical professional about using a traction device

MINI-MEDITATION BREAKS

Purpose: To ease your mind when you can't get to sleep, you have a big test, or you're in stressful situation. Or, you can use mini-meditation breaks (or what I call "waiting meditation") while standing in a busy line during shopping, waiting at a red light, or passing time in a doctor's or dentist's waiting area. I recommend putting down the phone and taking advantage of the golden opportunity to allow yourself to relax multiple times every day rather than waiting for your three sessions every week. I personally use the "waiting meditations" all the time and I am no longer impatient about waiting in line or waiting for an appointment. I now view it as my time to relax.

Positions: Sitting or lying down

Technique and Design:

- See the Diaphragmatic Breathing and Spine Decompression section above.

- Do 5 to 20 slow diaphragmatic breaths as you focus on pleasant scenery such as a beach or mountain overlook (or other relaxing mental images of your choice).

MINDFULNESS WALKING PROGRAM

A study by Gotink et al. (2016) concludes that "Mindful walking in nature may be an effective way to maintain mindfulness practice and further improve psychological functioning." Another study by Teut et al. (2013) indicates that a mindful walking program can help reduce psychological stress and improve quality of life.

Purpose: Mental and physical relaxation

Location: Pick a pleasant place to walk, such as a park, university campus, neighborhood, or local trail

 Technique and Design:

- Get familiar with your course. On a day prior to your relaxation walk, time the course you will be walking so there will be no need to look at a watch to know how long you have been walking. You can time a course for 15 minutes to an hour, depending on your fitness level and goals.
- Bring a small bottle of water flavored with some mint or basil leaves (or fruits like a cut strawberry).
- Take off your watch and turn off your phone before you start the walk.
- Direct your thoughts away from potential stressors. Ideally, during the relaxation walking program, you should make no judgments (about yourself or others), no decisions, and no plans.
- Start walking slowly, and continue walking at a pace your body is comfortable with for the day. Some days you might walk slowly and others days faster. This is not an aerobic routine for burning calories (although some calories will be burned). This program is for relaxation.
- Check your posture as you walk. How do you carry yourself? Are you tense or relaxed? Make small adjustments, such as walking tall and relaxed with your head up, for comfort and ease of movement.
- Focus on your feet. Feel each step for hardness or softness. Make small adjustments in your walking pattern for comfort and ease of movement.
- Notice your surroundings. What colors do you see? What shapes do you notice in the rocks and trees? How does the air smell? Do you hear or see any birds and animals? Do you feel the wind in your face? How do your clothes feel on your body? Take a small sip of your water. How does it taste?
- Notice your breathing. Is it slow or fast? Make small adjustments in your breathing pattern to see if you feel better, move freer, and breathe easier.
- Notice your thoughts. Where does your mind want to drift off to?

- Stop and perform the Calf Stretch exercise (see chapter 13) at the end of your walk. Instead of counting to 30, breathe in and out slowly 10 times as you stretch each leg.
- Sit or lie down in the grass. Close your eyes and relax. Feel the texture of the surface you are sitting or lying on. Is the surface firm or soft, warm or cool?
- Take 10 to 20 diaphragmatic breaths. Think about a color, sound, shape, taste, or feeling you experienced during your walk as you continue breathing diaphragmatically.
- Enjoy the rest of your day.

LABYRINTH WALKING PROGRAM

The labyrinth is an ancient meditative tool which has been in existence for thousands of years (Bigard 2009). Some of the ancient Nazca Lines in Peru may have been a labyrinth at one time for spiritual or meditation purposes (Ruggles et al. 2012). Labyrinth walking may be used in correctional facilities to improve coping (Maruca et al. 2016), mental health facilities for reflection, stress reduction, and the exploration of personal wellness (Heard et al. 2015) and be incorporated in healing gardens in cancer treatment centers (Griffith et al. 2002; Nicholson et al. 2002). A labyrinth is unlike a maze because a walking labyrinth has one path that brings you to the center and out again (Daniels 2008), while a maze generally has multiple paths and is designed to make you lose your way. A labyrinth, on the other hand, is designed to help a person find their way physically, mentally, and spiritually.

Purpose: Mental and physical relaxation. Also, a labyrinth may be used to train the vestibular system and help improve balance and coordination.

Locations:

- Find a labyrinth path in your community by checking the World-Wide Labyrinth Locator website (labyrinthlocator.com). A walking labyrinth may be found at public parks, schools, medical centers, rehabilitation centers, museums, or churches.
- Create your own labyrinth in your community or backyard by using stones, ropes, or a canvas.
- Create or use a paper or wood carving labyrinth for you to trace with your fingertip.
- Take a virtual labyrinth walk (labyrinthsociety.org/virtual-labyrinth -walk).

Technique:

- Take several diaphragmatic breaths to help clear your mind.

- Enter the labyrinth. Allow the walk or finger tracing on a paper labyrinth to take you on whatever mental and physical journey that is intended for that day.
- As you exit the labyrinth, take note of how you feel.

Additional Labyrinth Resources:
- A Maze Your Mind: Labyrinth Solutions, www.amazeyourmindlabyrinths.com
- Finger Labyrinths, www.bwatsonstudios.com
- Labyrinth Company, www.labyrinthcompany.com
- Labyrinthos, www.labyrinthos.net
- Relax4Life, www.relax4life.com
- The Labyrinth Society, labyrinthsociety.org
- Veriditas, www.veriditas.org

PROGRESSIVE RELAXATION TRAINING

"An anxious mind cannot exist in a relaxed body."

—Edmund Jacobson, MD, PhD

Relaxation slows heart rate, decreases blood pressure, and helps reduces anxiety and pain. Try the following two time-tested, adapted techniques of progressive relaxation created by pioneering psychiatrist Edmund Jacobson, MD, PhD (1888–1983).

Do these relaxation techniques while sitting in a chair, lying on your bed, reclining in the park on some soft grass, or relaxing at the beach (Jacobson 1962, 1964, 1964, 1967, 1976). Go *very* slowly through each two-and-a-half-minute routine, and breathe naturally. For best results, loosen tight clothing and remove shoes, lie on your back with a small towel under your lower back (if needed) with a small pillow under your knees, and close your eyes.

PHYSICAL PROGRESSIVE RELAXATION ROUTINE

This is a total body relaxation routine. You can have a therapist, trainer, or friend call out the relaxation sequences, or you can record the commands to play at your desired time intervals.

- To start, breathe in and out slowly three times using diaphragmatic breathing.
- Take a deep chest breath, and then relax with a diaphragmatic breath.
- Wrinkle up your forehead for five seconds, and then relax with two diaphragmatic breaths.
- Frown for five seconds, and then relax with two diaphragmatic breaths.

- Press your lips together for five seconds, and then relax with two diaphragmatic breaths.
- Shrug for five seconds, and then relax with two diaphragmatic breaths.
- Tighten your arm muscles for five seconds, and then relax with two diaphragmatic breaths.
- Make a fist for five seconds, and then relax with two diaphragmatic breaths.
- Tighten your abdominal muscles for five seconds, and then relax with two diaphragmatic breaths.
- Tighten your buttock muscles for five seconds, and then relax with two diaphragmatic breaths.
- Tighten your thigh muscles for five seconds, and then relax with two diaphragmatic breaths.
- Flex your toes toward you tightly for five seconds, and then relax with two diaphragmatic breaths.
- Point your toes away from you tightly for five seconds, and then relax with two diaphragmatic breaths.
- Squeeze your toes tightly for five seconds, and then relax with two diaphragmatic breaths.
- To end, smile lightly for five seconds, and then relax with two diaphragmatic breaths.

MENTAL PROGRESSIVE RELAXATION ROUTINE

This is a total body relaxation routine. You can have a therapist, trainer, or friend call out the relaxation sequences, or you can record the commands to play at your desired time intervals.

Refer to the above Physical Progressive Relaxation Routine, but in this case, apply the think-only technique. In other words, instead of actually wrinkling your forehead, simply think about doing it.

FACIAL RELAXATION ROUTINE

This is a facial relaxation routine. In my clinical experience relaxing the facial region alone can have a total body relaxation effect, reduce headaches, and decrease neck tension and temporomandibular joint (TMJ) pain. You can have a therapist, trainer, or friend call out the relaxation sequences, or you can record the commands to play at your desired time intervals. The seated version of the routine can be used in the office as a mini-relaxation break.

- To start, consider putting a little lavender essential oil on your shoulders or on a pillow. Also, you can put on some gentle and relaxing instrumental music.
- Now, lie down and rest your head on a pillow or sit with your head supported.

- Make sure you have a relaxed "neutral" jaw position. Your mouth should be closed lightly, with lips together and teeth not touching. Rest the upper part of the tip of your tongue against the hard palate just behind your upper central incisors (Flexner et al. 2018; Rocabado et al. 1991) and perform two diaphragmatic breaths.
- Relax your eye muscles (no squinting) and forehead muscles (no raised eyebrows).
- Close your eyes lightly and mentally "time travel" to your favorite place which provides you comfort and happiness and perform two diaphragmatic breaths.
- Breathe in and out slowly through your nose five times using diaphragmatic breathing.
- Smile partially and perform two diaphragmatic breaths.
- Keep your eyes closed the remainder of this routine. Now, mentally check your jaw and make sure the muscles are relaxed (no clenching of the teeth) and perform two diaphragmatic breaths.
- Mentally check your eyes and make sure the muscles are relaxed and perform two diaphragmatic breaths.
- Mentally check your eyebrows and make sure the muscles are relaxed with no tension in between the eyebrows and perform two diaphragmatic breaths.
- Mentally check your forehead and make sure the muscles are relaxed with no tension above your eyes and perform two diaphragmatic breaths.
- Mentally check your shoulders and make sure the muscles are relaxed and perform two diaphragmatic breaths.
- Thinks about your favorite place again and perform two diaphragmatic breaths.
- Slowly open your eyes and enjoy the rest of the day, or drift off to sleep if you perform this before you go to bed.

ADDITIONAL RESOURCES

- Carolyn McManus, PT, MS, MA, carolynmcmanus.com (search for Guided Relaxation & Meditation).

BOX 1: HOLISTIC HEALING

CONTROLLING TYPE A BEHAVIOR

According to cardiologists Meyer Friedman and Ray Rosenman, a Type A person may be considered someone who is impatient, aggressive, and very competitive. On the other hand, a Type B person may be viewed as being relaxed, patient, and easy going. A study by Friedman et al. (1986) indicates that "altering type A behavior reduces cardiac morbidity and mortality in post infarction patients." Although these findings about personality traits affecting health are considered controversial by some clinicians, it is a concept worth exploring. You can't necessarily change your personality, but you can certainly strive to make changes in unhealthy behavior patterns.

Consider the following:

- Observe and study successful type B personalities, and notice how they approach challenges and life in general.
- Live long and prosper, but don't annoy everyone around you with type A personality traits. Accept that not everyone has a perfectionist attitude.
- Don't feed the type A personality "beast" by engaging in high-intensity activities. Slow down to achieve balance. Try soothing activities such as yoga, tai chi, walking, and hiking, or hobbies like painting and music.
- Go home. Once you put in a reasonable amount of work for the day, relax or engage in a fun hobby. As some say, "Work to live and not live to work."
- Unplug. Limit daily time on blogs and social networks. Set aside a small amount of time every day to check in and connect, but focus on being creative and enjoying other aspects of life.
- Always watching your watch? Stop that! Learn to coexist with time, and don't let it rule your life.
- Rock 'n' roll on a rocking chair to relax and unwind.
- Be a classical music aficionado.
- Tame your temper, and cultivate calmness.
- Take regular vacations.
- Learn stress- and anger-management strategies.
- See a counselor to come to terms with unresolved personal issues.

MINDFULNESS AND MEDITATION TRAINING

"We take care of the future best by taking care of the present now."

—Jon Kabat-Zinn, PhD

A form of mindfulness-based stress reduction was developed by Jon Kabat-Zinn, PhD at the University of Massachusetts Medical School, Center for Mindfulness. A definition proposed by Kabat-Zinn (2003) for mindfulness meditation is "the awareness that emerges through paying attention on purpose, in the present moment, and nonjudgmentally to the unfolding of experience moment by moment."

For example, research shows that mindfulness meditation can reduce anxiety (Chen et al. 2012) and benefit some individuals with multiple sclerosis in terms of quality of life (Simpson et al. 2014). Also, combining cognitive behavioral therapy and mindfulness meditation might have long-term beneficial effects on insomnia (Ong et al. 2009).

A study by Fredrickson et al. (2008) concludes that "just as the broaden-and-build theory predicts, then, when people open their hearts to positive emotions, they . . . [make it possible to grow] in ways that transform them for the better."

TRANSCENDENTAL MEDITATION

Transcendental meditation (TM) is a form of meditation which may be used for stress relief, relieve anxiety, manage depression, cardiovascular health, weight management, and promote inner happiness. Transcendental meditation allows the mind to settle into a calm state of rest. It is beyond the scope of this book to outline the technique. I recommend you work with a qualified practitioner.

Let's See What Research Says . . .

- Practicing transcendental meditation may potentially reduce systolic and diastolic blood pressure (Ooi et al. 2017).
- Elder et al. (2014) find that "Transcendental Meditation program was effective in reducing psychological distress in teachers and support staff working in a therapeutic school for students with behavioral problems."

Transcendental Meditation Resources

- Transcendental Meditation, tm.org
- Transcendental Meditation for Women, tm-women.org

SELF-HYPNOSIS FOR REFRESHING YOUR MIND

Self-hypnosis may be used to promote healing, control stress, reduce anxiety, improve sleep, improve academic and athletic performance, help heal from trauma, and manage addictions. For further information, see the Additional Resources section at the end of this chapter. I highly recommend you work with a mental health professional trained in hypnosis and psychotherapy for a specific medical condition or concern. What is outlined in this section serves only as an introduction to self-hypnosis.

Let's See What Research Says . . .

- Forester-Miller (2017) finds that "the results support the inclusion of self-hypnosis in the multidisciplinary treatment plans for breast cancer patients and indicate the potential for increasing patient satisfaction ratings and improving patient care."
- Wolf et al. (2017) conclude that "Self-hypnosis can be used in clinical practice as an adjunct to the gold standard of local anesthesia for pain management."
- Elkins et al. (2013) find that "Guided self-hypnosis reduced perceived hot flashes in the pilot study with postmenopausal women."

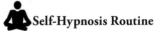**Self-Hypnosis Routine**

Perform this either in the morning or before you go to sleep:

- Start by getting comfortable in a quiet room.
- Perform five deep breaths using the abdomen. Try holding each breath for 3 to 5 seconds.
- Make sure your eyes are closed as you think of a relaxing place.
- Continue breathing. As you relax, think of a relaxing color (such as blue, green, or pink) for five breaths.
- Imagine the color slowly making its way from your head down to your feet.
- Slowly ease yourself into relaxation by counting down from 5 through 1 as you visualize large blue, green, or pink numbers in your head.
- Talk to yourself about positive things you want to reinforce such as
  » "My body is going to heal itself."
  » "I am going to get better."
  » "I am going to get an A on the exam."
  » "I am no longer fearful."
  Do the positive self-talk for least a minute or two (or 5 to 10 slow breaths).
- Slowly ease yourself back out of relaxation by counting up from 1 through 5 as you visualize the large blue, green, or pink numbers in your head.
- End by opening your eyes and enjoy the day. Or, close your eyes and go to sleep.

Hypnotherapy Resources

- American Hypnosis Association, hypnosis.edu
- American Society Of Clinical Hypnosis, asch.net
- Hypnotherapy Academy of America, hypnotherapyacademy.com
- International Hypnosis Association, hypnosiscredentials.com
- National Board for Certified Clinical Hypnotherapists, natboard.com
- National Hypnosis Association, nationalhypnosisassociation.com
- National Hypnotherapy Society, nationalhypnotherapysociety.org

MEASURING BODY-MIND APPROACHES

Clinicians may want to measure certain factors to determine if a particular body-mind approach is actually working. If you are not a healthcare provider, I recommend you work with one if you are interested in taking one of these tests. The following are three ways to measure mindfulness:

- Dragesund et al. (2017) find that using the revised *Body Awareness Rating Questionnaire* could be recommended for use with body-mind physical therapy approaches for musculoskeletal conditions. A sample item in the questionnaire is as follows: "I notice differences in the way my body reacts to various foods."

- Another measurement tool that could be is used is the *Mindful Attention Awareness Scale* to assess attention and awareness of ongoing events and experiences (Black et al. 2012; Brown et al. 2003; Carlson et al. 2005; Smith et al. 2017). A sample item in the questionnaire is as follows: "I find it difficult to stay focused on what's happening in the present."
- Finally, there is the *Five-Facet Mindfulness Questionnaire* to measure mindfulness skills we use in daily life (Lilja et al. 2011). A sample item in the questionnaire is as follows: "I don't pay attention to what I'm doing because I'm daydreaming, worrying, or otherwise distracted."

The measures can be used just prior to the beginning of a mindfulness program and then repeated again after a period of training (perhaps 8 to 12 weeks later or even after a year). A simple Google search of each test name will provide links for the actual tests and the questions used.

BOX 2: HOLISTIC HEALING

MONITORING YOUR BLOOD PRESSURE AT HOME

Measuring your blood pressure can be a key step to preventing heart attacks, strokes, and other cardiovascular problems. Use these guidelines for your portable digital blood-pressure unit:

- Before using your home unit for the first time, bring it to your physician's office so you can compare measurements on their equipment with your machine. The numbers should be very close. This is a good way to assess your machine's accuracy. I recommend doing this at least once a year. Now you are ready to use your home unit.
- Always make sure the batteries in your unit are working properly.
- For accurate measurements, take daily blood pressure readings at the same time of day. First thing in the morning is a good time since, ideally, you avoid food, drink, medications, smoking, and exercise for at least 30 minutes prior to your measurement.
- Avoid tobacco for 30 minutes and caffeine for 60 minutes before taking a blood pressure reading (Goodman et al. 2013). Ideally, do not smoke.
- Sit silently in a comfortable chair for five minutes before the measurement, your back supported and feet on the floor. Do not cross your legs or arms, or do anything to tax yourself mentally (like watching the news or completing a crossword puzzle) or physically (like tapping your feet nervously).
- Place the appropriate-size cuff (the wrong size will give you an inaccurate measurement) on your left upper arm as shown on the monitor diagram. Use your right arm if there is a medical reason you are unable to use your left. Place the cuff directly over your skin and not over a shirt or blouse and make sure the position of the arrow on the cuff is placed over the brachial artery (according to the diagram on the blood pressure cuff). Finally, make sure the lower edge of the cuff is approximately an inch above the crease where your elbow bends.

- Place your cuffed arm on a surface, such as a table or armrest, at about heart level. Don't leave your arm unsupported or attempt to hold it up at heart level. Your arm needs to be supported and relaxed for an accurate measure.
- Now relax your mind and body as well as the arm in the blood pressure cuff.
- Press the start button on the monitor; allow the cuff to automatically inflate.
- Once finished, the monitor will automatically display your blood pressure as two numbers (for example, 120/80). The top number is your systolic blood pressure and the bottom number is your diastolic blood pressure. Many units will also show your pulse (heart rate).
- Record your blood pressure for future reference and to share with your physician.
- Kudos for taking part in managing your own health!

The following is blood pressure monitor to consider for your home:

- Omron, omronhealthcare.com

ADDITIONAL MINDFULNESS RESOURCES

- Benson-Henry Institute for Mind Body Medicine, bensonhenryinstitute.org
- Center for Investigating Healthy Minds, investigatinghealthyminds.org
- Center for Mindfulness in Medicine, Health Care, and Society, umassmed.edu/cfm
- Institute for Mindful Leadership, instituteformindfulleadership.org
- Mind & Life Institute, mindandlife.org
- Mind Fitness Training Institute, mind-fitness-training.org
- Mindfulness Apps (Jon Kabat-Zinn), mindfulnessapps.com
- Mindfulness & Health, mindfulnesshealth.com
- Mindfulness in Education Network, mindfuled.org
- Mindful-Way Stress Reduction, mindful-way.com
- Norman Cousins Center for Psychoneuroimmunology at UCLA, www2.semel.ucla.edu/cousins
- The Center for Contemplative Mind in Society, contemplativemind.org
- UCLA Mindful Awareness Research Center, marc.ucla.edu
- UCSD Center for Mindfulness, ucsdcfm.wordpress.com
- Refer to the cards by Susan Kaiser Greenland *Mindful Games Activity Cards: 55 Fun Ways to Share Mindfulness with Kids and Teens* (2017).
- Refer to the book by Susan Kaiser Greenland *Mindful Games: Sharing Mindfulness and Meditation with Children, Teens, and Families* (2016).

ADDITIONAL INTEGRATIVE MEDICINE RESOURCES

- Academic Consortium for Integrative Medicine and Health, imconsortium.org
- Integrative Practitioner, integrativepractitioner.com

- National Center for Complementary and Integrative Health, nccih .nih.gov
- National Center for Integrative Primary Health Care, nciph.org
- Office of Cancer Complementary and Alternative Medicine, cam.cancer.gov
- Explore Integrative Medicine, exploreim.ucla.edu
- UCLA Center for East-West Medicine, cewm.med.ucla.edu

References

Bhatt SP, Luqman-Arafath TK, Gupta AK, et al. (2013). Volitional pursed lips breathing in patients with stable chronic obstructive pulmonary disease improves exercise capacity. *Chronic Respiratory Disease* 10 (1): 5–10.

Bigard M. (2009). Walking the labyrinth: An innovative approach to counseling center outreach. *Journal of College Counseling* 12 (2): 137–148.

Black DS, Sussman S, Johnson CA, et al. (2012). Psychometric assessment of the Mindful Attention Awareness Scale (MAAS) among Chinese adolescents. *Assessment* 19 (1): 42–52.

Brown KW, Ryan RM. (2003). The benefits of being present: Mindfulness and its role in psychological well-being. *Journal of Personality and Social Psychology* 84 (4): 822–848.

Carlson L.E, Brown KW. (2005). Validation of the Mindful Attention Awareness Scale in a cancer population. *Journal of Psychosomatic Research* 58 (1): 29–33.

Chaitow L, Bradley D, and Gilbert C. (2014). *Recognizing and Treating Breathing Disorders: A Multidisciplinary Approach,* 2nd ed. New York, NY: Churchill Livingstone Elsevier.

Chen KW, Berger CC, Manheimer E, et al. (2012). Meditative therapies for reducing anxiety: A systematic review and meta-analysis of randomized controlled trials. *Depression and Anxiety* 29 (7): 545–562.

Daniels M. (2008). An intrapersonal approach to enhance student performance. *Florida Communication Journal* 36 (2): 89–102.

Dragesund T, Strand LI, Grotle M. (2018). The revised Body Awareness Rating Questionnaire: Development into a unidimensional scale using Rasch analysis. *Physical Therapy.* 98 (2): 122–132.

Eason C. (2004). *The Complete Guide to Labyrinths.* Berkley, CA: The Crossing Press.

Eherer AJ, Netolitzky F, Hogenauer C, et al. (2012). Positive effect of abdominal breathing exercise on gastroesophageal reflux disease: A randomized, controlled study. *American Journal of Gastroenterology* 107 (3): 372–378.

Elder C, Nidich S, Moriarty F, et al. (2014). Effect of transcendental meditation on employee stress, depression, and burnout: A randomized controlled study. *Permanente Journal* 18 (1): 19–23.

Elkins G, Johnson A, Fisher W, et al. (2013). A pilot investigation of guided self-hypnosis in the treatment of hot flashes among postmenopausal women. *International Journal of Clinical and Experimental Hypnosis* 61 (3): 342–350.

Flexner LM, Hertling D. (2018). The temporomandibular joint. In: Brody LT, and Hall CM. *Therapeutic Exercise: Moving Toward Function,* 4th ed. Baltimore, MD: Wolters Kluwer.

Forester-Miller H. (2017). Self-hypnosis classes to enhance the quality of life of breast cancer patients. *American Journal of Clinical Hypnosis* 60 (1): 18–32.

Fredrickson BL, Cohn MA, Coffey KA, et al. (2008). Open hearts build lives: Positive emotions, induced through loving-kindness meditation, build consequential personal resources. *Journal of Personality and Social Psychology* 95 (5): 1045–1062.

Gotink RA, Hermans KS, Geschwind N, et al. (2016). Mindfulness and mood stimulate each other in an upward spiral: A mindful walking intervention using experience sampling. *Mindfulness (N Y)* 7 (5): 1114–1122.

Gotink RA, Chu P, Busschbach JJ, Benson H, et al. (2015). Standardised mindfulness-based interventions in healthcare: An overview of systematic reviews and meta-analyses of RCTs. *PLOS ONE* 10 (4).

Greenland SK, Harris A. (2017). *Mindful Games Activity Cards: 55 Fun Ways to Share Mindfulness with Kids and Teens.* Boulder, CO: Shambhala Publications. www.susankaisergreenland.com

Greenland SK. (2016). *Mindful Games: Sharing Mindfulness and Meditation with Children, Teens, and Families.* Boulder, CO: Shambhala Publications.

Griffith JS. (2002). Labyrinths: A pathway to reflection and contemplation. *Clinical Journal of Oncology Nursing* 6: 295–296.

Heard CP, Scott J, Yeo S. (2015). Walking the labyrinth: Considering mental health consumer experience, meaning making, and the illumination of the sacred in a forensic mental health setting. *Journal of Pastoral Care & Counseling* 69 (4): 240–250.

Hong Y, Jacinto G. (2012). Reality therapy and the labyrinth: A strategy for practice. *Journal of Human Behavior in the Social Environment* 22 (6): 619–634.

Jacobson E. (1962). *Progressive Relaxation,* 4th ed. Chicago, IL: University of Chicago Press.

Jacobson E. (1964). *Anxiety and Tension Control.* Philadelphia, PA: JB Lippincott.

Jacobson E. (1964). *Self-Operations Control Manual.* Chicago, IL: National Foundation for Progressive Relaxation.

Jacobson E. (1967). *Tension in Medicine.* Springfield, IL: Charles C Thomas.

Jacobson E. (1976). *You Must Relax,* 5th ed. New York, NY: McGraw-Hill Book Company, Inc.

Johnson DC, Thom NJ, Stanley EA, et al. (2014). Modifying resilience mechanisms in at-risk individuals: A controlled study of mindfulness training in Marines preparing for deployment. *American Journal of Psychiatry* 171 (8): 844–853.

Josefsson T, Ivarsson A, Lindwall M, et al. (2017). Mindfulness mechanisms in sports: Mediating effects of rumination and emotion regulation on sport-specific coping. *Mindfulness* 8 (5): 1354–1363.

Kabat-Zinn J. (2003). Mindfulness-based interventions in context: Past, present, and future. *Clinical Psychology: Science and Practice* 10: 144–56.

Kabat-Zinn J. (2005). *Wherever You Go, There You Are: Mindfulness Meditation in Everyday Life,* 10th ed. New York, NY: Hyperion.

Kabat-Zinn J. (2005). *Coming to Our Senses: Healing Ourselves and the World Through Mindfulness.* New York, NY: Hyperion.

Kabat-Zinn J. (2007). *Arriving at Your Own Door: 108 Lessons in Mindfulness.* New York, NY: Hyperion.

Kisner C, Colby LA, Borstad J. (2018). *Therapeutic Exercise: Foundations and Techniques,* 7th ed. Philadelphia, PA: FA Davis.

Lilja J, Frodi-Lundgren A, Hanse JJ, et al. (2011). Five Facets Mindfulness Questionnaire—Reliability and factor structure: A Swedish version. *Cognitive Behaviour Therapy* 40 (4): 291–303.

Marturano J. (2014). *Finding the Space to Lead: A Practical Guide to Mindful.* New York, NY: Bloomsbury Press.

Maruca AT, Shelton D. (2016). Correctional nursing interventions for incarcerated persons with mental disorders: An integrative review. *Issues in Mental Health Nursing* 37 (5): 285–292.

Molholt R. (2011). Roman labyrinth mosaics and the experience of motion. *Art Bulletin* 93 (3): 287–303.

Nicholson M. (2002). Ask an expert: Constructing labyrinths for patients with cancer. *Clinical Journal of Oncology Nursing* 6: 296–297.

Ong JC, Shapiro SL, Manber, R. (2009). Mindfulness meditation and cognitive behavioral therapy for insomnia: A naturalistic 12-month follow-up. *Explore (NY)* 5 (1): 30–36.

Ooi SL, Giovino M, Pak S C. (2017). Transcendental meditation for lowering blood pressure: An overview of systematic reviews and meta-analyses. *Complementary Therapies in Medicine* 34: 26–34.

Rocabado M, Iglarsh ZA. (1991). *Musculoskeletal Approach to Maxillofacial Pain.* Philadelphia, PA: JB Lippincott.

Ruggles C, Saunders NJ. (2012). Desert labyrinth: Lines, landscape and meaning at Nazca, Peru. *Antiquity* 86 (334): 1126–1140.

Sarno J. (1991). *Healing Back Pain: The Mind-Body Connection.* New York, NY: Warner Books.

Savel RH, Munro CL. (2017). Quiet the mind: Mindfulness, meditation, and the search for inner peace. *American Journal of Critical Care* 26 (6): 433–436.

Schechter D. (2014). *Think Away Your Pain: Your Brain is the Solution to Your Pain.* Culver City, CA: MindBody Medicine Publications.

Simpson R, Booth J, Lawrence M, et al. (2014). Mindfulness based interventions in multiple sclerosis—A systematic review. *BMC Neurology* 14: 15.

Smith ORF, Melkevik O, Samdal O, et al. (2017). Psychometric properties of the five-item version of the Mindful Awareness Attention Scale (MAAS) in Norwegian adolescents. *Scandinavian Journal of Public Health* 45 (4): 373–380.

Teut M, Roesner EJ, Ortiz M, et al. (2013). Mindful walking in psychologically distressed individuals: A randomized controlled trial. *Evidence-Based Complementary and Alternative Medicine* 2013: 489856.

UCLA Mindful Awareness Research Center. 2017). Benefits of mindfulness. Retrieved on November 4, 2017 from http://marc.ucla.edu.

Venes D. (Ed.) (2017). *Taber's Cyclopedic Medical Dictionary,* 23rd ed. Philadelphia, PA: FA Davis.

Wilhelm R. (commentary by CG Jung). (1962). *The Secret of the Golden Flower: A Chinese Book of Life* (a translation). San Diego, CA: A Harvest Book.

Wolf TG, Wolf D, Below D, et al. (2016). Effectiveness of self-hypnosis on the relief of experimental dental pain: A randomized trial. *International Journal of Clinical and Experimental Hypnosis* 64 (2): 187–199.

Zucker D, Sharma A. (2012). Labyrinth walking in corrections. *Journal of Addictions Nursing* 23 (1): 47–54.

Holistic Healing Boxes

Controlling Type A Behavior

Friedman M, Thoresen CE, Gill JJ, et al. (1986). Alteration of Type A behavior and its effect on cardiac recurrences in post myocardial infarction patients: Summary results of the recurrent coronary prevention project. *American Heart Journal* 112 (4): 653–665.

Monitoring Your Blood Pressure at Home

Goodman CC, Snyder TE. (2013). *Differential Diagnosis for Physical Therapists: Screening for Referral,* 5th ed. St. Louis, MO: Elsevier. www.differentialdiagnosisforpt.com.

CHAPTER 2

MANAGING YOUR STRESS

"It's not stress that kills us, it is our reaction to it."

—Hans Selye, MD, PhD

Some causes of stress include chronic overstimulation of the senses (excessive noise or overcrowding), lack of sleep, poor diet, overtraining with exercise, information overload (due in large part to cellular phones and the Internet), and constant barrage of news via various media outlets, financial concerns, relationship problems, or job issues.

Hans Selye, MD, PhD (1907-1982), an endocrinologist known for his research on the effects of stress on the human body, stated that "activity and rest must be judiciously balanced, and every person has his own characteristic requirements for rest and activity." Consider looking into the three books (Selye 1974,1976,1976) that Dr. Selye wrote on the subject for additional information.

In my clinical practice as a physical therapist, I recommend my patients find the root causes of their stress and try to find strategies to correct or manage their triggers. A trigger for one person may not even register as stress in another person. For example, some individuals consider standing in long lines or being stuck in freeway traffic as a high level of stress. Other individuals may look at these situations as a way to slow down their hectic life or listen to soothing music. Our bodies cannot be in a constant state of "fight or flight" (sympathetic nervous system) where the stress hormones are dominant. We need to have balance where we are in a state of "rest and digest" (parasympathetic nervous system) to allow for digestion, healing, and recovery.

LET'S SEE WHAT RESEARCH SAYS . . .

- "Contact with natural outdoor environments benefits mental health. Our results also suggest that having contact with natural outdoor environments that can facilitate stress reduction could be particularly beneficial" (Triguero-Mas et al. 2017).

- Poor nutrition in the evening or consuming empty calories for break-fast resulted in increased stress levels (Widaman 2016).
- Stress and depression can promote obesity (Kiecolt-Glaser et al. 2015).
- Stress management for individuals with type 2 diabetes mellitus has a beneficial role for stress levels and glycemic control (Koloverou et al. 2014).
- Stress can accelerate cellular aging (Epel 2008).
- Stress can have harmful effects on the heart (Dimsdale 2008).
- Stress from hostile or abrasive relationships can affect physiological functioning and health dynamics such as wound healing (Kiecolt-Glaser et al. 2005).
- Stress can slow wound healing (Kiecolt-Glaser et al. 1995).

 Use the following strategies to help reduce your stress levels:

- Smile a lot! Smiling tends to relax the facial muscles (compared to frowning) and may improve your mood. Smile and others will smile with you (Abel 2002; Hess et al. 2001; Niedenthal 2007). Give it a try.
- Exercise. Go for a walk, hike, or bike ride.
- Take a yoga class (Kiecolt-Glaser et al. 2010).
- Try tai chi or qigong.
- Relax in a hammock under a shady tree.
- Engage in music, art, and hobbies.
- Play with your pets.
- Yawn while stretching your face and body as a wake-up cue or relaxation technique throughout the day. Some clinicians believe yawning might increase arousal (Gupta et al. 2013), while others feel it can reduce anger, anxiety, and stress.
- Try acupuncture.
- Get a massage or use self-massage to relax upper- and lower-body muscles.
- Close your eyes lightly for a 10-second mini-break after close-up work on a computer.
- Create a daily "to do" list each morning so you don't have to stress over having to remember simple things you need to take care of throughout your day.
- Use a reading stand while sitting in a chair or on a bed to relieve neck strain and shoulder tension.
- Try aromatherapy. The smells of lavender, rose, vanilla, and lemongrass can put you in a relaxed mood (Murad 2010).
- Try the Emotional Freedom Technique (EFT) (Church et al. 2012). The Tapping Solution Foundation website www.tappingsolutionfoundation.org indicates that "The basic technique requires you to focus on the negative emotion at hand: a fear or anxiety, a bad memory, an unresolved problem, or anything that's bothering you. While maintaining

your mental focus on this issue, use your fingertips to tap 5-7 times each on 9 of the body's meridian points."

- Try attending a Japanese Tea Ceremony. An article by Keenan (1996) indicates that "Serious practitioners of tea develop a mind set and body control that enables them to transform tension-producing details of everyday life into moments of beauty, meaningfulness and tranquility." A study by Shiah et al. (2013) indicates that "Tea treated with good intentions improved mood more than ordinary tea derived from the same source."

- Reduce work (or school) stress by glancing away frequently from close visual tasks and training yourself to "look easy" to reduce physiological stress. To "look easy" simply means to keep your facial muscles, jaw, and mind relaxed enough to accomplish and concentrate on the task with ease and purpose (Birnbaum 1985).

- Go outside for a walk to get fresh air and natural light and to look off into the distance. For example, look at the clouds, distant trees, or out over the ocean or lake without squinting. Gazing into the distance tends to relax while prolonged close-up work can lead to stress (Birnbaum 1984,1985).

- Keep forehead muscles relaxed. While on the phone or computer, periodically touch your forehead muscles to feel if they are activated. If eyebrows are raised or forehead crinkled, practice relaxing your facial muscles.

- See the Facial Relaxation Routine in chapter 1.

- Relax in a reclining chair. This can relieve pressure on your low-back region. Or, relax in a rocking chair. A study shows that individuals with Alzheimer's disease who *actively* use a rocking chair for one to two hours per day show significant improvements in anxiety, depression, and balance, and also a reduction in pain medication usage (Pierce et al. 2009). Another study indicates that active rocking might be a good form of low-exertion exercise for frail, elderly individuals (Houston 1993).

- Try a fidget spinner to perhaps relax and reduce stress. To the best of knowledge, there is no hard-core research to support its use, but they are kind of fun to play with. Just be aware that they may be a choking hazard in young children (Schecter et al. 2017).

- Limit unnecessary decision making. An article by Vohs et al. (2008) indicates that "making choices led to reduced self-control (i.e., less physical stamina, reduced persistence in the face of failure, more procrastination, and less quality and quantity of arithmetic calculations)."

- Try providing a helping hand to those in need but at some point consider distancing yourself from perpetually negative individuals.

- Consider gardening.

- Consider learning to cook. Take professional classes.

- Stop relationships which are not going anywhere and bringing you down.
- Finally, think positive. Your body believes what your brain tells it.

Box 3: Holistic Healing

Pain Management Information

If you have pain, I recommend you first contact your healthcare provider for an evaluation. The following are some resources to consider for pain management:

- American Academy of Pain Management, aapainmanage.org
- American Academy of Pain Medicine, painmed.org
- American Chronic Pain Association, theacpa.org
- American Pain Foundation, painfoundation.org
- American Pain Society, americanpainsociety.org
- Arthritis Foundation, arthritis.org
- International Association for the Study of Pain, iasp-pain.org
- International Headache Society, ihs-headache.org
- International Pelvic Pain Society, pelvicpain.org
- International Spine & Pain Institute, ispinstitute.com
- Neuro Orthopaedic Institute, gradedmotorimagery.com
- NIH Pain Consortium, painconsortium.nih.gov
- PainEDU, painedu.org
- Practical Pain Management, practicalpainmanagement.com
- Refer to google.com for a spine decompression routine by physical therapist Sarah Meeks, PT, MS, GCS (search for Sarah Meeks Realignment Routine).
- Thoracic Outlet Syndrome Information, tosinfo.com (from James D. Collins, MD of UCLA Radiology).
- Refer to the book *Back Mechanic* (McGill, 2015), backfitpro.com.
- Refer to the book *Complementary Therapies for Pain Management: An Evidence-Based Approach* (Ernst et al. 2007).
- Refer to the book *Explain Pain* (Butler et al. 2003), noigroup.com.
- Refer to the book *Goodbye Back Pain: A Sufferer's Guide to Full Back Recovery* (Faye 2008).
- Refer to the book *Low Back Disorders* (McGill 2016).
- Refer to the book *Manual Therapy for Musculoskeletal Pain Syndromes* (Fernandez-de-las-Penas 2016).
- Refer to the book *Mechanisms and Management of Pain for the Physical Therapist* (Sluka 2016).
- Refer to the book *The End of Back Pain: Access Your Hidden Core to Heal Your Body* (Roth 2014).

- Refer to the books *Dissolving Pain: Simple Brain-Training Exercises for Overcoming Chronic Pain* (2010) and *The Open-Focus Brain: Harnessing the Power of Attention to Heal Mind and Body* (2007).
- Refer to the book *Thoracic Outlet Syndrome* (Illig et al. 2013).
- Refer to the book *Wall and Melzack's Textbook of Pain* (McMahon et al. 2013).
- Refer to the booklet *Everyone Has Back Pain* (Louw et al. 2015).
- Refer to the booklet *Sex and Back Pain* (Hebert 1997), www.impaccusa.com.
- Refer to the booklet *Treat Your Own Back* (McKenzie 2011).
- Refer to the booklet *Treat Your Own Neck* (McKenzie 2011).
- Refer to the booklet *Treat Your Own Shoulder* (McKenzie et al. 2009).
- Refer to the booklet *Why Do I Hurt?* (Louw 2013).
- Refer to the article by Sidorkewicz et al. (2015) titled "Documenting Female Spine Motion During Coitus with a Commentary on the Implications for the Low Back Pain Patient."
- Refer to the article by Sidorkewicz et al. (2014) titled "Male Spine Motion During Coitus: Implications for the Low Back Pain Patient."

PRACTICAL STRESS-RELIEVING BREATHING TECHNIQUES

Work with a healthcare provider to help you determine which type of breathing technique(s) may be best for your needs to reduce stress and anxiety. The following are some types of breathing techniques which may be used in different situations:

- **Chest breathing**—features breathing into the chest and allowing the ribs to expand. This type of deep breathing technique may be used with individuals who have osteoporosis (Kaplan 1995).
- **Diaphragmatic breathing** (also called belly breathing)—features either breathing in through the nose and exhaling through the mouth, or breathing in and out through the nose. This is a standard technique used in many type of stress reduction and anxiety management programs (Haff et al. 2016). Diaphragmatic breathing may also stimulate intestinal activity (McMillan 1921) and may be used to help treat individuals with constipation. This breathing pattern may also be used for managing pain, lymphedema, and thoracic outlet syndrome (Kisner et al. 2018) and to manage panic attacks or a panic disorder (Yamada et al. 2017). Finally, variations of diaphragmatic breathing are used in yoga, tai chi, qigong exercises, mindfulness, and Transcendental Meditation.
- **Pursed-lip breathing**—features unresisted inspiration followed by active oral exhalation through a narrowed (pursed) mouth opening. May be used for patient with chronic obstructive pulmonary disease (COPD) (Bhatt et al. 2013; O'Sullivan et al. 2014).

- **Unilateral Nostril Breathing**—in unilateral nostril breathing, one nostril is closed at a time. Used to reduce anxiety (Gerberg et al. 2017), oxygenating the prefrontal cortex (Singh et al. 2016), and improving recall of memory (Garg et al. 2016). One study by Bhavanani et al. (2014) states that "air flow through right nostril (surya nadi and pingala swara) is activatory in nature, whereas the flow through left nostril (chandra nadi and ida swara) is relaxatory." Another study by Thakur et al. (2011) concludes that "right nostril breathing enhances numerical data retrieval mostly as a result of left brain activation."

- **Alternate Nostril Breathing**—in alternate nostril breathing, alternate nostrils (right and then left) are closed. Used to reduce anxiety (Gerberg et al. 2017).

- **Coherent Breathing** (also called resonant breathing)—natural breathing in and out through the nose with equal length on the inspiration and expiration. Used for emotional calmness and mental alertness (Gerberg et al. 2017).

- **Qigong Breath** 4-4-6-2—breathe in on a count of 4, hold breath for a count of 4, exhale on a count of 6, and hold for a count of 2 and then repeat. Used to reduce anxiety and rage (Gerberg et al. 2017).

- **Voicing Strategies and Movement**—for example, this type of breathing may involve counting out loud to 4 or 7 as a weak patient sits down to gain increased control of the activity. See the work of physical therapist Mary Massery, PT, DPT, DSc at masserypt.com.

- **Resistance Breathing**—singing and chanting are forms of resistance breathing (Gerberg et al. 2017).

- **Breath Moving**—with the eyes closed, a person imagines moving the breath to the top of the head and then to base of the spine. This technique may be used in individuals who have pain or asthma. Refer to the website www.robertpeng.com for more information (Gerberg et al. 2017).

- **Pilates Breathing**—features deep breathing while keeping the abdomen pulled in by means of active contraction of the transverse abdominal and pelvic floor muscles (Cancelliero-Gaiad et al. 2014).

- **Valsalva Maneuver in Athletics**—features a brief breath hold and may be used during max strength training exercises. However, problems such as an aneurysm, blackout, increased blood pressure, or dizziness may result. Therefore, this technique is typically for high performance athletes (Haff et al. 2016).

Practical Stress-Relieving Self-Massage

Let's See What Research Says . . .

- Self-massage to the lateral thigh, lateral torso and the bottom of the foot appears to be effective in improving performance of the Functional Movement Screen overhead deep squat (Monteiro et al. 2017).
- Self-massage to lower body with a foam roller reduced delayed-onset muscle soreness and enhanced muscle recovery after an intense exercise protocol (Pearcey et al. 2015).
- A self-massage stick helped reduce upper back pain associated with myofascial trigger points (Wamontree et al. 2015).
- Self-massage to the thigh muscle and around the knee with the hands may help manage knee pain and stiffness in individuals who have knee osteoarthritis (Atkins et al. 2013).

In conclusion, some studies show that self-massage may be used to help relieve pain and improve recovery. So, give it a try and see how you feel.

The following are some easy stress-relieving self-massage techniques you can perform for one to two minutes in the comfort of your home. Consult with a physical therapist or massage therapist to learn additional self-massage techniques. Also, see the book *The TB12 Method* by Tom Brady, an NFL quarterback with five Super Bowl wins, for more excellent self-massage techniques for the entire body (Brady 2017).

- **Foot Massage**—you can use a Rubz ball under your foot to relieve tension and recover after intense or weight-bearing activity (Figure 2-1). Check out the website www.rubzmassage.com.
- **Knee Massage**—you can use your hands to gently knead out the tension in your thigh muscle and around your knees by rubbing in a small circular pattern (Figure 2-2).

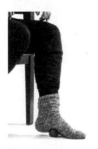 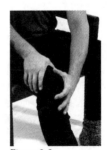

Figure 2-1   Figure 2-2

- **Shoulder/Neck Massage**—you can use your hand to gently knead out the tension in your neck and shoulders by squeezing your muscles with your hand (Figure 2-3).

- **Thera Cane Massage**—you can use a Thera Cane on your upper and lower back to relieve tension, cooldown after a workout, and recover after intense activity (Figure 2-4). Check out the website www.thera-cane.com for more information.
- **Stick Massage**—you can use a massage stick on your lower back, calf muscles, hamstrings, and upper back to relieve tension, cooldown after a workout, and recover after intense activity (Figure 2-5). Check out the website www.thestick.com for more information.

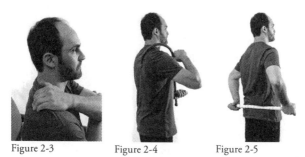

Figure 2-3   Figure 2-4   Figure 2-5

SELF-MASSAGE AND MOBILIZATION

(This section was contributed by Derek Plonka, DPT, MTOM, L.Ac, CSCS, Doctor of Physical Therapy / Licensed Acupuncturist at Insight Wellness Clinic in Santa Monica, California, www.insightwellnessclinic.com)

DISCLAIMER: In the event that you have a medical condition, such as osteoporosis, a herniated disc, or an compromise of your spinal/ pelvic structural integrity, please consult a medical professional to determine if this is the appropriate treatment for you. When implementing treatment, it is recommended you work with a healthcare practitioner (such as a licensed physical therapist) who is familiar with using foam rolls for self-massage.

A small foam roll (approximately two inches in diameter) can be used to restore normal soft tissue and joint mobility of the spine, which are typically addressed with manual treatment from a licensed physical therapist

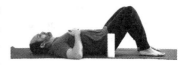

Figure 2-6

(Figure 2-6). The use of a small foam roller allows the body to receive a self-directed treatment while being in a relaxed position.

Starting Position: Lying on the floor with the knees bent. If the floor is uncomfortable or the foam roller is too intense, you may begin on a bed.

1. **Pelvic Region:**
   » Hold the foam roller and place a corner of it under one of your buttocks (Figure 2-7).
   » Allow your body to relax under the pressure of the foam roller.

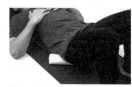

Figure 2-7

» As you relax, begin to notice any of the **3Ts (Tenderness, Tightness, or Tension).** Use this time to look for any areas that feel different than the rest of your body.

» Once a **3T** is found, just stay there. Allow your body to relax and soften to the pressure of the foam roller. Stay there until the intensity of the **3T is 50% less than what you began with**. It may take 30 seconds. It may take 2 minutes, but just relax and allow the muscle to release under the pressure of the foam roller.

» Once a release has occurred, gently roll or move to another **3T**, seeking to soften the muscles of both buttocks before moving to the lower back and the rest of the spine.

2. **Lumbar—Cervical Region:**

» Once the pelvic region has released enough to feel 50% less intense, move to the lower back by placing the small foam roller horizontally across the pelvic region.

» Once your sacrum (lower end of the spine) is resting on the foam roller, gently walk your body downward with your feet and allow the small foam roller to move up your spine.

» You will notice a point where your buttocks drop off of the small foam roller, which is where your lower back (lumbar spine) begins (Figure 2-8).

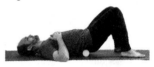

Figure 2-8

» Again, notice the **3Ts** as you slowly walk the small foam roller up the spine, stopping at each point to address the **3Ts** and allow it to become **50% less Tender, Tight, or Tense.**

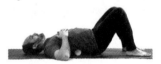

Figure 2-9

» Continue to slowly walk the small foam roller up (Figure 2-9), until you have touched every section of your spine, up to the base of your skull or until an area that is too tender or does not release is reached. This **3T-Barrier** should not be skipped over. This is an area that must be slowly worked into and may not release during this session. It may take several sessions, days, or weeks to obtain a release of that area.

» Once you have walked the small foam roller as high as it will go, *without your body bracing from too much pain*, begin the return by slowly and gently walking it back down the spine.

» On the return, address each **3T** again and notice that they may have changed in placement or quality.

» With the small foam roller now back under the sacrum, lift your pelvis and remove the foam roller. Allow the pelvic region to return back to the floor and relax. **NEVER GET UP WITH THE FOAM ROLLER UNDER YOUR BODY.**

» Now gently drop your knees to the left, then to the right, and then back to the left, allowing the rest of your body to follow. Assuming a side-lying position, slowly rise up to a sitting position. This will reduce the possibility of a muscle spasm after the small foam roller mobilization has been performed.

The small foam roller mobilization requires consistency and time to make sustainable changes to your spine by improving the mobility. Many of my (Derek Plonka) patients, as well as myself, have made a commitment to performing this routine for 10 minutes in the morning and 20 to 30 minutes before bed to restore as much symmetrical mobility (both sides feel equally loose) to the spine as possible. Over time, my clients and I have been able to increase mobility and symmetry of our bodies.

PRACTICAL STRESS-RELIEVING PARTNER FACE MASSAGE

This is a fantastic way to relax. I use similar facial massage techniques for my patients who are experiencing headaches, migraines, temporomandibular joint (TMJ) pain, cervical pain, Bell's palsy (a form of facial paralysis), and difficulty with relaxation, stress, and anxiety. A study by Gomes et al. (2014) finds that massage therapy on the masticatory muscles helped individuals with a temporomandibular disorder open their jaw better and a study by Hatayama et al. (2008) concludes that a facial massage might reduce psychological distress.

Have your spouse or friend perform a gentle massage to your face. I recommend performing this massage without gel or creams. Start by lying on your back and breathing diaphragmatically. Have your spouse or friend perform the following sequence:

- Using both index fingers, gently and slowly pull upward from the upper ridge of your nose to the top of your forehead. Repeat 3 to 5 times.
- Using all of your fingers, place them just above the eyebrows (like playing a piano) and gently pull upward with all the fingers. Repeat 3 to 5 times.
- Using the index and middle fingers, perform a gentle circular massage to the temple regions. Repeat 3 to 5 times.
- Using the index fingers, perform a gentle, sweeping upward and outward motion from the inner and bottom of the eyes to the side of the eyebrows. Repeat 3 to 5 times.
- Using the index fingers, perform a gentle outward pulling motion from the outer and bottom part of the nostrils. Repeat 3 to 5 times.
- Using the index and middle fingers, perform a gentle circular massage to the outer jaw muscles. Repeat 3 to 5 times.
- Repeat the forehead massage (piano touch) and this simple facial massage routine is finished.

If you need any additional training in this technique, please see a massage therapist or a physical therapist. Also, be sure to check out chapter 1: Mindfulness and Relaxation Training for additional techniques which may help you manage and relieve stress.

PRACTICAL GUIDE FOR YOUR STRESS MANAGEMENT

- Do you have any medical conditions you need to adjust your lifestyle for (such as anxiety, depression, or post-traumatic stress disorder)? If yes, you should work with your primary healthcare provider and with a counselor, psychologist, or psychiatrist.
- Go to credible websites (or apps) (such as The American Institute of Stress) and obtain more information about stress.
- Go to PubMed.gov (www.pubmed.gov) and enter the medical condition along with the word "stress" (for example, search as "anxiety AND stress") to search for the latest information. Speak with your healthcare provider if you need help interpreting the studies.
- Identify your stress trigger factors (such as busy traffic, long commutes, relationship concerns, financials worries, or career concerns). Determine what steps you are taking to improve your stress trigger(s).
- Identify your stress relievers from past experiences (such as a massage, walking, aromatherapy, or engaging in hobbies). If you have not identified any stress relievers for yourself, consider making a list of things you would like to try to relieve stress (such as yoga, labyrinth walking, meditation, or a new hobby).
- Determine if you may have any food sensitivities or triggers (as outlined in this book) which may be contributing to your anxiety.
- Determine if you may have any nutrient deficiencies (such as folic acid, magnesium, selenium, vitamin B complex, vitamin D, or zinc) which may be contributing to your anxiety or mood disorder (Gerbarg et al. 2017).
- Determine if you have an appropriate exercise program to help you manage and overcome stress and anxiety.
- Determine if you are getting adequate sleep every night to ensure you are waking up feeling refreshed.
- Determine if you have any habits (such as drinking beverages with sugar and additives or caffeine, smoking, or consuming an excess of alcohol) which may be contributing to your anxiety or stress.
- Determine what type of meditation style fits your needs. Do you prefer static meditation, such as sitting in one place performing guided imagery, or moving meditation, such as labyrinth walking, yoga, tai chi, or qigong?

Enjoy the calmness!

Tips to Reduce Anxiety and Stay Calm

As with any unusual symptom, *if in doubt, get it checked out*. The following are some practical tips for you to consider for helping you reduce anxiety and stay calm (Cohen 2014; Wentz 2013,2017):

- Get a full medical checkup to rule out any medical conditions (such as Hashimoto's thyroiditis or post-traumatic stress disorder)
- Get help from a psychologist or counselor to learn personalized strategies
- See your doctor about trying some magnesium supplements
- See a dietitian to identify any potential food or nutrient deficiencies (such as magnesium, selenium, or Vitamin B complex)
- Minimize or avoid **common trigger foods or substances** (such as sugar, fruits, dairy, wheat, gluten, grains, eggs, nuts, seeds, soy, shellfish, peanuts, chocolate, processed meats, nightshades like potatoes and tomatoes, caffeine, alcohol, lectins, and canola oil) which may be sensitizing your system
- Try some probiotics to prevent constipation (which may also lead to the body holding on to toxins)
- Maintain normal blood sugar levels
- Try smelling some lavender oil scent
- Meditate or pray
- Go for a walk or do some form of exercise
- Play with your pets
- Keep a diary or journal
- Listen to soothing music
- Paint or draw
- Try yoga, tai chi, or qigong
- Get some fresh air and outdoor bright light
- Get a massage
- Get enough sleep every night
- Try singing, humming, or whistling
- Drive slowly and in a safe and respectful manner
- Avoid smoking
- For a **panic attack** (or **panic disorder**), try diaphragmatic breathing (Yamada et al. 2017), see a specialist about slow breathing training (Meuret et al. 2009; Meuret et al. 2010), perform regular aerobic exercise along with cognitive behavioral therapy (CBT) (Gaudlitz et al. 2015), perform yoga in combination with CBT (Vorkapic et al. 2014), and use other multimodal interventions focusing on self-care behaviors, such as self- and/or partner-assisted massage with scented oils, journaling, nutrition counseling, and exercise (McPherson et al. 2013).

Additional Massage Resources

- American Massage Therapy Association, amtamassage.org
- Deep tissue massagers, massagers.wahl.com
- GRID Foam Rollers and GRID STK, tptherapy.com
- Hyperice, hyperice.com
- Massage Bar and RumbleRoller, roguefitness.com
- Massage tools, performbetter.com
- Massage tools, optp.com
- RAD Rounds, radroller.com
- Twin Ball Massager, thebodyshop.com
- MeyerPT, meyerpt.com

Additional Resources

- American Psychological Association, apa.org
- Stress Management Society, stress.org.uk
- The American Institute of Stress, stress.org
- UCLA Center for Neurobiology of Stress and Resilience, uclacns.org

References

Abel MH. (2002). *An Empirical Reflection on the Smile (Mellen Studies in Psychology* (Volume 4). Lewiston, NY: Edwin Mellen Press.

Atkins DV, Eichler D A. (2013). The effects of self-massage on osteoarthritis of the knee: A randomized, controlled trial. *International Journal of Therapeutic Massage & Bodywork* 6 (1): 4-14.

Bhatt SP, Luqman-Arafath TK, Gupta AK, et al. (2013). Volitional pursed lips breathing in patients with stable chronic obstructive pulmonary disease improves exercise capacity. *Chronic Respiratory Disease* 10 (1): 5–10.

Bhavanani AB, Ramanathan M, Balaji R, et al. (2014). Differential effects of uninostril and alternate nostril pranayamas on cardiovascular parameters and reaction time. *International Journal of Yoga* 7 (1): 60–65.

Birnbaum MH. (1984). Nearpoint visual stress: A physiological model. *Journal of the American Optometric Association* 55 (11): 825–835.

Birnbaum MH. (1985). Nearpoint visual stress: Clinical implications. *Journal of the American Optometric Association* 56 (6): 480–490.

Block SH, Block CB. (2014). *Mind-Body Workbook for Anxiety: Effective Tools for Overcoming Panic, Fear, and Worry.* Oakland, CA: New Harbinger Publications, Inc.

Brady T. (2017). *The TB12 Method: How to Achieve a Lifetime of Sustained Peak Performance.* New York, NY: Simon & Schuster.

Cancelliero-Gaiad KM, Ike D, Pantoni CB, et al. (2014). Respiratory pattern of diaphragmatic breathing and Pilates breathing in COPD subjects. *Brazilian Journal of Physical Therapy* 18 (4): 291–299.

Church D, Yount G, Brooks AJ. (2012). The effect of emotional freedom techniques on stress biochemistry: A randomized controlled trial. *Journal of Nervous and Mental Disease* 200 (10): 891–896.

Dimsdale JE. (2008). Psychological stress and cardiovascular disease. *Journal of the American College of Cardiology* 51 (13): 1237–1246.

Epel ES. (2009). Psychological and metabolic stress: A recipe for accelerated cellular aging? *Hormones* 8 (1): 7–22.

Flexner LM, Hertling D. (2018). The temporomandibular joint. In: Brody LT, and Hall CM. *Therapeutic Exercise: Moving Toward Function,* 4th ed. Baltimore, MD: Wolters Kluwer.

Garg R, Malhotra V, Tripathi Y, et al. (2016). Effect of left, right and alternate nostril breathing on verbal and spatial memory. *Journal of Clinical and Diagnostic Research* 10 (2): CC01-3.

Gerbarg PL, Muskin PR, Brown RP. (2017). *Complementary and Integrative Treatments in Psychiatric Practice.* Arlington, VA: American Psychiatric Association Publishing.

Gomes CA, Politti F, Andrade DV, et al. (2014). Effects of massage therapy and occlusal splint therapy on mandibular range of motion in individuals with temporomandibular disorder: A randomized clinical trial. *Journal of Manipulative and Physiological Therapeutics* 37 (3): 164–169.

Gupta S, Mittal S. (2013). Yawning and its physiological significance. *International Journal of Applied & Basic Medical Research* 3 (1): 11–15.

Haff GG, Triplett NT. (Eds.). (2016). *Essentials of Strength Training and Conditioning,* 4th ed. Champaign IL: Human Kinetics.

Hatayama T, Kitamura S, Tamura C, et al. (2008). The facial massage reduced anxiety and negative mood status, and increased sympathetic nervous activity. *Biomedical Research* 29 (6): 317–320.

Hess U, Blairy S. (2001). Facial mimicry and emotional contagion to dynamic emotional facial expressions and their influence on decoding accuracy. *International Journal of Psychophysiology* 40 (2): 129–141.

Houston KA. (1993). An investigation of rocking as relaxation for the elderly. Does rocking elicit in the elderly the physiologic changes of the relaxation response? *Geriatric Nursing* 14 (4): 186–189.

Kaplan FS. (1995). *Clinical Symposia: Prevention and Management of Osteoporosis.* Summit, NJ: Ciba-Geigy Corporation 47 (1): 1–32.

Keenan J. (1996). The Japanese Tea Ceremony and stress management. *Holistic Nursing Practice* 10 (2): 30–37.

Kiecolt-Glaser JK, Christian L, Preston H, et al. (2010). Stress, inflammation, and yoga practice. *Psychosomatic Medicine* 72 (2): 113–121.

Kiecolt-Glaser JK, Habash DL, Fagundes CP, et al. (2015). Daily stressors, past depression, and metabolic responses to high-fat meals: A novel path to obesity. *Biological Psychiatry* 77 (7): 653–660.

Kiecolt-Glaser JK, Loving TJ, Stowell JR, et al. (2005). Hostile marital interactions, proinflammatory cytokine production, and wound healing. *Archives General Psychiatry* 62 (12): 1377–1384.

Kiecolt-Glaser K, Marucha PT, Malarkey WB, et al. (1995). Slowing of wound healing by psychological stress. *Lancet* 346 (8984): 1194–1196.

Kisner C, Colby LA, Borstad J. (2018). *Therapeutic Exercise: Foundations and Techniques,* 7th ed. Philadelphia, PA: FA Davis.

Koloverou E, Tentolouris N, Bakoula C, et al. (2014). Implementation of a stress management program in outpatients with Type 2 diabetes mellitus: A randomized controlled trial. *Hormones (Athens, Greece)* 13 (4): 509–518.

McMillan M. (1921). *Massage and Therapeutic Exercise.* Philadelphia, PA: WB Saunders.

Monteiro ER, SkarabotJ, Vigotsky AD, et al. (2017). Acute effects of different self-massage volumes on the FMS overhead deep squat performance. *International Journal of Sports Physical Therapy* 12 (1): 94–104.

Murad H. (2010). *The Water Secret: The Cellular Breakthrough to Look and Feel 10 Years Younger.* Hoboken, NJ: John Wiley & Sons, Inc.

Niedenthal, PM. (2007). Embodying emotion. *Science* 316 (5827): 1002–1005.

O'Sullivan SB, Schmitz TJ, Fulk GD. (2014). *Physical Rehabilitation,* 6th ed. Philadelphia, PA: FA Davis Company.

Pearcey GE, Bradbury-Squires DJ, Kawamoto JE, et al. (2015). Foam rolling for delayed-onset muscle soreness and recovery of dynamic performance. *Journal of Athletic Training* 50 (1): 5–13.

Pierce C, Pecen J, McLeod KJ. (2009). Influence of seated rocking on blood pressure in the elderly: A pilot clinical study. *Biological Research for Nursing* 11 (2): 144–151.

Sapolsky RM. (2004). *Why Zebras Don't Get Ulcers: The Acclaimed Guide to Stress, Stress-Related Diseases, and Coping,* 3rd ed. New York, NY: St Martin's Griffin.

Schecter RA, Shah J, Fruitman K, et al. (2017). Fidget spinners: Purported benefits, adverse effects and accepted alternatives. *Current Opinion in Pediatrics* 29 (5): 616–618.

Selye H. (1974). *Stress without Distress.* Philadelphia, PA: Lippincott.

Selye H. (1976). *Stress in Health and Disease.* Boston, MA: Butterworths.

Selye H. (1976). *The Stress of Life,* revised edition. New York, NY: McGraw-Hill.

Shiah YJ, Radin D. (2013). Metaphysics of the tea ceremony: A randomized trial investigating the roles of intention and belief on mood while drinking tea. *Explore (NY)* 9 (6): 355–360.

Singh K, Bhargav H, Srinivasan TM. (2016). Effect of uninostril yoga breathing on brain hemodynamics: A functional near-infrared spectroscopy study. *International Journal of Yoga* 9 (1): 12–19.

Thakur GS, Kulkarni DD, Pant G. (2011). Immediate effect of nostril breathing on memory performance. *Indian Journal of Physiology and Pharmacology* 55 (1): 89–93.

Triguero-Mas M, Donaire-Gonzalez D, Seto E, et al. (2017). Natural outdoor environments and mental health: Stress as a possible mechanism. *Environmental Research* 159: 629–638.

Vohs KD, Baumeister RF, Schmeichel BJ, et al. (2008). Making choices impairs subsequent self-control: A limited-resource account of decision making, self-regulation, and active initiative. *Journal of Personality and Social Psychology* 94 (5): 883–898.

Wamontree P, Kanchanakhan N, Eungpinichpong W, et al. (2015). Effects of traditional Thai self-massage using a Wilai massage stick(TM) versus ibuprofen in patients with upper back pain associated with myofascial trigger points: A randomized controlled trial. *Journal of Physical Therapy Science* 27 (11): 3493–3497.

Widaman AM, Witbracht MG, Forester SM, et al. (2016). Chronic stress is associated with indicators of diet quality in habitual breakfast skippers. *Journal of the Academy of Nutrition and Dietetics* 116 (11): 1776–1784.

Yamada T, Inoue A, Mafune K, et al. (2017). Recovery of percent vital capacity by breathing training in patients with panic disorder and impaired diaphragmatic breathing. *Behavior Modification* 41 (5): 665–682.

Holistic Healing Boxes

Pain Management Information

Butler D. (1991). *Mobilisation of the Nervous System.* New York, NY: Churchill Livingstone.

Butler D. (2005). *The Neurodynamic Techniques.* Adelaide City West, South Australia: Noigroup Publications.

Butler DS, Moseley GL. (2003). *Explain Pain.* Adelaide, Australia: Noigroup Publications.

Ernst E, Pittler MH, Wider B. (Eds.). (2007). *Complementary Therapies for Pain Management: An Evidence-Based Approach.* St. Louis, MO: Mosby Elsevier.

Faye L. (2008). *Goodbye Back Pain: A Sufferer's Guide to Full Back Recovery,* 2nd ed. Charleston, SC: BookSurge.

Fehmi L, Robbins J. (2007). *The Open-Focus Brain: Harnessing the Power of Attention to Heal Mind and Body.* Boston, MA: Trumpeter Books.

Fehmi L, Robbins J. (2010). *Dissolving Pain: Simple Brain-Training Exercises for Overcoming Chronic Pain.* Boston, MA: Trumpeter Books.

Fernandez-de-las-Penas C, Cleland JA, Dommerholt J. (2016). *Manual Therapy for Musculoskeletal Pain Syndromes.* United Kingdom: Elsevier.

Hebert L. (1997). *Sex and Back Pain,* 3rd ed. Greenville, ME: Impacc USA. www.impaccusa.com.

Illig KA, Thompson RW, Freischlag JA, et al. (Eds.). (2013). *Thoracic Outlet Syndrome.* London, England: Springer-Verlag.

Louw A. (2013). *Why Do I Hurt? A Patient Book About the Neuroscience of Pain.* Minneapolis, MN: Orthopedic Physical Therapy Products.

Louw A, Flynn T, Puentedura E. (2015). *Everyone Has Back Pain.* Story City, IA: International Spine and Pain Institute.

McGill SM. (2014). *Ultimate Back Fitness and Performance,* 5th ed. Waterloo, Ontario, Canada: Backfitpro Inc. (formerly Wabuno Publishers).

McGill SM. (2015). *Back Mechanic.* Waterloo, Ontario, Canada: Backfitpro Inc. www.backfitpro.com.

McGill SM. (2016). *Low Back Disorders,* 3rd ed. Champaign IL: Human Kinetics.

McKenzie R. (2011). *Treat Your Own Back,* 9th ed. Minneapolis, MN: Orthopedic Physical Therapy Products.

McKenzie R. (2011). *Treat Your Own Neck,* 5th ed. Minneapolis, MN: Orthopedic Physical Therapy Products.

McKenzie R, Watson G, Lindsay R. (2009). *Treat Your Own Shoulder.* Minneapolis, MN: Orthopedic Physical Therapy Products.

McMahon SB, Koltzenburg M, Tracey I, et al. (Eds.). (2013). *Wall and Melzack's Textbook of Pain,* 6th ed. Philadelphia, PA: Elsevier Saunders.

Melzack R, Wall PD. (2008). *The Challenge of Pain,* Updated 2nd edition. London, England: Penguin Books.

Mulligan BR. (2006). *Manual Therapy: NAGS, SNAGS, MWMS etc.,* 5th ed. Wellington, New Zealand: Plane View Service, Ltd.

Mulligan BR. (2012). *Self-Treatments for Back, Neck, and Limbs,* 3rd ed. Wellington, New Zealand: Plane View Service, Ltd.

Roth PA. (2014). *The End of Back Pain: Access Your Hidden Core to Heal Your Body.* New York, NY: HarperCollins Publishers.

Sidorkewicz N, McGill S. (2014). Male spine motion during coitus: Implications for the low back pain patient. *Spine* 39 (20): 1633–1639. www.ncbi.nlm.nih.gov/pmc/articles/PMC4381984/.

Sidorkewicz N, McGill SM. (2015). Documenting female spine motion during coitus with a commentary on the implications for the low back pain patient. *European Spine Journal* 24 (3): 513–520. www.ncbi.nlm.nih.gov/pubmed/25341806.

Sluka KA. (2016). *Mechanisms and Management of Pain for the Physical Therapist,* 2nd ed. Philadelphia, PA: Wolters Kluwer.

Turk DC, Melzack R. (2011). *Handbook of Pain Assessment.* New York, NY: Guilford Press.

Waddell G. (2004). *The Back Pain Revolution,* 2nd ed. London, England: Churchill Livingstone.

Tips to Reduce Anxiety and Stay Calm

Cohen S. (2014). *Thyroid Healthy: Lose Weight, Look Beautiful and Live the Life You Imagine.* Dear Pharmacist, Inc.

Gaudlitz K, Plag J, Dimeo F, et al. (2015). Aerobic exercise training facilitates the effectiveness of cognitive behavioral therapy in panic disorder. *Depression and Anxiety,* 32 (3): 221–228.

McPherson F, McGraw L. (2013). Treating generalized anxiety disorder using complementary and alternative medicine. *Alternative Therapies in Health and Medicine* 19 (5): 45–50.

Meuret AE, Rosenfield D, Hofmann SG, et al. (2009). Changes in respiration mediate changes in fear of bodily sensations in panic disorder. *Journal of Psychiatric Research* 43 (6): 634–641.

Meuret AE, Rosenfield D, Seidel A, et al. (2010). Respiratory and cognitive mediators of treatment change in panic disorder: Evidence for intervention specificity. *Journal of Consulting and Clinical Psychology* 78 (5): 691–704.

Vorkapic CF, Range B. (2014). Reducing the symptomatology of panic disorder: The effects of a yoga program alone and in combination with cognitive-behavioral therapy. *Frontiers in Psychiatry* 5: 177.

Wentz I. (2017). *Hashimoto's Protocol: A 90-Day Plan for Reversing Thyroid Symptoms and Getting Back Your Life.* New York, NY: HarperOne.

Wentz I, Nowosadzka M. (2013). *Hashimoto's Thyroiditis: Lifestyle Interventions for Finding and Treating the Root Cause.* Izabella Wentz (publisher).

Yamada T, Inoue A, Mafune K, et al. (2017). Recovery of percent vital capacity by breathing training in patients with panic disorder and impaired diaphragmatic breathing. *Behavior Modification* 41 (5): 665–682.

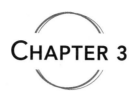

CHAPTER 3

GETTING ENOUGH SLEEP

"Sleep is the best meditation."

—Dalai Lama

Even though scientists do not know the exact purpose of sleep, we do know that getting enough sleep every night is essential for good health. Chronic sleep problems can increase your risk of heart attack, stroke, high blood pressure, diabetes, depression, and other medical problems. A person could lose sleep because he or she is experiencing pain, taking certain medications, or undergoing hormonal changes (such as menopause). Uncontrolled stress and worry, recent surgery, or poor sleeping habits (such as eating a heavy meal or doing intense exercise just prior to sleep) may also contribute to a person losing sleep. Quality of sleep is considered good when a person can fall asleep relatively quickly (within 5 to 15 minutes), wake up easily, stay asleep almost continuously, and sleep long enough to feel refreshed the next day (Akerstedt et al. 1997).

The following list sheds light on potential results of sleep deprivation (Ancoli-Israel et al. 2005; Cohen et al. 2009; Kundermann et al. 2004; Stone et al. 2008; UCLA Conference 2009, 2010; Walker 2009):

- Daytime fatigue, low energy, physical and mental tiredness, and weariness
- Mood disturbances
- Impaired cognitive functioning
- Impaired memory and concentration
- Difficulty sustaining attention with tasks
- Slowed response times (good reaction times are critical for safe driving, safety at work, and preventing falls)
- Increased incidence of colds and viruses, and a weakened immune system
- Increased pain perception
- Increased risk of falls
- Decreased job performance

- Reduced quality of life and inability to enjoy social relationships
- A possible role in the current obesity epidemic
- Decreased safety on the road, leading to car crashes

LET'S SEE WHAT RESEARCH SAYS . . .

- Programmed exercise improved sleep quality in middle-aged women but had no significant effect on the severity of insomnia (Rubio-Arias et al. 2017).
- Mindfulness meditation improves sleep quality in older adults (Black et al. 2015).
- Grigsby-Toussaint et al. (2015) indicate that talking a walk through a park, on a trail, or through your local neighborhood may help facilitate quality sleep.
- Prather et al. (2015) find that sleeping seven or more hours may help reduce susceptibility to the common cold.
- Cai et al. (2014) indicate that regular moderate- to high-intensity step aerobics training "can improve sleep quality and increase the melatonin levels in sleep-impaired postmenopausal women."
- Elite athletes should consider the fact that early-morning training programs reduce sleep duration and increase pre-training fatigue levels (Sargent et al. 2014).
- Al-Sharman et al. (2013) indicate that "sleep facilitates learning clinically relevant functional motor tasks."
- Neurotoxic waste removal (such as removal of potentially neurotoxic waste products that accumulate in the awake central nervous system) may be one of the fundamental purposes for sleep (Xie et al. 2013).
- Siengsukon et al. (2009) indicate that despite certain unanswered questions in sleep research, "therapists should consider encouraging sleep following therapy sessions as well as promoting healthy sleep in their patients with chronic stroke to promote offline motor learning of the skills practiced during rehabilitation."

25 RULES FOR CHOOSING SNOOZING

Here's a list of rules to follow to help you improve sleep habits and nighttime rituals for a good night's sleep:

RULE 1: GET ENOUGH SLEEP EVERY NIGHT

The American Academy of Sleep Medicine (AASM) recommends that "Adults should sleep 7 or more hours per night on a regular basis to promote optimal health." The consensus statement from the AASM also indicates that "Sleeping less than 7 hours per night on a regular basis is associated with adverse health outcomes, including weight gain and obesity, diabetes, hypertension, heart disease and stroke, depression, and increased risk of death. Sleeping less than 7 hours per night is also associated with impaired immune function, increased pain, impaired performance, increased errors, and greater risk of accidents." Finally, the AASM recommendations indicate that "Sleeping more than 9 hours per night on a regular basis may be appropriate for young adults, individuals recovering from sleep debt, and individuals with illnesses. For others, it is uncertain whether sleeping more than 9 hours per night is associated with health risk" (Watson et al. 2015).

The American Academy of Sleep Medicine recommends the following sleep guidelines for specific age groups in a 24-hour period to promote optimal health (Paruthi et al. 2016):

- Infants one to twelve months of age should sleep 12 to 16 hours (including naps)
- Children one to two years of age should sleep 11 to 14 hours (including naps)
- Children three to five years of age should sleep 10 to 13 hours (including naps)
- Children six to twelve years of age should sleep 9 to 12 hours
- Teenagers thirteen to eighteen years of age should sleep 8 to 10 hours

RULE 2: ESTABLISH BEDTIME HABITS

Have regular bedtime and waking hours by going to bed when sleepy, at a relatively consistent time, and getting up at the same time each day to synchronize your body clock.

RULE 3: CREATE A COMFY ROOM

Make sure your room is dark, quiet, and cool but comfortable. In most cases, room temperatures below 54 degrees Fahrenheit and above 75 degrees Fahrenheit will disrupt sleep (National Sleep Foundation 2013). Also, keep the room well ventilated.

RULE 4: SLEEP IN A COMFY BED

Make sure your bed, blankets, sheets, and pillows feel comfortable to you. Also, be sure you have a mattress that meets your needs.

RULE 5: DON'T WATCH THE CLOCK

Don't be a clock watcher (Bloom et al. 2009). Turn your alarm clock so it does not face your bed, since time pressure of clock watching might contribute to poor sleep (Ancoli-Israel 1996). This also keeps the clock light from disturbing you.

Rule 6: Embrace Mindlessness Before Bed

Allow at least one hour to unwind before bedtime (Kryger et al. 2016) by avoiding, during that time, stimulating activities such as watching a movie, reading an intense book, having emotional discussions, or playing competitive games like chess.

Rule 7: Tone Down the Music

Avoid intense or fast-paced music close to bedtime since it acts as a stimulant. However, do listen to music that is soothing and relaxing. Go to bed with a relaxed mind.

Rule 8: Stay Off Your Devices

A study shows that computer use between 7:00 p.m. and midnight increases risk of poor sleep among young adults (Mesquita et al. 2010).

Rule 9: Turn Off the Radio and Television before Falling Asleep

Keeping the radio and television turned on to help a person fall asleep can ultimately disrupt sleep (Gooneratne et al. 2011). The external stimuli of sound and light does not allow for relaxation. A quiet, dark room is best for falling asleep—and staying asleep.

Rule 10: Do What's Relaxing, Not Taxing

Engage in relaxing activities 20 to 30 minutes before sleep (Attarian 2010). Try gentle yoga, tai chi, qigong, relaxation techniques, or mindfulness training (see chapter 1). Teach your mind and body that your bed is for relaxation, not frustration.

Rule 11: Exercise Regularly

A study by Reid et al. (2010) indicates that engaging in moderate aerobic physical activity generally improves "sleep quality, mood, and quality of life in older adults with chronic insomnia." Another study indicates that vigorous late-night exercise on a stationary bicycle did not disturb sleep in young and fit individuals without sleep disorders (Myllymäki et al. 2011). However, sleep researchers typically agree that intense exercise close to bedtime acts as a stimulant and might prevent you from getting a good night's sleep. Get regular exercise in the afternoon or early evening, but avoid it close to bedtime (Kryger et al. 2016).

Rule 12: Absorb Bright Morning Light

Early bright light exposure is very helpful in synchronizing your body clock and helping to wake you in the morning—the best source is sunlight (Ancoli-Israel et al. 2005). If you can't get outdoors early in the morning, have breakfast near a window or on a balcony, porch, or patio. The timing of bright light exposure might be adjusted to late afternoon or evening by a sleep medicine physician if a patient has certain difficulties, such as falling asleep too early, working late shifts, or traveling by air frequently (Zee et al. 2010).

Rule 13: Make Your Bed a Sleep-Only Zone

Do not watch television, read, write, eat, talk on the telephone, use your laptop, or play board games on your bed.

Rule 14: Use Caution with Naps

Consider avoiding daytime naps if you have difficulty with nighttime sleep. If you are unsure about napping during the day, discuss the benefits with your physician. However, avoid naps close to bedtime. If you do take a nap, try to keep it around 10 to 30 minutes in the afternoon (Brooks et al. 2006; Milner et al. 2009).

Rule 15: Pass Up Certain Foods

Avoid foods such as aged cheeses, spicy foods, smoked meats, and ginseng tea near bedtime since they might keep you awake. On the other hand, a study shows that eating two kiwifruits one hour before bedtime might help individuals with sleep disturbances fall asleep (Lin et al. 2011).

Rule 16: Cut Out Caffeine

Avoid caffeinated foods and beverages (coffee, tea, chocolate, sodas, or colas) close to bedtime since caffeine is a stimulant and disturbs sleep (Attarian 2010). The effects of caffeine can remain in the body for three to five hours (Ancoli-Israel 1996).

Rule 17: Bid Bye-Bye to Tobacco

Avoid smoking and other tobacco products within two hours of bedtime since nicotine is a stimulant that disturbs sleep (Kryger et al. 2016). Better yet, give up smoking altogether for a variety of health benefits.

If you do smoke, talk to your doctor about quitting. They can recommend various methods others have used successfully, such as nicotine replacement therapy, which can come in the form of patches, gum, lozenges, inhalers, or nasal spray. You can also visit www.Smokefree.gov to create a Quitting Plan and to receive daily, free texts of encouragement, advice, and tips. It may take you a few tries—however—many others have quit smoking, and you can, too.

Rule 18: Nix the Nightcap

Consuming alcohol near bedtime fragments and disrupts sleep (Kryger et al. 2016; Van Reen et al. 2011). Also, a study indicates that stopping alcohol consumption at bedtime can improve sleep conditions (Morita et al. 2012). Another study by Jefferson et al. (2005) indicates that some "insomniacs do engage in specific poor sleep hygiene practices, such as smoking and drinking alcohol just before bedtime."

Rule 19: Eat Dinner in the Early Evening

Avoid late, heavy meals within three hours of bedtime. The key is not to go to bed hungry or too full. A heavy meal can cause indigestion or heartburn and, thus, keep you awake.

Rule 20: Air Out Your Bedroom

Make sure your bedroom air is free of disturbing irritants or odors. Consider opening the bedroom windows for a short period to air out the room before you go to sleep.

Rule 21: Take Meds Like Clockwork

Since many prescription and over-the-counter medicines can affect sleep, take your medications according to your physician's instructions. Don't vary your medication times unless directed by your physician or pharmacist.

Rule 22: Go Easy on the Fluids and Take a Bedtime Bathroom Break

Avoid excess consumption of fluids within two hours of bedtime to prevent frequent bathroom trips at night (Attarian 2010). Also, empty your bladder (and bowels, if necessary) before going to sleep to prevent bathroom trips that can interfere with sleep.

Rule 23: Can't Sleep? Get Up

Getting to sleep should be effortless and not forced. If you don't fall asleep within 20 minutes, get out of bed and do something relaxing. Counting sheep to sleep is unlikely to help. Try gentle stretching, 5 to 10 minutes of yoga, mindfulness meditation, or listening to soothing music. You can also try imagery distraction (Harvey et al. 2002), which entails imagining a situation you find interesting and engaging (such as relaxing at the beach with your feet in warm sand, sitting in a cozy chair on top of a mountain overlooking a distant lake, or swinging in a hammock between two palm trees and listening to the gentle waves breaking on the shore).

Rule 24: Be Careful with Sharing

Sharing your bed with your children or pets can disturb your (and their) sleep.

Rule 25: Say No to Sleeping Pills

Always consult with your physician before using over-the-counter sleeping pills.

 ## Sleep Preparation Routine

In practical terms, I personally think that 16 hours of reality is enough. There is a time for pleasant dreams and quiet time. In fact, I look forward to sleep since many of my most creative ideas come to me during sleep and my productive creative time is as soon as I awaken. Besides, the body needs patterns and cycles to thrive. Even my cats know the benefit of sleep because when I say "It's sleepy time," they both do a mad dash to the bedroom. The following is a simple sleep routine you can use to help get a good night's sleep. Please feel free to change the order and elements according to your needs:

- Power down all your electronic devices.
- Take care of toilet needs.
- Wash your hands and face and brush and floss your teeth.
- Groom and talk to your pet. He/she has been waiting all day to hear about your adventures.
- Smell a little scent of lavender oil to relax. You can place a drop of lavender oil on your pillow (Faydali et al. 2018).
- Gently massage your neck, back, and foot for one minute.
- Turn off all the lights.
- Feel your back on your cozy bed and the warm blankets over you.
- Take a moment of silence through prayer or personal reflection to be grateful for another day.
- Sleep tight.

 ## Acupressure Routine for Relaxation

If you still need additional relaxation strategies to help you relax before sleep, try some self-acupressure. See an acupuncturist for more detailed instructions. Try the following points for three minutes each to help you relax (Harris et al. 2005) (Table 3-1):

TABLE 3-1: SELF-ACUPRESSURE FOR RELAXATION

Anmian point	Lightly tap behind the ear (posterior to the mastoid process)
Yin Tang point	Massage the area between your eyebrows
HT 7 point	Massage with your thumb on the palm and little finger side where your wrist forms a crease with your hand
LV 3 point	Massage the middle top portion of your foot between the first and second toes
SP 6 point	Massage the inside of your lower leg about four fingers above your inner ankle bone, behind the shin bone

For further information about healthy sleep habits, talk to your family physician and obtain information from a local sleep disorders clinic. If you have severe difficulty with sleeping, your physician might recommend treatment using biofeedback therapy or cognitive behavioral therapy, or refer you to a sleep lab to obtain more information.

 ## PRACTICAL GUIDE FOR YOUR SLEEP ROUTINE

- Do you have any medical condition you need to adjust your lifestyle for (such as sleep apnea, arthritis, anxiety, depression, or post-traumatic stress disorder)? If yes, you should work with your primary healthcare provider and with a sleep specialist, counselor, psychologist, or psychiatrist.
- Go to credible websites (or apps) (such as the National Sleep Foundation) to obtain more information about sleep.
- Go to PubMed.gov (www.pubmed.gov) and enter the medical condition along with the word "sleep" (for example, search as "arthritis AND sleep") to search for the latest information. Speak to your healthcare provider if you need help interpreting the studies.
- Identify factors which may be preventing you from getting a good night's sleep (such as stress, late night eating, or late night computer use). Determine what steps you are taking to improve these factors.
- Identify your sleep enhancers from past experiences (such as a massage, walks, aromatherapy, or engagement in hobbies). If you have not identified any stress relievers for yourself, consider making a list of things you would like to try to relieve stress (such as meditation, self-hypnosis, or a new, calming hobby like painting).
- Determine if you may have any food sensitivities or triggers which may be contributing to your difficulty in sleeping.

- Determine if you may have any nutrient deficiencies (such as folic acid, magnesium, selenium, vitamin B complex, vitamin D, or zinc) which may be contributing to your sleep disorder.
- Determine if you have an appropriate exercise program to help you improve your sleep.
- Determine if you have a nighttime ritual to help you sleep. If not, see the sample Sleep Preparation Routine outlined in this chapter.
- Determine if you have any habits (such as ingesting sugar and additives from soft drinks or caffeine, smoking, or consuming an excess of alcohol consumption) which may be contributing to your difficulty in falling asleep.
- Determine what type of meditation style fits your needs. Do you prefer static meditation, such as sitting in one place performing guided imagery, or moving meditation, such as labyrinth walking, yoga, tai chi, or qigong?

Enjoy your pleasant dreams!

Box 5: Holistic Healing

Healthful Habits

Look at how you can make amazing changes in your life by making one healthy choice!

- Purchase the best health insurance you can afford in order to access quality medical services when needed.
- Get a yearly checkup by your family physician.
- Get appropriate vaccinations.
- Get regular checkups from your dentist and dental hygienist.
- Get periodic checkups from your eye physician.
- Go to sleep at a consistent time every night.
- Exercise daily by taking part in fun activities.
- Avoid sitting for prolonged periods.
- Frequently get outside for fresh air and sunshine.
- Eat a healthful breakfast, lunch, and dinner.
- Choose healthful snacks.
- Give up smoking.
- Minimize alcohol consumption.
- Take medications as prescribed.
- Brush and floss your teeth after meals.
- Wash your hands as necessary throughout the day.
- Sit, stand, and walk with good posture.
- Take regular vacations to unwind and relax.
- Minimize unpaid overtime hours when possible.
- Focus on your goals.

- Save your money and try to reduce debts to prevent stress.
- Strive to make a positive contribution to your surroundings.
- Smile and laugh more often.
- Log off, tune out, or power down your computer, phone, or tablet for extended periods.
- Give a family member a hug or word of encouragement.
- Remember to pet your cat or dog more frequently.
- Avoid gossip and negative talk.
- Complain less and compliment more.
- Minimize drama and look for the lighter side of life.

ADDITIONAL RESOURCES

- American Academy of Sleep Medicine, aasmnet.org
- American Sleep Association, sleepassociation.org
- National Sleep Foundation, sleepfoundation.org
- Sleep Education, sleepeducation.org
- Sleep to Live Institute, sleeptoliveinstitute.com
- Sleepnet.com, sleepnet.com
- The Better Sleep Council, bettersleep.org
- Refer to the National Institutes of Health, nih.gov (search for Sleepless in America).
- Refer to the article "Sleep Health Promotion: Practical Information for Physical Therapists" in the *Physical Therapy* journal (Siengsukon et al. 2017).

REFERENCES

Akerstedt T, Hume K, Minors D, et al. (1997). Good sleep—its timing and physiological sleep characteristics. *Journal of Sleep Research* 6 (4): 221–229.

Al-Sharman A, and Siengsukon CF. (2013). Sleep enhances learning of a functional motor task in young adults. *Physical Therapy* 93 (12): 1625–1635.

Ancoli-Israel S. (1996). *All I Want Is a Good Night's Sleep.* St. Louis, MO: Mosby-Yearbook.

Ancoli-Israel S, Cooke JR. (2005). Prevalence and comorbidity of insomnia and effect on functioning in elderly populations. *Journal of the American Geriatrics Society* 53 (Supplement 7): S264–71.

Attarian HP. (2010). *Sleep Disorders in Women: A Guide to Practical Management.* Totowa, New Jersey: Humana Press.

Black DS, O'Reilly GA, Olmstead R, et al. (2015). Mindfulness meditation and improvement in sleep quality and daytime impairment among older adults with sleep disturbances: A randomized clinical trial. *JAMA Internal Medicine* 175 (4): 494–501.

Bloom HG, Ahmed I, Alessi CA, et al. (2009). Evidence-based recommendations for the assessment and management of sleep disorders in older persons. *Journal of the American Geriatrics Society* 57 (5): 761–789.

Brooks A, Lack L. (2006). A brief afternoon nap following nocturnal sleep restriction: Which nap duration is most recuperative? *Sleep* 29 (6): 831–840.

Cai ZY, Wen-Chyuan Chen K, Wen HJ. (2014). Effects of a group-based step aerobics training on sleep quality and melatonin levels in sleep-impaired postmenopausal women. *Journal of Strength and Conditioning Research* 28 (9): 2597–2603.

Cohen S, Doyle WJ, Alper CM, et al. (2009). Sleep habits and susceptibility to the common cold. *Archives of Internal Medicine* 169 (1): 62–67.

Epstein L, Mardon S. (2007). *Harvard Medical School Guide to a Good Night's Sleep.* New York, NY: McGraw-Hill.

Faydali S, Cetinkaya F. (2018). The effect of aromatherapy on sleep quality of elderly people residing in a nursing home. *Holistic Nursing Practice* 32 (1): 8–16.

Gerbarg PL, Muskin PR, Brown RP. (2017). *Complementary and Integrative Treatments in Psychiatric Practice.* Arlington, VA: American Psychiatric Association Publishing.

Gooneratne NS, Tavaria A, Patel N, et al. (2011). Perceived effectiveness of diverse sleep treatments in older adults. *Journal of the American Geriatrics Society* 59 (2): 297–303.

Grigsby-Toussaint DS, Turi KN, Krupa M, et al. (2015). Sleep insufficiency and the natural environment: Results from the US Behavioral Risk Factor Surveillance System survey. *Preventive Medicine* 78: 78–84.

Harris RE, Jeter J, Chan P, et al. (2005). Using acupressure to modify alertness in the classroom: A single-blinded, randomized, cross-over trial. *Journal of Alternative and Complementary Medicine* 11 (4): 673–679.

Harvey AG, Payne S. (2002). The management of unwanted pre-sleep thoughts in insomnia: Distraction with imagery versus general distraction. *Behaviour Research and Therapy* 40 (3): 267–277.

Hereford JM. (2014). *Sleep and Rehabilitation: A Guide for Health Professionals.* Thorofare, NJ: SLACK.

Jefferson CD, Drake CL, Scofield HM, et al. (2005). Sleep hygiene practices in a population-based sample of insomniacs. *Sleep* 28 (5): 611–615.

Kryger MH, Roth T, Dement WC. (2016). *Principles and Practice of Sleep Medicine,* 6th ed. Philadelphia, PA: Elsevier.

Kundermann B, Krieg JC, Schreiber W, et al. (2004). The effect of sleep deprivation on pain. *Pain Research & Management* 9 (1): 25–32.

Kushida CA (Ed.). (2008). *Handbook of Sleep Disorders,* 2nd ed. Boca Raton, FL: CRC Press.

Lin HH, Tsai PS, Fang SC, et al. (2011). Effect of kiwifruit consumption on sleep quality in adults with sleep problems. *Asia Pacific Journal of Clinical Nutrition.* 20 (2): 169–174.

Mednick SC, Ehrman M. (2006). *Take a Nap! Change Your Life.* New York, NY: Workman Publishing Company, Inc.

Mesquita G, Reimao R. (2010). Quality of sleep among university students: Effects of nighttime computer and television use. *Arquivos de Neuro-Psiquiatria* 68 (5): 720–725.

Milner CE, Cote KA. (2009). Benefits of napping in healthy adults: Impact of nap length, time of day, age, and experience with napping. *Journal of Sleep Research* 18 (2) 272–281.

Morita E, Miyazaki S, Okawa M. (2012). Pilot study on the effects of a 1-day sleep education program: Influence on sleep of stopping alcohol intake at bedtime. *Nagoya Journal of Medical Science* 74 (3–4): 359–365.

Myllymäki T, Kyröläinen H, Savolainen K, et al. (2011). Effects of vigorous late-night exercise on sleep quality and cardiac autonomic activity. *Journal of Sleep Research* 20 (1 Part 2): 146–153.

National Sleep Foundation. (2013). *Sleeping smart.* National Sleep Foundation. Retrieved on November 4, 2017 from www.sleepfoundation.org.

Paruthi S, Brooks LJ, D'Ambrosio C, et al. (2016). Recommended amount of sleep for pediatric populations: A consensus statement of the American Academy of Sleep Medicine. *Journal of Clinical Sleep Medicine* 12 (6): 785–786.

Prather AA, Janicki-Deverts D, Hall MH, et al. (2015). Behaviorally assessed sleep and susceptibility to the common cold. *SLEEP* 38 (9): 1353–1359.

Reid KJ, Baron KG, Lu B, et al. (2010). Aerobic exercise improves self-reported sleep and quality of life in older adults with insomnia. *Sleep Medicine* 11 (9): 934–940.

Rubio-Arias JA, Marin-Cascales E, Ramos-Campo DJ, et al. (2017). Effect of exercise on sleep quality and insomnia in middle-aged women: A systematic review and meta-analysis of randomized controlled trials. *Maturitas* 100: 49–56.

Sargent C, Lastella M, Halson SL, et al. (2014). The impact of training schedules on the sleep and fatigue of elite athletes. *Chronobiology International* 31 (10): 1160–1168.

Siengsukon CF, Al-Dughmi M, Stevens S. (2017). Sleep health promotion: Practical information for physical therapists. *Physical Therapy* 97 (8): 826–836.

Siengsukon CF, Boyd LA. (2009). Does sleep promote motor learning? Implications for physical rehabilitation. *Physical Therapy* 89 (4): 370–383.

Stone KL, Ancoli-Israel S, Blackwell T, et al. (2008). Actigraphy-measured sleep characteristics and risk of falls in older women. *Archives of Internal Medicine* 168 (16): 1768–1775.

Van Reen E, Tarokh L, Rupp TL, et al. (2011). Does timing of alcohol administration affect sleep? *Sleep* 34 (2): 195–205.

Walker MP. (2009). The role of sleep in cognition and emotion. *Annals of the New York Academy of Sciences* 1156: 168–197.

Watson NF, Badr MS, Belenky G, et al. (2015). Recommended amount of sleep for a healthy adult: A joint consensus statement of the American Academy of Sleep Medicine and Sleep Research Society. *Journal of Clinical Sleep Medicine* 11 (6): 591–592.

Wilk KE, Joyner D. (2014). *The Use of Aquatics in Orthopedic and Sports Medicine Rehabilitation and Physical Conditioning.* Thorofare, NJ: SLACK.

Xie L, Kang H, Xu Q, et al. (2013). Sleep drives metabolite clearance from the adult brain. *Science* 342 (6156): 373–377.

Zee PC, Goldstein CA. (2010). Treatment of shift work disorder and jet lag. *Current Treatment Options in Neurology* 12 (5): 396–411.

CHAPTER 4

NUTRITION FOR LIFE

"Eat food. Not too much. Mostly plants."

—Michael Pollan

Please speak with a registered dietitian to obtain specific nutritional guidelines for your needs. The following is not intended to be a complete coverage of nutrition information. There are many excellent books covering nutrition for health. I also recommend you start with the American Academy of Nutrition and Dietetics website www.eatright.org for solid evidence-based information. Therefore, the focus on this chapter is on covering some specialty topics in nutrition and the health benefits of fruits and vegetables.

Here is another example from my dad which conveys the importance of nutrition as a part of a lifestyle program. He was always trying to pass on his years of knowledge he acquired in medicine so I could be a good clinician. One day, just before I graduated from my physical therapy program at the University of Pittsburgh, he challenged me to consider the most important factors for our well-being. I think at the time I said exercise was the key, since this is what I was going to do for a living. He nodded and said perhaps I might want to reconsider my position. He asked me, how long can an average person go without breathing? We agreed it was about a minute or so. Then, he asked how long someone can go without drinking water? We agreed it would be a matter of days. He asked how long someone can go without eating any food. Again, we agreed it would be a matter of weeks. He asked the same about sleep. Once again, we agreed it would be a week or more before some harm came to the body as a result of no sleep. Then, he asked how long a person could go without exercising. Well, we agreed that as long as a person was moving around to some degree (and not bedridden), then the person could go for many years without formal exercise. And many individuals do. Of course, it may not be quality years due to all the problems which can occur as a result of being sedentary (such as stiffness, perhaps pain, weakness, and potentially the onset of various diseases), but nevertheless, formal exercise is not on the same level of significance for the body to stay alive as breathing, drinking water, eating food, or sleeping. And to this day, I use a similar hierarchy when I educate my patients about wellness. I focus on the breath for relaxation and recovery, hydration, nourishing and healing foods, quality sleep, and of course, fun and meaningful movements and exercise. In terms of nutrition, I consider food to be medicine. Foods can not only nourish us but also help heal our mind and body.

MINDFUL EATING

Why are we as a culture so obsessed with fast food and instant messaging? Why are many of us in such a rush? Is there a finish line somewhere? It would be best if we focus on eating home-cooked meals in a peaceful manner and going to a local café to enjoy good conversation with friends and family instead of staring at a screen. I personally cannot wait until they have Internet-free and cellphone-free cafes. Maybe, in this way, we can rekindle the lost art of enjoyable and creative conversation.

A study by Miller et al. (2014) states that "mindful eating may be an effective intervention for increasing awareness of hunger and satiety cues, improving eating regulation and dietary patterns, reducing symptoms of depression and anxiety, and promoting weight loss." The following are aids to help you include mindful eating as a part of your lifestyle:

- Avoid emotional eating.
- Sit in a firm and supportive chair during meals.
- Turn off all electronic devices.
- Avoid talking while chewing your food not only to enjoy the satisfying tastes, but also to prevent choking.
- Chew your food slowly. Jeannette Hyde (www.jeannettehyde.com), a registered nutritional therapist and the author of *The Gut Makeover* (2017), recommends you chew each bite of food 20 times to stimulate the production of stomach acid and enzymes. Eating slowly can help you improve digestion and lose weight since it takes about 20 minutes for the satiety hormones to kick in after eating.
- Sit in a location that allows you to look at nature or pleasant scenery.
- Avoid discussing business or personal problems while eating to allow for relaxed digestion.

Engage your five senses as you eat your healing meals:
- **Observe** the colors in your food (such as the red, orange, green, and yellow colors).
- **Feel** your food's textures (the shape of a berry or carrot).
- **Listen** to the sounds your foods make (the crunching of celery or an apple).

- **Smell** your food's delicious aromas (the scent of mint or cinnamon).
- **Taste** the sweet, salty, bitter, sour, or spice in your foods (such as the tartness of a lemon).

MINDFUL EATING LESSON

To start the lesson, pick your favorite fruit and have a seat in a comfortable chair. I'll pick a banana for this example. Now, let's engage all your senses as you eat the banana (or the fruit you chose). First, observe the color. It has a relaxing yellow color. Now, slowly peel back your banana and listen to the sound it makes. To me, it sounds like a tearing-type noise. Next, feel the texture of the peeled banana. It feels squishy to me. Okay, now smell your banana. Mine smells sweet and pleasant. Finally, take a small bite of your banana and taste. Mine tastes very sweet and mushy. So that is one example of mindful eating. Imagine eating all of your meals in a slow and deliberate manner. More than likely you would have less indigestion, enjoy your meal, and perhaps lose some weight. For more information about mindful eating, check out the book *Mindful Eating: A Guide to Rediscovering a Healthy and Joyful Relationship with Food (Revised Edition)* by Jan Chozen Bays (Shambhala Publications, 2017).

WHAT ARE FUNCTIONAL FOODS?

The concept of "Functional Food" was first used in Japan in the 1980s. A review article by Motohashi et al. (2017) states that "functional foods are extremely beneficial components found naturally in foods or added to the regular diet which include secondary metabolites, prebiotics, probiotics, synbiotics in addition to the usual vitamins, minerals, and amino acids. Functional food ingredients contain biologically beneficial carotenoids, fatty acids, flavonoids, betalains, phenols, phenolic acids, phytosterols, alkaloids, phytoestrogens, and dietary fibre." The authors go on to state that functional foods "help fight disease, boost immune system, energy, maintain healthy skin, maintain joints and strong bones, improve healthy digestion and promote longevity. Certain components in functional foods exhibit antioxidant, cardioprotective, antidiabetic, hepato and neuroprotective, antimicrobial activities and constipation improvement." For additional information, refer to the following websites:

- Functional Food Center, functionalfoodscenter.net
- Institute of Food Technologists, ift.org
- Institute for Functional Medicine, ifm.org

YOU CANNOT OUTRUN A BAD DIET

An editorial article by Malhotra et al. (2015) states that "It is time to wind back the harms caused by the junk food industry's Public Relations machinery. Let us bust the myth of physical inactivity and obesity. You cannot outrun a bad diet." For instance, if you eat half a large pizza most every night but exercise for 30 minutes a day, you will probably still be unhealthy. This is especially true if you have food sensitivities to the grains, gluten, dairy, or tomatoes (foods classified as nightshades) contained in the pizza. It's not a matter of just exercising or running off the calories we consume from food to lose weight or stay fit, but consuming foods which help to nourish and repair the body.

The foods we consume should not contain harmful ingredients (such as additives, preservatives, or dyes) which can harm your body. No food we eat should contain a list of chemicals we cannot even pronounce. Then, there is the matter of sugar and how it is disguised in all of the foods at the supermarket. Why does anyone need *high*-fructose *corn syrup, sucrose,* barley malt, dextrose, maltose, or rice syrup? If you want to learn more about sugar, then I suggest you go to the Sugar Science website http://sugarscience.ucsf.edu to learn more. And, next time you are at the market, look at the ingredients in all of the soft drinks. I sincerely hope that the evidence clearly shows that no soft drink (diet or otherwise) belongs in the human body. How about a nice glass of water or a cup of soothing tea instead?

My feeling is that junk food is consumed because that is what we see in all of the advertising. If we think about the consequences of the foods we eat and plan our snacks better, then we can dramatically minimize bringing harm to our bodies. For example, my favorite go-to snacks when I have a craving or while I'm traveling are easy-to-eat foods such as avocados, bananas, kiwis or perhaps, a nutrition bar such as an EPIC bar (www.epicbar.com) or LARABAR (www.larabar.ca). Other healthy snacks could be a little dark chocolate and almonds (or walnuts). In terms of beverages, I either opt for water or tea. This will usually keep me happy until I can sit down and have a nice meal with good conversation. So, what's on your healthful snack list?

WHAT FOODS SHOULD YOU CHOOSE?

Good nutrition is a balance of healthful proteins (such as fish, grass-fed beef or lamb, chicken, yogurt, cheese, nuts, seeds, or legumes), healthful fats (such as nuts, seeds, olive oil, or avocados), healthful carbohydrates (such as vegetables, fruits, or whole grains if your body tolerates grains), and healthful beverages (such as water or herbal tea). Good nutrition also is knowing about **common trigger foods or substance**s (such as sugar, fruits, dairy, wheat, gluten, grains, eggs, nuts, seeds, soy, shellfish, peanuts, chocolate, processed meats, and night-shades like potatoes and tomatoes, caffeine, alcohol, lectins, and canola oil) which may affect your system. In my opinion, this is where the concept of moderation breaks down. Go for moderation if you want to feel moderate. Go for precision if you want to feel excellent. Okay, but how does a person know if a certain food is a trigger for some symptom? The key is to pay attention to your body and see if you get any reactions to food while you eat or after you eat. Ideally, it is better to isolate a single food (such as a tomato, milk for dairy, or bread for gluten sensitivity) instead of a combination of ingredients in a meal (such as pizza which has tomatoes, dairy, gluten, oil, etc.). If you suspect a food allergy or sensitivity, it is best to work with a registered dietitian and a physician specializing in food allergies. I have personally worked with a dietitian and saw several allergists over the years, and I obtained very useful information about my body. Consider eliminating certain foods or all allergens for a period of time (for example, two to three months) and then gradually add them back. Do a quick screen on yourself after each meal or on a daily basis to see how you react to certain foods and determine if any cause the following symptoms: headache or migraine, congestion, sneezing, coughing, abdominal bloating, abdominal pain or cramping, increased heart rate, hyperactivity, nausea, diarrhea, flushed face, itching or rash, poor concentration, or fatigue.

The remainder of this chapter will hopefully help you fine-tune your food choices during grocery trips.

PRACTICAL NUTRITION

Consider looking at nutrition this way: Could you pick or catch the foods you are currently eating? In other words, could you have picked that box of cookies from a tree or caught those doughnuts fishing in a lake or ocean? The best wholesome foods for your body will typically be those that give you enough calories, allow your body to heal and maintain itself, and do not cause stomach irritation, nausea, cramping, bloating, or allergies. The more you speak with people around you the more you will realize that almost any food may cause an adverse reaction in someone. Therefore, the right food choices for each individual are critical for optimal health.

Individual dietary choices are influenced by habits, culture, nutritional knowledge, price, availability, taste, and convenience. A study by Imamura et al. (2015) systematically assessed different dietary patterns across 187 nations in 1990 and 2010 and the authors conclude that "Increases in unhealthy patterns are outpacing increases in healthy patterns in most world regions." Our multicultural and global society needs to find ways to reduce the financial barriers to healthful eating, which in turn can reduce illness and disease (Rao et al. 2013).

Also, food is not only important for human health, but the health of the planet since agriculture impacts environmental sustainability (Tilman et al. 2014).

Also, a person can eat in a healthful manner whether he or she is a vegetarian or a non-vegetarian. Healthfully eating can come in a variety of packages. The key to good nutrition is not only choosing foods that agree with your body, but also selecting foods that are processed as little as possible and closest to the way nature intends for us to eat.

Choosing Wisely

Every purchase we make or don't make influences the marketplace. If a significant percentage of the population chose healthful foods and snacks, then the fast-food, soft drink, and junk food industries would eventually either have to change their approach or become obsolete. After all, "we are what we eat."

Consider choosing quality foods which adhere to the following fresh farm-to-table approach:

- Produced as eco-friendly and with recyclable materials
- Produced in a sustainable manner
- Product claims are 100% truthful. Consider checking the Food and Drug Administration (FDA) website fda.gov as one source of verification
- Product is truly all-natural. In other words, it's not a product like a soft drink where it takes an army of chemists to create. For example, an apple is something you pick from a tree, and it is consumed in its natural state and as food that is considered safe and natural for the body.
- Free of genetically modified organisms (GMO-free)
- Antibiotic-free
- Pesticide-, additive-, and chemical-free
- Free of artificial colors, flavors, sweeteners, or preservatives
- Free of artificial growth hormones
- Locally grown
- Organic
- Animals are pasture-raised (chicken and eggs)
- Animals are grass-fed
- Fish are wild caught

For additional good health, try the following:

- Shop at farmers markets
- Eat a variety of colors and seasonal fruits and vegetables
- Eat in moderate amounts
- Eat slow
- Vary the brands of products you are using, such as bottled water and olive oil. This way, you are getting a variety of nutrients in your body and helping to prevent imbalances and deficiencies.

We all know good nutrition is not about "cookies and cakes and pies, oh my!" A calorie is not just a calorie. Your source of food has a tremendous impact on your health. Calories from doughnuts do not carry the same life-sustaining nutrients as berries or green leafy vegetables. The calories might be the same, but nutritional content and the life-giving effect is not.

Food First Approach

Proper nutrition should be an accessible concept available to all groups of people. Everyone can eat healthfully without spending tons of money on supplements and specialized foods. Supplements typically come in handy when there is a deficiency or some specific need, such as low levels of calcium or vitamin D. Nourish yourself with food first, and then supplement only if necessary.

Water for Health

We know we should drink water for good health but how much is enough? Again, I recommend you consult the American Academy of Nutrition and Dietetics website www.eatright.org and search for "water." Another good source to learn more about water safety is the Food and Drug Administration website www.fda.gov.

Finally, I will mention a study about alkaline water. A review article by Fenton et al. (2016) states that a "systematic review of the literature revealed a lack of evidence for or against diet acid load and/or alkaline water for the initiation or treatment of cancer. Promotion of alkaline diet and alkaline water to the public for cancer prevention or treatment is not justified." Perhaps future research will have a conclusion one way or another regarding the general health and wellness benefits of drinking alkaline water and not solely focus on hydration after exercise (Weidman et al. 2016). Refer to the Precision Nutrition website www.precisionnutrition.com and search for "alkaline water" for a review about alkaline water. In the meantime, you may want to consider periodically changing water brands to include natural spring water (such as Evian, Fiji, or Icelandic Glacial) and other brands (such as Aquafina, Dasani, or Essentia) so that you get a variety of minerals and nutrients in your diet. Also check the Fluoride Action Network www.fluoridealert.org if you want to learn more about fluoride in your water.

Let's See What Research Says . . .

- "Individuals with type 2 diabetes improved their glycemic control and lost more weight after being randomized to a very **low-carbohydrate ketogenic diet** and lifestyle online program rather than a conventional, low-fat diabetes diet online program" (Saslow et al. 2017). For additional information about the ketogenic diet, see the article in JAMA (Abbasi 2018).

- Lis et al. (2017) find that "short-term **FODMAP** [fermentable oligosaccharide, disaccharide, monosaccharide, and polyols] reduction may be a beneficial intervention to minimize daily GI symptoms in runners with exercise-related GI distress." For example, the FODMAPs eliminate certain foods containing fructose (such as apples, pears, dried fruit, fruit juice, honey, and corn syrup), lactose (such as milk, ice cream, yogurt, and cheese), fructans (such as broccoli, cabbage, eggplant, garlic, leeks, onions, wheat, breads, and pasta), galactans (such as beans, chickpeas, kidney beans, lentils, and soybeans), and polyols (such as avocadoes, blackberries, cherries, peaches, plums, green bell peppers, mushrooms, and corn). For further information about FODMAPs, please see chapter 17: Sustainable Weight Loss Guide.

- Marum et al. (2016) find that **FODMAP** restrictions may reduce gastrointestinal disorders and fibromyalgia (a chronic, rheumatic disease characterized by widespread myofascial pain) symptoms, including pain sores.

- The **Mediterranean diet** "decreases inflammation and improves endothelial function" (Schwingshackl et al. 2014). The Mediterranean diet is characterized by foods such as cereals, vegetables, legumes, nuts, fish, fresh fruits, and olive oil as the principal sources of fat, and by low meat consumption and low-to-moderate consumption of milk, dairy products, and wine (Mattioli et al. 2017).

- The MIND (**M**editerranean-DASH Diet **In**tervention for **N**eurodegenerative **D**elay) Diet study, which is based on the Mediterranean and DASH diets, concludes that this diet "substantially slows cognitive decline with age." The authors indicate that the "MIND diet components are 10 brain healthy food groups (green leafy vegetables, other vegetables, nuts, berries, beans, whole grains, seafood, poultry, olive oil, and wine) and five unhealthy food groups (red meats, butter and stick margarine, cheese, pastries and sweets, and fried/fast food) (Morris et al. 2015)."

- A traditional **Mediterranean diet** "could modify markers of heart failure toward a more protective mode" (Fito et al. 2014).

- "A **Paleolithic diet** improved glycemic control and several cardiovascular risk factors compared to a diabetes diet in patients with type 2 diabetes" (Jonsson et al. 2013). A review article by Manheimer et al. (2015) states that "there was no single Paleolithic nutritional pattern. Food choices critically depended on the geographical latitude and climate." A book by Cordain (2011) and a review article by Cordain et al. (2005) go into further detail about the origins and practical applications of the Paleolithic diet.

- "A **low-fat plant-based diet** in a corporate setting improved body weight, plasma lipids, and, in individuals with diabetes, glycemic control" (Mishra et al. 2013).
- A study called the **Dietary Approaches to Stop Hypertension** (DASH) indicates that individuals with hypertension can lower their blood pressure through lifestyle and behavioral changes consisting of weight loss, sodium reduction, increased physical activity, and limited alcohol consumption (Appel et al. 2003).

FINDING THE IDEAL DIET

Every year many nutrition books promising to lead us down the path to perfect health are published. Each one is an answer for some or a source of controversy for others. As a consumer, I am no different than anyone else. I have purchased and tried many of the varied approaches to nutrition.

So which diet is best? The answer is, it depends. It depends on your body's physiology, your philosophy, and the results that are obtained. A one-size-fits-all approach does not work. Each book can provide a person another tool to try, and ultimately, that individual has to determine if it works for their needs or not.

This reminds me of a story my mother told me when I was about ten years old. When she was my age, several of her friends were challenging her beliefs and she was trying to determine the right way to do something. Her father asked her, "What is the best way to arrive at the number 10?" Mom gave him a blank stare. Her father prompted her to list off all the mathematical possibilities for arriving at the number 10. So Mom replied, "9 + 1 = 10, 5 + 5 = 10, 2 x 5 = 10, 20 / 2 = 10, and 20 − 10 = 10." After pausing a moment to think, she said they were all correct. As the story goes, her father smiled and encouraged her to remember that lesson later in life when she had her views challenged again.

In my mind, this is why different diets work for some groups of people for losing weight or regaining health but do not work for everyone. For this reason, each person has to go through some trial and error to find the best diet for their body. Of course, this same trial- and-error method extends to finding the ideal exercise, sleep duration, stress management strategy, and meditation technique for that individual. One person feels great on a vegetarian diet, while another person only feels great on a Paleo diet. It sounds to me like the same lesson Mom learned when she was 10 years old.

FOOD ALLERGIES AND SENSITIVITIES

Specialized diets might come into play for individuals with certain medical conditions (such as diabetes or hypertension), celiac disease (gluten allergy), food allergies (such as to eggs, fish, shellfish, soy, peanuts, tree nuts, or milk), or food intolerances (such as lactose or fructose) and sensitivities (such as to additives, preservatives, corn, or yeast). For individuals with food allergies or sensitivities, it's best to try an elimination diet and also to work with a registered dietitian and allergist.

PHYTONUTRIENTS AND YOUR HEALTH

Eating 400 grams to 600 grams (as an example, an average apple is between 70 and 100 grams) a day of fruits and vegetables is associated with reduced incidence of various forms of cancer, heart disease, and many chronic diseases (Heber et al. 2006; Pennington et al. 2010). This is consistent with the recommendation of the World Health Organization that increasing individual fruit and vegetable consumption to approximately 600 grams per day could reduce ischemic stroke worldwide (Lock et al. 2005).

In the book *What Color Is Your Diet?*, David Heber, MD, PhD, and Susan Bowerman, MS, RD, state that "foods can be classified according to color—red, red/purple, orange, orange/yellow, green, yellow/green, and white/green—based on the specific chemicals that absorb light in the visible spectrum and thus create the different colors. These chemicals are called 'phytonutrients' or 'phytochemicals,' and each of these colored compounds works in different ways to protect your genes and your DNA." The authors further state that "there are 150,000 edible plant species on earth, and we have just listed about 60 or so varieties in our Color Code. While this is a big improvement over the few servings per day the average American eats, there is still a long way to go" to become a healthier society.

The Rainbow Nutrition Guide (Table 4-1) outlines one way to organize your eating plan so you include more healthful fruits and vegetables into your diet. Why eat all this variety? Look at it like this: You are simply stacking the odds in your favor for maintaining good health. However, keep in mind what health author and registered dietitian Tracy Olgeaty Gensler MS, RD (Altug and Gensler 2006), states that "While it's tempting to champion the well-researched fruits or vegetables over the others, every single fruit and vegetable offers you some health benefit."

Table 4-1: Rainbow Nutrition Guide

Groups	Compounds	Some Research Areas	Food Sources
Green Group	sulforaphane, isothiocyanate, indole	· Sulforaphane inhibits breast cancer stem cells (Li et al. 2010) · Broccoli may reduce risk of prostate cancer (Traka et al. 2008)	bok choy, broccoli, Brussels sprouts, cabbage, Chinese cabbage, kale, watercress
Yellow/ Green Group	lutein, zeaxanthin	· Lutein and zeaxanthin have a potential role in the prevention and treatment of certain eye diseases, such as age-related macular degeneration, cataract, and retinitis pigmentosa (Ma et al. 2010)	avocado, collard greens, green beans, green peas, green and yellow peppers, mustard greens, romaine lettuce, spinach, turnip greens, yellow corn, zucchini honeydew melon, kiwifruit
White/ Green Group	allyl sulfide (allicin), flavonoid (quercetin and kaempferol	· Has antibacterial, antiviral, and antitumor effects (Heber 2001; Venes 2017) · Lowers blood cholesterol levels (Venes 2017) · Garlic-derived compounds are effective to inhibit a variety of human cancers, such as prostate, breast, colon, skin, lung, and bladder cancers (Wang et al. 2010)	asparagus, celery, chives, endive, garlic, leek, mushroom, onion, shallot pear
Orange/ Yellow Group	beta-cryptoxanthin	· Helps fight heart disease · Fruits high in antioxidant nutrients appear to be associated with reduced risk of incident squamous intraepithelial lesions of the cervix (Siegel et al. 2010)	guava, kumquat, nectarine, orange, papaya, peach, pineapple, star fruit, tangelo, tangerine

Orange Group	alpha- and beta-carotene	· A diet rich in beta-carotene and lutein/zeaxanthin may play a role in renal cell carcinoma prevention (Hu et al. 2009) · Beta-carotene and lycopene were associated with a lower prevalence of metabolic syndrome (Sluijs et al. 2009)	acorn squash, butternut squash, carrot, orange pepper, pumpkin, sweet potato, winter squash, yellow squash apricot, cantaloupe, mango, persimmon
Red Group	lycopene	· Can protect the cells in the body from oxidative damage · Lycopene inhibits in vitro cell growth and induces apoptosis (programmed cell death) in breast and prostate cancer cells (Gullett et al. 2010)	pink grapefruit, pink grapefruit juice, tomato (cooked and raw), tomato juice, tomato paste, tomato sauce, tomato soup, watermelon
Red/Purple Group	anthocyanin	· May have a beneficial effect on heart disease by inhibiting blood clot formation and are anti-inflammatory (Heber 2001) · May help with age-related declines in mental function · Pomegranate may retard prostate cancer progression and inhibit growth of breast cancer cells (Gullett et al. 2010)	cooked beets, purple cabbage blackberry, blueberry, cherry, cranberry, cranberry juice, cranberry sauce, fig, grape juice, pear, plum, pomegranate, prune, purple passion fruit, raspberry, red apple, red grapes, strawberry

Adapted from Heber D, and Bowerman S. (2001). *What Color is Your Diet?* New York: Harper Collins/Regan; Altug and Gensler 2006; Heber et al. 2006; Steinmetz et al. 1991, 1991, 1996.

REASONING FOR SEASONING

A variety of spices (Table 4-2) have been shown to help inflammatory diseases such as cancer, atherosclerosis, myocardial infarction, diabetes, allergy, asthma, arthritis, Crohn's disease, multiple sclerosis, Alzheimer's disease, osteoporosis, psoriasis, septic shock, and AIDS (Aggarwal et al. 2004, 2008).

An article by Gupta et al. (2010) states that "It is now believed that 90 percent to 95 percent of all cancers are attributed to lifestyle, with the remaining 5 percent to 10 percent attributed to faulty genes." The medical profession is now turning its focus to the use of plant-derived dietary agents called nutraceuticals.

We know that pharmaceuticals pertain to drugs or the pharmacy. The authors of this article explain that "A nutraceutical (a term formed by combining the words 'nutrition' and 'pharmaceutical') is simply any substance considered to be a food or part of a food that provides medical and health benefits."

Another article discusses nutraceuticals such as curcumin, carotenoids, acetyl-L-carnitine, coenzyme Q_{10}, vitamin D, and polyphenols, all natural substances that might help reduce the expression of disease-promoting genes (Virmani et al. 2013). Perhaps very soon, all major supermarkets will display the healing and prevention properties, based on research, of every single fruit and vegetable in the store.

The Foods and Spices Guide (Table 4-2) helps you to understand the benefits of various foods and spices. Always consult with your physician or healthcare provider before using spices, herbs, or supplements for medical purposes. If you take medications, there could be adverse reactions (Stargrove et al. 2008).

TABLE 4-2: FOODS AND SPICES GUIDE

FOOD SOURCE	ACTIVE COMPOUND	SOME AREAS OF BENEFIT
Aloe	Emodin	Antioxidant, anti-inflammatory, antifungal, immunoprotective (El-Shemy et al. 2010)
Basil and rosemary	Ursolic acid	Chemopreventive activity (Aggarwal et al. 2004)
Black pepper	Piper nigrum	Anti-inflammatory, antioxidant, and anticancer activities (Liu et al. 2010)
Cloves	Eugenol	Antioxidant and anti-inflammatory activities (Aggarwal et al. 2004)
Fennel, anise, coriander	Anethol	Antioxidant and anti-inflammatory activities (Aggarwal et al. 2004)
Garlic	Diallyl sulfide, ajoene, S-ally cysteine, allicin	Chemopreventive and anti-inflammatory activities (Aggarwal et al. 2004; Mehta et al. 2010)
Ginger	Gingerol	Chemopreventive potential, treatment of nausea with motion or chemotherapy, anti-inflammatory (Aggarwal et al. 2004; Mehta et al. 2010)
Gingko biloba	Ginkgolides	Chemoprevention, antioxidant, anti-inflammatory activities (Mehta et al. 2010; Ye et al. 2007)
Ginseng	Ginsenoside	Antiviral against influenza A virus (Lee et al. 2014)
Green tea	Catechins	Chemopreventive potential (Gullett et al. 2010)
Honey-bee propolis	Caffeic acid	Anti-inflammatory and antimicrobial effects (Khayyal et al.1993; Sherlock et al. 2010)

Oleander	Oleanderin	Chemopreventive potential (Afaq et al. 2004)
Parsley	Apigenin	Antioxidant capacity (Henning et al. 2011; Meeran et al. 2008)
Red chili pepper	Capsaicin	Chemopreventive potential (Aggarwal et al. 2004)
Soybean	Genistein	Antioxidant (Gullett et al. 2010)
Sumac (spice)	Rhus coriaria	Hypoglycemic and antioxidant activity (Candan et al. 2004; Giancarlo et al. 2006)
Turmeric	Curcumin	Chemopreventive, anti-inflammatory, lowers blood cholesterol, improves arthritis associated symptoms (Aggarwal et al. 2004; Gullett et al. 2010; Panahi et al. 2014)

PRACTICAL GUIDE FOR YOUR DIET SELECTION

Do you have any medical condition you need to adjust your lifestyle for (such as hypertension, osteoporosis, osteoarthritis, thyroid condition, diabetes, or cancer)? If yes:

- First, work with your primary healthcare provider and a registered dietitian to optimize your diet.
- Second, go the Academy of Nutrition and Dietetics website www.eatright.org and search for your medical condition.
- Third, go to credible websites (or apps) for each condition (such as the National Osteoporosis Foundation for bone-related inquiries) to obtain more information.
- Fourth, read good nutrition textbooks to obtain basic and advanced nutrition information for your needs. Consider books such as the *Academy of Nutrition and Dietetics Complete Food and Nutrition Guide* by Robert Duyff; *Nutrition Diagnosis-Related Care* by Sylvia Escott-Stump; *Krause's Food & The Nutrition Care Process* by L. Kathleen Mahan and Janice Raymond. Use these sources along with information from your healthcare provider.
- Fifth, go to the Academy of Nutrition and Dietetics website eatright.org and the National Institutes of Health: Office of Dietary Supplements website ods.od.nih.gov/factsheets (Table 4-3) to find information about specific nutrients from foods.
  - » **Recipes:** You can also go the Academy of Nutrition and Dietetics website eatright.org for additional recipes.
- Sixth, before you start taking supplements, go to the Office of Dietary Supplements website ods.od.nih.gov and the US Food and Drug Administration website fda.gov

- Finally, go to PubMed.gov (pubmed.gov) and enter the medical condition of concern to you along with the word "diet" (for example, search as "osteoporosis AND diet") to search for the latest information. Speak with your healthcare provider if you need help interpreting the studies.

TABLE 4-3: SELECTED SOURCES OF NUTRIENTS

VITAMINS	· Vitamin A—ods.od.nih.gov/factsheets/list-all/VitaminA · Vitamin B1 (Thiamine)—ods.od.nih.gov/factsheets/list-all/Thiamin · Vitamin B2 (Riboflavin)—ods.od.nih.gov/factsheets/list-all/Riboflavin · Vitamin B12—ods.od.nih.gov/factsheets/list-all/VitaminB12 · Folate—ods.od.nih.gov/factsheets/Folate-Consumer · Vitamin C—ods.od.nih.gov/factsheets/list-all/VitaminC · Vitamin D—ods.od.nih.gov/factsheets/list-all/VitaminD · Vitamin E—ods.od.nih.gov/factsheets/list-all/VitaminE
MINERALS	· Calcium—https://ods.od.nih.gov/factsheets/list-all/Calcium · Iron—https://ods.od.nih.gov/factsheets/list-all/Iron · Magnesium—https://ods.od.nih.gov/factsheets/list-all/Magnesium · Selenium—https://ods.od.nih.gov/factsheets/list-all/Selenium · Zinc—https://ods.od.nih.gov/factsheets/list-all/Zinc

- Consider keeping a daily journal or diary to help you determine potential sources of food sensitivities, intolerances, or allergens. Refer to chapter 14: Tracking Your Progress.
- Consider looking at your cultural background to determine if certain foods may be more tolerable to your system.
- Consider avoiding foods you already have sensitivities or reactions to.
- To obtain more information about various vitamins and minerals, go to the USDA National Nutrient Database for Standard Reference website ndb.nal.usda.gov.
- If you have irritable bowel syndrome, look into the FODMAP diet website and App, monashfodmap.com
- If you are trying to lose weight, refer to chapter 17: Sustainable Weight Loss Guide.

Enjoy eating healthy meals!

BOX 6: HOLISTIC HEALING

HASHIMOTO'S THYROIDITIS HEALTH GUIDE

Hashimoto's thyroiditis is named after Hakaru Hashimoto (1881-1934), a Japanese surgeon. This autoimmune disease is characterized by inflammation, destruction, and fibrosis of the thyroid gland, and ultimately results in hypothyroidism. In other words, there are inadequate levels of thyroid hormone in the body. Thyroid deficiencies cause diminished basal metabolism, cold intolerance, fatigue, mental apathy, physical sluggishness, constipation, muscle aches, dry hair and skin, decreased metabolism, and weight gain (Porter et al. 2011; Venes 2017).

Additional Resources

- American Association of Clinical Endocrinologists, aace.com
- American Autoimmune Related Diseases Association, aarda.org
- American Thyroid Association, thyroid.org
- Dr. Izabella Wentz, PharmD, thyroidpharmacist.com
- Dr. Izabella Wentz, PharmD, rootcology.com
- *EmPower* magazine, empoweryourhealth.org
- Endocrine Society, endocrine.org
- European Thyroid Association, eurothyroid.com
- Society for Endocrinology, endocrinology.org
- Suzy Cohen, RPh, suzycohen.com
- The Hashimoto's Institute, hashimotosinstitute.com
- Thyroid Disease Manager, thyroidmanager.org
- Thyroid Federation International, thyroid-fed.org/tfi-wp
- Refer to the book *Hashimoto's Protocol* (Wentz 2017).
- Refer to the book *Hashimoto's Thyroiditis* (Wentz 2013).
- Refer to the book *Thyroid Healthy* (Cohen 2014).

ADDITIONAL RESOURCES

- American Academy of Allergy, Asthma & Immunology, aaaai.org
- American Academy of Nutrition and Dietetics, eatright.org
- American Botanical Council, abc.herbalgram.org
- Celiac Disease Foundation, celiac.org
- Eatwild.com, eatwild.com
- Herb Research Foundation, herbs.org
- HerbMed, herbmed.org
- Living Without's Gluten Free & More, livingwithout.com
- Monterey Bay Aquarium's Seafood Watch, seafoodwatch.org
- Office of Dietary Supplements, ods.od.nih.gov
- Phenol-Explorer, phenol-explorer.eu
- Sports, Cardiovascular, and Wellness Nutrition, scandpg.org
- USDA National Nutrient Database for Standard Reference, ndb.nal .usda.gov

REFERENCES

Abbasi J. (2018). Interest in the ketogenic diet grows for weight loss and Type 2 diabetes. *JAMA* 319 (3):215–217.

Afaq F, Saleem M, Aziz MH, et al. (2004). Inhibition of 12-O-tetradecanoylphorbol-13-acetate-induced tumor promotion markers in CD-1 mouse skin by oleandrin. *Toxicology and Applied Pharmacology* 195 (3): 361–369.

Aggarwal BB, Kunnumakkara AB, Harikumar KB, et al. (2008). Potential of spice-derived phytochemicals for cancer prevention. *Planta Medica* 74 (13): 1560–1569.

Aggarwal BB, Shishodia S. (2004). Suppression of nuclear factor-kappa B activation pathway by spice-derived phytochemicals: Reasoning for seasoning. *Annals of the New York Academy of Sciences* 1030: 434–441.

Altug Z, Gensler TO. (2006). *The Anti-Aging Fitness Prescription: A Day-by-Day Nutrition and Workout Plan to Age-Proof Your Body and Mind*. New York, NY: Healthy Living Books.

Appel LJ, Champagne CM, Harsha DW, et al. (2003). Effects of comprehensive lifestyle modification on blood pressure control: Main results of the premier clinical trial. *JAMA* 289 (16): 2083–2093.

Bays JC. (2017). *Mindful Eating: A Guide to Rediscovering a Healthy and Joyful Relationship with Food (Revised Edition)*. Boston, MA: Shambhala Publications.

Candan F, Sokmen A. (2004). Effects of Rhus coriaria L (Anacardiaceae) on lipid peroxidation and free radical scavenging activity. *Phytotherapy Research* 18 (1): 84–86.

Clark N. (2014). *Nancy Clark's Sports Nutrition Guidebook*, 5th ed. Champaign IL: Human Kinetics.

Cullum-Dugan D, Pawlak R. (2015). Position of the Academy of Nutrition and Dietetics: Vegetarian diets. *Journal of the Academy of Nutrition and Dietetics* 115 (5): 801–810. www.andjrnl.org/article/S2212-2672%2815%2900261-0/pdf.

Duyff RL. (2012). *The American Dietetic Association's Complete Food & Nutrition Guide*, 4th ed. New York, NY: Houghton Mifflin Harcourt Publishing Company.

Eaton SB, Konner M. (1985). Paleolithic nutrition. A consideration of its nature and current implications. *New England Journal of Medicine* 312 (5): 283–289.

El-Shemy HA, Aboul-Soud MA, Nassr-Allah AA, et al. (2010). Antitumor properties and modulation of antioxidant enzymes' activity by aloe vera leaf active principles isolated via supercritical carbon dioxide extraction. *Current Medicinal Chemistry* 17 (2): 129–138.

Fito M, Estruch R, Salas-Salvado J, et al. (2014). Effect of the Mediterranean diet on heart failure biomarkers: A randomized sample from the PREDIMED trial. *European Journal of Heart Failure* 16 (5): 543–550.

Fuhrman J. (2011). *Eat to Live: The Amazing Nutrient Rich Program for Fast and Sustained Weight Loss*. New York, NY: Little, Brown and Company.

Giancarlo S, Rosa LM, Nadjafi F, et al. (2006). Hypoglycaemic activity of two spices extracts: Rhus coriaria L. and Bunium persicum Boiss. *Natural Product Research* 20 (9): 882–886.

Gullett NP, Amin ARMR, Bayraktar S, et al. (2010). Cancer prevention with natural compounds. *Seminars in Oncology* 37 (3): 258–281.

Gupta SC, Kim JH, Prasad S, et al. (2010). Regulation of survival, proliferation, invasion, angiogenesis, and metastasis of tumor cells through modulation of inflammatory pathways by nutraceuticals. *Cancer and Metastasis Reviews* 29 (3): 405–434.

Heber D, Blackburn GL, Go VLW, et al. (Eds.). (2006). *Nutritional Oncology,* 2nd ed. Boston, MA: Academic Press.

Heber D, Bowerman S. (2001). *What Color is Your Diet?* New York, NY: HarperCollins.

Henning SM, Zhang Y, Seeram NP, et al. (2011). Antioxidant capacity and phytochemical content of herbs and spices in dry, fresh and blended herb paste form. *International Journal of Food Sciences and Nutrition* 62 (3): 219–225.

Hu J, La Vecchia C, Negri E, et al. (2009). Dietary vitamin C, E, and carotenoid intake and risk of renal cell carcinoma. *Cancer Causes & Control* 20 (8): 1451–1458.

Imamura F, Micha R, Khatibzadeh S, et al. (2015). Dietary quality among men and women in 187 countries in 1990 and 2010: A systematic assessment. *Lancet Global Health* 3 (3): e132–142.

James JM, Burks W, Eigenmann P. (2012). *Food Allergy.* St. Louis, MO: Elsevier Saunders.

Jonsson T, Granfeldt Y, Ahren B, et al. (2009). Beneficial effects of a Paleolithic diet on cardiovascular risk factors in Type 2 diabetes: A randomized cross-over pilot study. *Cardiovascular Diabetology* 8: 35.

Kohn JB. (2014). Is there a diet for histamine intolerance? *Journal of the Academy of Nutrition and Dietetics* 114 (11): 1860.

Khayyal MT, el-Ghazaly MA, el-Khatib AS. (1993). Mechanisms involved in the anti-inflammatory effect of propolis extract. *Drugs under Experimental and Clinical Research* 19 (5): 197–203.

Lee JS, Hwang HS, Ko EJ, et al. (2014). Immunomodulatory activity of red ginseng against influenza A virus infection. *Nutrients* 6 (2): 517–529.

Li Y, Zhang T, Korkaya H, et al. (2010). Sulforaphane, a dietary component of broccoli/broccoli sprouts, inhibits breast cancer stem cells. *Clinical Cancer Research* 16 (9): 2580–2590.

Lis DM, Stellingwerff T, Kitic CM, et al. (2018). Low FODMAP: A preliminary strategy to reduce gastrointestinal distress in athletes. *Medicine and Science in Sports and Exercise* 50 (1):116–123.

Liu Y, Yadev VR, Aggarwal BB, et al. (2010). Inhibitory effects of black pepper (Piper nigrum) extracts and compounds on human tumor cell proliferation, cyclooxygenase enzymes, lipid peroxidation and nuclear transcription factor-kappa-B. *Natural Product Communications* 5 (8): 1253–1257.

Lock K, Pomerleau J, Causer L, et al. (2005). The global burden of disease attributable to low consumption of fruit and vegetables: Implications for the global strategy on diet. *Bulletin of the World Health Organization* 83: 100–108.

Ma L, Lin XM. (2010). Effects of lutein and zeaxanthin on aspects of eye health. *Journal of the Science of Food and Agriculture* 90 (1): 2–12.

Mahan LK Raymond JL. (2017). *Krause's Food & the Nutrition Care Process,* 14th ed. St. Louis, MO: Elsevier.

Manheimer EW, van Zuuren EJ. (2015). Paleolithic nutrition for metabolic syndrome: Systematic review and meta-analysis. *American Journal of Clinical Nutrition* 102 (4): 922–932.

Marum AP, Moreira C, Saraiva F, et al. (2016). A low fermentable oligo-di-mono saccharides and polyols (FODMAP) diet reduced pain and improved daily life in fibromyalgia patients. *Scandinavian Journal of Pain* 13: 166–172.

Mattioli AV, Palmiero P, Manfrini O, et al. (2017). Mediterranean diet impact on cardiovascular diseases: A narrative review. *Journal of Cardiovascular Medicine (Hagerstown)* 18 (12): 925–935.

Meeran SM, Katiyar SK. (2008). Cell cycle control as a basis for cancer chemoprevention through dietary agents. *Frontiers in Bioscience* 13: 2191–2202.

Mehta RG, Murillo G, Naithani R, et al. (2010). Cancer chemoprevention by natural products: How far have we come? *Pharmaceutical Research* 27 (6): 950–961.

Mishra S, Xu J, Agarwal U, et al. (2013). A multicenter randomized controlled trial of a plant-based nutrition program to reduce body weight and cardiovascular risk in the corporate setting: The GEICO study. *European Journal of Clinical Nutrition* 67 (7): 718–724.

Morris MC, Tangney CC, Wang Y, et al. (2015). MIND diet slows cognitive decline with aging. *Alzheimer's & Dementia: The Journal of the Alzheimer's Association* 11 (9): 1015–1022.

Motohashi N, Gallagher R, Anuradha V, et al. (2017). Functional foods and their importance in geriatric nutrition. *Journal of Clinical Nutrition and Metabolism* 1 (1).

Panahi Y, Rahimnia AR, Sharafi M, et al. (2014). Curcuminoid treatment for knee osteoarthritis: A randomized double-blind placebo-controlled trial. *Phytotherapy Research* 28 (11): 1625–1631.

Pennington JAT, Spungen J. (2010). *Bowes & Church's Food Values of Portions Commonly Used,* 19th ed. Baltimore, MD: Lippincott Williams & Wilkins.

Pollan M. (2006). *The Omnivore's Dilemma.* New York, NY: Bloomsbury.

Pollan M. (2008). *In Defense of Food: An Eater's Manifesto.* New, NY: Penguin Press.

Pollan M. (2009). *Food Rules: An Eater's Manual.* New, NY: Penguin Press.

Rao M, Afshin A, Singh G, et al. (2013). Do healthier foods and diet patterns cost more than less healthy options? A systematic review and meta-analysis. *BMJ Open* 3 (12): e004277

Saslow LR, Mason AE, Kim S, et al. (2017). An online intervention comparing a very low-carbohydrate ketogenic diet and lifestyle recommendations versus a plate method diet in overweight individuals with type 2 diabetes: A randomized controlled trial. *Journal of Medical Internet Research* 19 (2): e36.

Schwingshackl L, Hoffmann G. (2014). Mediterranean dietary pattern, inflammation and endothelial function: A systematic review and meta-analysis of intervention trials. *Nutrition, Metabolism & Cardiovascular Diseases* 24 (9): 929–939.

Shanahan C, Shanahan L. (2009). *Deep Nutrition: Why Your Genes Need Traditional Food.* Lawai, HI: Big Box Books.

Sherlock O, Dolan A, Athman R, et al. (2010). Comparison of the antimicrobial activity of Ulmo honey from Chile and Manuka honey against methicillin-resistant Staphylococcus aureus, Escherichia coli and Pseudomonas aeruginosa. *BMC Complementary and Alternative Medicine* 10: 47.

Siegel EM, Salemi JL, Villa LL, et al. (2010). Dietary consumption of antioxidant nutrients and risk of incident cervical intraepithelial neoplasia. *Gynecologic Oncology* 118 (3): 289–294.

Sluijs I, Beulens JW, Grobbee DE, et al. (2009). Dietary carotenoid intake is associated with lower prevalence of metabolic syndrome in middle-aged and elderly men. *Journal of Nutrition* 139 (5): 987–992.

Stargrove M, Treasure J, McKee D. (2008). *Herb, Nutrient, and Drug Interactions: Clinical Implications and Therapeutic Strategies.* St. Louis, MO: Mosby Elsevier.

Steinmetz KA, Potter JD. (1991). Vegetables, fruit, and cancer. I. Epidemiology. *Cancer Causes & Control* 2 (5): 325–357.

Steinmetz KA, Potter JD. (1991). Vegetables, fruit, and cancer. II. Mechanisms. *Cancer Causes & Control* 2 (6): 427–442.

Steinmetz KA, Potter JD. (1996). Vegetables, fruit, and cancer prevention: A review. *Journal of the American Dietetic Association* 96 (10): 1027–1039.

Tilman D, Clark M. (2014). Global diets link environmental sustainability and human health. *Nature* 515: 518–522.

Traka M, Gasper AV, Melchini A, et al. (2008). Broccoli consumption interacts with GSTM1 to perturb oncogenic signaling pathways in the prostate. *PloS One* 3 (7): e2568.

Venes D. (Ed.) (2017). *Taber's Cyclopedic Medical Dictionary,* 23rd ed. Philadelphia, PA: FA Davis.

Villacorta M. (2013). *Peruvian Power Foods.* Deerfield, FL: Health Communications, Inc.

Virmani A, Pinto L, Binienda Z, et al. (2013). Food, nutrigenomics, and neurodegeneration-neuroprotection by what you eat! *Molecular Neurobiology* 48 (2): 353–362.

Wang YB, Qin J, Zheng XY, et al. (2010). Diallyl trisulfide induces Bcl-2 and caspase-3-dependent apoptosis via downregulation of Akt phosphorylation in human T24 bladder cancer cells. *Phytomedicine* 17 (5): 363–368.

Weidman J, Holsworth RE, Brossman B, et al. (2016). Effect of electrolyzed high-ph alkaline water on blood viscosity in healthy adults. *Journal of the International Society of Sports Nutrition* 13: 45.

Ye B, Aponte M, Dai Y, et al. (2007). Ginkgo biloba and ovarian cancer prevention: Epidemiological and biological evidence. *Cancer Letters* 251 (1): 43–52.

HOLISTIC HEALING BOX

Hashimoto's Thyroiditis Health Guide

Cohen S. (2014). *Thyroid Healthy: Lose Weight, Look Beautiful and Live the Life You Imagine.* Dear Pharmacist, Inc.

Nikolaidou C, Gouridou E, Ilonidis G, et al. (2010). Acute renal dysfunction in a patient presenting with rhabdomyolysis due to hypothyroidism attributed to Hashimoto's disease. *Hippokratia* 14 (4): 281–283.

Porter RS, Kaplan JL. (Eds.). (2011). *The Merck Manual of Diagnosis and Therapy,* 19th ed. Whitehouse Station, NJ: Merck Research Laboratories.

Venes D. (Ed.). (2017). *Taber's Cyclopedic Medical Dictionary,* 23rd ed. Philadelphia, PA: FA Davis.

Wentz I. (2017). *Hashimoto's Protocol: A 90-Day Plan for Reversing Thyroid Symptoms and Getting Back Your Life.* New York, NY: HarperOne.

Wentz I, Nowosadzka M. (2013). *Hashimoto's Thyroiditis: Lifestyle Interventions for Finding and Treating the Root Cause.* Izabella Wentz (publisher).

Xiang G, Xiang L, Xiang L, et al. (2012). Change of plasma osteoprotegerin and its association with endothelial dysfunction before and after exercise in Hashimoto's thyroiditis with euthyroidism. *Experimental and Clinical Endocrinology and Diabetes* 120 (9): 529–534.

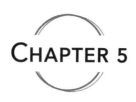

CHAPTER 5

SUSTAINABLE EXERCISE

"If we could give every individual the right amount of
nourishment and exercise, not too little and not too much,
we would have found the safest way to health."

—Hippocrates

Sustainable exercise is *not* about promising miracle cures or quick-fix solutions, trying to sell a specific product, or finding a one-size-fits-all exercise routine. Every person has the freedom of choice to pursue whatever lifestyle, activity, sport, or exercise he or she wishes. This book is about outlining guidelines for making healthful choices. Therefore, sustainable exercise, as I see it, is about being adaptable and finding balance and enjoyment in the exercises, sports, or movements you are engaging in. The key for sustainable exercise is to train, play, and exercise wisely so you can be back another day to do the same. Following proper training strategies allows you to train and maintain physical independence over your lifespan. Remember, the "no pain, no gain" philosophy for general fitness is out and the "train smart and have fun" approach is in!

BENEFITS OF EXERCISE

Evidence-based exercise can be used therapeutically to improve activities of daily living, quality of life, and conditions such as osteoporosis, osteoarthritis, diabetes, hypertension, scoliosis, low back pain, and obesity. The following are some of the benefits of exercise:

- Increases endurance (stamina) and strength
- Reduces stress, anxiety, and depression
- Decreases blood pressure
- Lowers low-density lipoprotein (LDL) cholesterol (bad cholesterol)
- Raises high-density lipoprotein (HDL) cholesterol (good cholesterol)
- Improves sleep
- Improves control of blood sugar levels
- Improves flexibility, balance, coordination, agility, and reaction time

- Improves mood, self-confidence, cognitive processing speed, and attention span
- Improves posture and daily function (such as the ability to get out of a chair with ease)
- Improves pelvic floor strengthening before and after pregnancy
- Improvement in musculoskeletal issues (for example, knee or shoulder pain)
- Improvement after orthopedic surgery, such as after total knee or hip replacement surgery, rotator cuff surgery, or back and neck surgery
- Improvement and control of medical conditions, such as asthma, diabetes, facial palsy, stroke, or peripheral neuropathy
- Alleviates back pain, especially when associated with decreased body weight
- Slows age-related decline in bone mineral density and improves bone density
- Slows age-related decline in muscle mass and strength, as well as improves muscle mass and strength
- Less risk of falling
- Less body fat and excess weight

LIFESTYLE AND FUNCTIONAL EXERCISE

Lifestyle exercise is the performance of daily routine activities such as chores, errands, work, or hobbies. Functional exercise includes activities like rolling side to side in bed, moving from sitting in a chair to standing, squatting to lift a package, or carrying groceries. Here are some suggestions for increasing lifestyle and functional exercise:

- Park your car in the spot farthest from the store each time you shop.
- Take the stairs at work instead of the elevator.
- Walk to and from work if you live close enough.
- If you can, ride your bicycle to work or part of the way.
- While you watch your favorite television show, walk in place instead of sitting on the couch.
- Work in your garden.
- Vacuum the house.
- Rake leaves.
- Sweep the floor.
- Wash and vacuum your car.
- Walk up and down all the aisles in the grocery store before you shop.
- Walk while meeting with a work colleague.
- Walk around the mall from one end to the other before or after shopping.
- Walk to pick up lunch at work instead of ordering delivery.
- Take breaks at work and walk around the office from one end to the other.
- Walk once around the block before entering your house or apartment building.
- Take your dog for a walk, or take a walk with another friend.

Exercise Guidelines

Please be aware that this chapter outlines some of my humble (and perhaps biased) opinions for training. When beginning a fitness routine, most people ask the following questions:

- "How many days a week should I train?"
- "How much weight should I use?"
- "How many sets or reps should I perform?"
- "How much rest should I take between sets and workouts?"

The answer to all of the above questions is this: It depends. There are no magic formulas—only guidelines. These statements refer to general fitness, but the same holds true for elite athletes in a variety of sports. Each person is unique and requires different movements at varied intervals. A football player does not train the same way a tennis player or swimmer trains. There are similar training strategies, but workouts are completely different to accommodate varied demands.

Training for fitness is different for each person and should be based on the following:

- What is the person's level of experience—beginner, intermediate, or advanced?
- How well does the person feel on training day?
- How much rest did the person get the previous night?
- How well-nourished and hydrated is the person on training day?
- Is the person mentally focused or are there distractions?

There's also no rule that says every workout should be the same. Train with variety and train to feel good—not to tear yourself down.

Box 7: Holistic Healing

Scoliosis Information

Scoliosis can be defined as an "abnormal lateral curvature of the vertebral column" (Kisner et al. 2018). The following are resources you can use to find more information about scoliosis treatment and prevention:

- American Academy of Orthopaedic Surgeons, orthoinfo.aaos.org (search scoliosis)
- Katharina Schroth's Three-Dimensional Scoliosis Treatment, scoliosistreatment-schroth.com
- National Scoliosis Foundation, scoliosis.org
- Scoliosis Rehab Inc., scoliosisrehab.com
- Scoliosis Research Society, srs.org
- *Scoliosis and Spinal Disorders*, scoliosisjournal.com

21 BODY RULES FOR EXERCISING

This section outlines basic concepts to keep in mind when performing exercises. I take no credit for coming up with the body rules because top clinicians, trainers, and coaches have been using these principles for many years.

Many of these rules might not apply to elite athletes, who take risks and push the limits of their bodies for purposes of competition. If your primary goal is improving or maintaining good health and you are not an elite athlete, don't think about training like one. Instead focus on good health and keeping your body fit and mobile.

Activity is for everyone, from young to old. A study by Pahor et al. (2014) indicates that "a structured, moderate-intensity physical activity program compared with a health education program reduced major mobility disability over 2.6 years among older adults at risk for disability. These findings suggest mobility benefit from such a program in vulnerable older adults." The physical activity in this study included walking, and also strength, flexibility, and balance training.

I suggest you keep the following body rules in mind as you exercise:

RULE 1: FIRST DO NO HARM

Hippocrates, an ancient Greek physician known as the "father of medicine" (Venes 2017), is reported to have said, "First do no harm." Exercise is meant to make you feel better and improve your mind and body. The purpose of exercise is not to create injury or pain. Therefore, train without pain.

RULE 2: LISTEN TO YOUR BODY

Take your time figuring out which movements are best for your body. For example, some people might not be able to squat deeply due to their hip joint structure and soft-tissue limitations. You might need a wide squat stance while your workout partner does better with a narrow stance. Learn the natural patterns of your body.

RULE 3: RESPECT PAIN AND ITS SYMPTOMS

Be mindful of your body's signals. If an exercise hurts, modify it to a pain-free motion or skip it. Take charge of your pain by knowing which movements create discomfort and modifying activities and motions as necessary. Also, avoid movements and exercises that cause burning, tingling, numbness, and shooting or radiating pain.

Rule 4: Think and Move

Think about the movements as you perform a skill or activity. This way, you are learning to move more efficiently and you are staying in the moment.

Rule 5: Train Your Brain

Mentally practicing a task or skill before doing the movement or exercise might help your body perform better. However, mentally practicing a skill is incomplete without performing the physical action as well.

Rule 6: Slow Down

Consider not training with weights or body weight exercises when you are in a rush to finish or are distracted with other personal matters. Injuries can happen when you are in a hurry or not focused.

Rule 7: Understand Risk Versus Reward

Minimize or avoid risky exercises. Once again, if you are an elite athlete, there are certain assumed risks with training and competition. If you're not an athlete, then why risk breaks, tears, and injury? Train for longevity and sustainability.

Rule 8: Don't Overtrain

Exercise just enough to get good results, but don't overtrain. Some signs of overtraining include fatigue, apathy, depression or irritability, decreased desire for and enjoyment of training, decline in performance, loss of muscle strength, weight loss or loss of appetite, sleep disturbances, and gastrointestinal disturbances.

Rule 9: Be Aware of Your Posture

Train with good form and body awareness to build and maintain good posture.

Rule 10: Focus on Form

Train with good form and think about your movement patterns so you imprint these into your brain.

Rule 11: Breathe Properly

Breathe freely, even when you are stiffening your core muscles during exercises such as push-ups and squats.

Rule 12: Spare Your Spine

Stiffen your core muscles only enough for the task at hand. Professor Stuart McGill, PhD states that "It takes sufficient stability and no more" (McGill 2014). If you are lifting a pencil off the ground, you will stiffen your core some but not maximally. However, if you are bending to lift and carry two heavy suitcases, you will stiffen the core to a much higher degree. How hard? It depends. It takes practice to determine how much you can lift and carry in real life or during exercise. Professional weight lifters take many years to learn how to safely lift, pull, push, and carry heavy loads. Go slow and learn the limitations of your body. Also, protect your spine during exercise by maintaining the normal spine curves.

Rule 13: Recover and Recuperate

Rest and recover thoroughly after workouts. Stay clear of training approaches that constantly push you and tear you down without respecting pain, recovery, and meaningful progress. Listen to your body. Also, periodically take time off from training to allow your body to fully recuperate from repetitive movements. This includes getting enough sleep every night. Even a good thing like exercise can be done in excess, so breaks are needed. After an extended vacation of one to four weeks, consider backing off to body weight exercises (meaning no additional resistance) for your strength workouts and cut back to around half the intensity on your other training. This allows your mind and body to ease back into your daily schedule.

Rule 14: Train with Variety

Vary workouts to prevent injury and mental burnout. Don't get focused on one type of training. By varying your exercises with movements, such as weight training, sports, qigong, tai chi, yoga, Pilates, and walking, you are helping to prevent muscle imbalances and overuse injuries.

Rule 15: Be Adaptable

No two days are the same in a person's life. Modify your exercise routine (and nutrition program) when you have illness, pain, injury, high stress levels, restricted sleep, or surgery.

Rule 16: Be Open-Minded

Stay abreast of the latest information and be willing to modify your program as new research is presented.

Rule 17: Monitor Your Training Load

Discuss with your fitness professional or healthcare provider ways you can monitor your exercise and training loads to prevent injury. For example, you might use methods such as heart rate, blood pressure, rating of perceived exertion (RPE), and also questionnaires, diaries, and journals (Halson 2014).

Rule 18: Control Your Mental Stress

Uncontrolled stress can sap your energy and delay healing. See chapter 2: Managing Your Stress for more information on how to control stress.

Rule 19: Nourish Your Body

Provide your body with needed nutrients for repair and maintenance before, during, and after workouts.

Rule 20: Include Some Rotational Exercises

Include some rotational movement into your workouts since sports (such as golf, tennis, and basketball) and daily activities (such as reaching overhead or bending to tie your shoe) involve rotation of various body regions. Try rotational activities such as yoga, tai chi, qigong, or other martial arts.

RULE 21: SIMPLIFY

Even some strength and conditioning professionals who work with elite athletes question the current trend of overtraining and high-risk exercises. But trends come and go, and this one is changing not only in the athletic population, but also in the general fitness population, with the focus now centering on the least amount of training for maximum results. If five exercises give you the same results as 10, which program would you choose? Choosing the five-exercise program is a no-brainer. It's all about precision training versus a shotgun approach.

DID YOU KNOW?

- "The human body is about 40% skeletal muscle and 10% smooth and cardiac muscle" (Hall 2011).
- Muscle mass is 70 percent to 75 percent water, whereas water in fat tissue can vary between 10 percent and 40 percent (Institute of Medicine of the National Academies 2005).
- One pound of lean body mass (muscle) burns 14 calories per day and one pound of fat burns two calories per day (Heber 1999; Heber et al. 2001). As you increase your lean body mass, you burn more calories at rest and during activity.
- Naci et al. (2013) state that for certain conditions, including diabetes prevention, heart disease prevention, and stroke recovery, exercise can be just as beneficial as pharmaceutical drugs.
- Natural muscle mass and strength can decrease dramatically with age. For example, after age 30, muscle mass declines between 3% and 8% each decade and after age 50, this rate increases to 5–10% per decade (Westcott 2012).
- Neumann (2010) states that "periods of reduced muscle activity lead to atrophy and usually marked reductions in strength, even in the first few weeks of inactivity. The loss in strength can occur early, up to 3% to 6% per day in the first week alone. After only 10 days of immobilization, healthy individuals can experience up to a 40% decrease of initial one-repetition maximum (1-RM)" (Appell 1990; Thom et al. 2001).

So what is the take-home message of all these facts? Stay active throughout your life!

 ## PRACTICAL GUIDE FOR YOUR EXERCISE ROUTINE

- Do you have any medical condition or pre-existing injuries you need to adjust your lifestyle for (such as hypertension, osteoporosis, osteoarthritis, thyroid condition, diabetes, or cancer)? If yes:

- » First, work with your primary healthcare provider and a physical therapist (or occupational therapist) to optimize your movement patterns.
- » Second, work with a fitness trainer or mind body practitioner (such as someone who specializes in yoga, Pilates, Feldenkrais Method, or Alexander Technique) to further develop your fitness routine.
- » Third, go the American Physical Therapy Association website www.apta.org and search for your medical condition.
- » Fourth, go to credible websites (or apps) for each condition (such as the National Osteoporosis Foundation for bone-related inquiries) and obtain more information.
- » Fifth, go to good exercise textbooks to obtain basic and advanced exercise information. Consider books such as the *Essentials of Strength Training and Conditioning* by G Gregory Haff and N. Travis Triplett; *Therapeutic Exercise* by Carolyn Kisner, Lynn Colby, and John Borstad; *Therapeutic Exercise* by Lori Brody and Carrie Hall; *ACSM's Guidelines for Exercise Testing and Prescription* by the American College of Sports Medicine. Use these sources along with information from your healthcare provider.
- » Finally, go to PubMed.gov and enter the medical condition along with the word "exercise" (for example, search as "osteoporosis AND exercise") to search for the latest information. Speak with your healthcare provider if you need help interpreting the studies.
- Identify if you prefer to exercise alone (for example, at home, at a park, or on a trail) or in a group setting (for example, a gym, fitness studio, or mall walking group).
- Identify if you are under stress or a Type A personality who may need yoga, tai chi, qigong, or Pilates. Or, do you need to engage in more competitive sports such as soccer, softball, tennis, or golf to add excitement to your life?
- To obtain more information about exercise, go to the American College of Sports Medicine website (acsm.org) and the National Strength & Conditioning Association website (nsca.com).
- If you are engaging in sporting activities, refer to the Stop Sport Injuries website, stopsportsinjuries.org.

Have fun moving!

Box 8: Holistic Healing

Natural Bright Light for Good Health

Light exposure through sunshine has been an integral part of human development. Our current society is severely lacking in outdoor light exposure since so many of us work indoors, some without windows or any adequate light exposure. Light exposure is essential for preventing depression and sleep disorders, and improving mood, alertness, reaction time, performance, and sleep quality (Levandovski et al. 2013; Turner et al. 2008).

For good health, light exposure needs to be at a sufficient intensity (greater than 2,500 lux), for an optimal length of time, and from a specific source of light (particularly bluer light sources such as outdoor daylight, which is in the 440–500 nanometer wavelength range, with skylight having a dominant wavelength of 477 nanometers). Adequate light exposure is especially important in the morning upon wakening and also during the day since outdoor light is necessary for increasing alertness, cognition, core body temperature, as well as improving nocturnal sleep quality, reducing or eliminating depression, and increasing the brain's mood-elevating serotonin levels (Lehrl et al. 2007; Turner et al. 2008).

Try the following strategies to increase bright light exposure:

- Open your curtains to let in as much outdoor light as possible, especially in the morning.
- If you can't get outdoors in the morning, have your breakfast near a window or on a balcony, porch, or patio.
- Eat your lunch outdoors, even if you sit under a tree or in the shade. After eating, take a 15-minute walk.
- At work, try to sit near a window, especially if you work on a computer. Being able to look away from your monitor and into the distance can also reduce eye strain.
- Go outdoors during work breaks. Even an overcast day, which has 2,000 to 10,000 lux, provides more light than the typical indoor lighting of an office building.
- Exercise outdoors before work, during lunch, or after work. For example, try walking, or stretch on your balcony or porch.
- Plan outdoor activities during the weekends.
- Take winter vacations in sunny climates.
- Remodel your home to add more windows or skylights.
- Place your home computer so it faces a window (but avoid direct glare).

ADDITIONAL RESOURCES

- American College of Sports Medicine, acsm.org
- American Physical Therapy Association, apta.org
- National Strength and Conditioning Association, nsca.com

REFERENCES

American College of Sports Medicine. (2014). *ACSM's Resource Manual for Guidelines for Exercise Testing and Prescription*, 7th ed. Philadelphia, PA: Wolters Kluwer Lippincott Williams & Wilkins.

American College of Sports Medicine. (2018). *ACSM's Guidelines for Exercise Testing and Prescription*, 10th ed. Philadelphia, PA: Wolters Kluwer Lippincott Williams & Wilkins.

Appell HJ. (1990). Muscular atrophy following immobilisation. A review. *Sports Medicine* 10 (1): 42–58.

Astrand PO, Rodahl K, Dahl HA, et al. (2003). *Textbook of Work Physiology: The Physiological Bases of Exercise*, 4th ed. Champaign, IL: Human Kinetics.

Hall JE. (2011). *Guyton and Hall Textbook of Medical Physiology*, 12th ed. Philadelphia, PA: Saunders Elsevier.

Halson SL. (2014). Monitoring training load to understand fatigue in athletes. *Sports Medicine* 44 (Supplement 2): 139–147.

Heber D. (1999). *The Resolution Diet: Keeping the Promise of Permanent Weight Loss.* Garden City Park, NY: Avery Publishing Group.

Heber D, Bowerman S. (2001). *What Color is Your Diet? The 7 Colors of Health.* New York, NY: HarperCollins.

Hettinger T. (1961). *Physiology of Strength.* Springfield, IL: Charles C Thomas Publishers.

Hettinger T, Muller EA. (1953). Muscle capacity and muscle training. *Arbeitsphysiologie* 15 (2): 111–126.

Institute of Medicine of the National Academies. (2005). *Water, Dietary Reference Intakes for Water, Sodium, Chloride, Potassium, and Sulfate.* Washington, DC: National Academy Press.

Kisner C, Colby LA, Borstad J. (2018). *Therapeutic Exercise: Foundations and Techniques,* 7th ed. Philadelphia, PA: FA Davis.

McGill SM. (2014). *Building the Ultimate Back: From Rehabilitation to Performance* (course manual). Los Angeles, CA, April 26–27.

McGill SM. (2014). *Ultimate Back Fitness and Performance,* 5th ed. Waterloo, Canada: Wabuno Publishers (Backfitpro Inc.). www.backfitpro.com.

McGill SM. (2016). *Low Back Disorders,* 3rd ed. Champaign IL: Human Kinetics.

McGill SM, Hughson RL, Parks K. (2000). Lumbar erector spinae oxygenation during prolonged contractions: Implications for prolonged work. *Ergonomics* 43 (4): 486–493.

Naci H, Ioannidis JP. (2013). Comparative effectiveness of exercise and drug interventions on mortality outcomes: Metaepidemiological study. *BMJ* 347: f5577.

Neumann DA. (2010). *Kinesiology of the Musculoskeletal System: Foundations for Rehabilitation,* 2nd ed. St. Louis: Mosby Elsevier.

Pahor M, Guralnik JM, Ambrosius WT, et al. (2014). Effect of structured physical activity on prevention of major mobility disability in older adults: The life study randomized clinical trial. *JAMA* 311 (23): 2387–2396.

Thom JM, Thompson MW, Ruell PA, et al. (2001). Effect of 10-day cast immobilization on sarcoplasmic reticulum calcium regulation in humans. *Acta Physiologica Scandinavica* 172 (2): 141–147.

Venes D. (Ed.) (2017). *Taber's Cyclopedic Medical Dictionary,* 23rd ed. Philadelphia, PA: FA Davis.

Verkhoshansky Y, Siff M. (2009). *Supertraining,* 6th ed. Rome, Italy: Verkhoshansky. www.verkhoshansky.com.

Verkhoshansky Y, Verkhoshansky N. (2011). *Special Strength Training Manual for Coaches.* Rome Italy: Verkhoshansky SSTM. www.verkhoshansky.com.

Westcott WL. (2012). Resistance training is medicine: effects of strength training on health. *Current Sports Medicine Reports* 11 (4): 209–216.

Holistic Healing Boxes

Scoliosis Information

Kisner C, Colby LA, Borstad J. (2018). *Therapeutic Exercise: Foundations and Techniques,* 7th ed. Philadelphia, PA: FA Davis.

Natural Bright Light for Good Health

Lehrl S, Gerstmeyer K, Jacob JH, et al. (2007). Blue light improves cognitive performance. *Journal of Neural Transmission* 114 (4): 457–460.

Levandovski R, Pfaffenseller B, Carissimi A, et al. (2013). The effect of sunlight exposure on interleukin-6 levels in depressive and non-depressive subjects. *BMC Psychiatry* 13: 75.

Turner PL, Mainster MA. (2008). Circadian photoreception: ageing and the eye's important role in systemic health. *British Journal of Ophthalmology* 92 (11): 1439–1444.

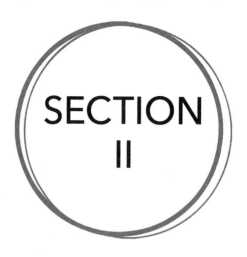

SECTION II

MIND BODY HEALTH AND INTEGRATIVE MOVEMENT

This section introduces you to a variety of mind body fitness and integrative movement systems. I have personally taken workshops and seminars in each of these areas involving integrative movement. The primary purpose of this section is not to show extensive poses and training programs for each system. The main goal of this section is to show you some of the research for each of the topics and outline a basic routine you can use in the comfort of your home. Hopefully, this can guide you into which areas you would like to explore for your personal health. The truth is that there are many outstanding books outlining each topic in great detail. I personally think the best way to learn any one of these systems is to work with a qualified practitioner in your area and read the specialty books they recommend as a supplement to their instruction.

Photos / Videos: Please note that the author decided to place additional photos and videos regarding yoga, tai chi, qigong, Pilates, the Feldenkrais Method, and the Alexander Technique on his social media sites identified in this book.

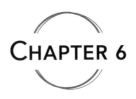

CHAPTER 6

YOGA FOR HEALTH

This chapter was completed with the assistance of Romy Phillips, MFA, E-RYT 500, C-IAYT. Romy is a certified yoga instructor who has been teaching since 2001. She has studied many styles of yoga, but primarily Ashtanga and Iyengar. She teaches group classes regularly and leads teacher trainings, workshops, and intensives in the United States and internationally. Anatomy, kinesiology, and injury management, are the highlight of her trainings. She currently teaches in Los Angeles, California at various studios (YogaWorks and Santa Monica Yoga) and also in numerous cities throughout Japan, China, and Vietnam, including Tokyo, Osaka, Beijing, Shenzhen, and Saigon. Finally, Romy is very excited about taking all her years of experience studying movement in dance (ballet, modern, and jazz) and yoga and sharing it in her new book *Yoga Forma: A Visual Resource Guide for the Spine and Lower Back* (Cedar Fort Publishing, 2018). Her book is available on Amazon, Barnes & Noble, and Books & Things (booksandthings.com).

Romy Phillips, MFA, E-RYT 500, C-IAYT
Certified Yoga Therapist / Yoga Practitioner
Yogathology
Los Angeles, California
www.yogathology.com
Author of *Yoga Forma: A Visual Resource Guide for the Spine and Lower Back* (Cedar Fort Publishing, 2018)
Author of *Level 1, Level ½, Level 2, Level 2/3, and Sequences for Specialty Classes* for teachers (Yogathology, 2017)
Author of *Yoga Sessions with Romy Phillips DVD* (Parts 1 and 2) (Amazon, 2006)

"Yoga is like music. The rhythm of the body, the melody of the mind, and the harmony of the soul create the symphony of life."

—B.K.S. Iyengar

Yoga is a science and art that has evolved over the years to be recognized for its health benefits. "In its technical sense, yoga refers to that enormous body of spiritual values, attitudes, precepts, and techniques that have developed in India over at least five millennia and that may be regarded as the very foundation of ancient Indian civilization" (Feuerstein 2001). Over the years, there have proven to be many physical and physiological benefits to practicing yoga. Currently, there are many relevant studies conducted by the Western community highlighting the significance of yoga for healing.

The medical dictionary now has a definition of yoga (Venes 2017) citing in its origins, yoga's aim was to primarily calm the mind and prepare the body for meditation. This is true. If you look deeper, you will discover the methods and techniques associated with the practice of yoga provide the subtle link between mind and body. There are many classical texts that refer to yoga. Some teach that yoga is the skill of "effortless effort." Unfortunately, in our contemporary Western world, yoga tends to place an emphasis on the physical postures (called asanas) and coordinated breathing and less on its meditative aspects.

Yoga is first mentioned in the Vedas, which are ancient and sacred books of Hinduism. Many texts historically associated with yoga's origins clearly state that the primary focus of yoga was to quiet the mind and the physical practice itself was to prepare the body for meditation. The yoga asanas were meant to prepare the body to sit comfortably in meditation. For example, many of the asanas address stiffness in the lower body—the hips, knees, and ankles as well as strengthen the spine, allowing one to successfully feel at ease in their bodies so that they could refine their breathing, thus calming and focusing the mind for meditation. The numerous yoga asanas practiced today stem from many lineages and styles, but what we primarily practice in the West has its direct influence from Tirumalai Krishnamacharya, an Indian yoga teacher who systemized many of the asanas associated with modern Hatha yoga. Some of his renowned students included B.K.S. Iyengar (founder of Iyengar yoga), K. Patthibi Jois (developed the vinyasa style of yoga and referred to as Ashtanga yoga), and T.K.V. Desikachar (developed Viniyoga). There are many more popular styles, such as Kundalini, Bikram, and Sivananda and contemporary versions such as, Yin Yoga, Vinyasa Flow and Acro Yoga. All of these styles are considered Hatha yoga, but taught with a different emphasis.

In this chapter we will focus on the contributions of B.K.S Iyengar, Patthibi Jois, and Desikachar because of the stylistic and fundamental qualities that are a practical resource for learning and building awareness. For example, Iyengar Yoga tends to be alignment based and therapeutic and highly accessible for many practitioners of all levels, ages and conditions. Restoratives are a traditional therapeutic element unique to the Iyengar practice that helps calm the nervous system. In addition, many of the props we use today were created by B.K.S. Iyengar as a means to help the practitioner go deeper into a pose or modify or enhance a pose. Blocks, straps, rope walls, chairs, bolsters, and more evolved from the Iyengar system. Furthermore, Restorative Yoga with a primary benefit of calming the nervous system, has gained in popularity, but many practitioners may not be aware that restoratives are a traditional therapeutic element unique to the Iyengar practice. Whereas, Ashtanga is a six-set series of asanas consisting of primary, intermediate, and four advanced programs, each progressing in difficulty and practiced with vinyasa which synchronizes movement and breath and challenges the practitioner to stay focused as they move dynamically through linked postures. With Viniyoga, sequences are developed utilizing asana, breath (pranayama), meditation and other elements, that are more specific to the an individual's needs. There can be dynamic movement that is gentle as well as therapeutic.

Z Altug's Perspective for Doing Yoga

In my clinical practice as a physical therapist, I typically recommend yoga to patients and clients who need to manage stress, improve core stability and balance, and work on posture and mobility. Other general reasons to try yoga include:

- Relieve stress and tension
- Improve overall health
- Improve flexibility
- Improve breathing
- Improve strength
- Improve balance
- Improve posture
- Improve circulation
- Help manage pain
- Help prevent falls
- Help manage weight
- Help find inner peace

Romy Phillips's Perspective for Doing Yoga

I've noticed from my experience as a teacher many people initially approach yoga either to relax and relieve stress, or for fitness, unaware of the magnitude and scope of yoga's benefits on a physical, emotional, and even spiritual level. There are styles of yoga, such as restoratives and Yin Yoga, that primarily encourage relaxation, and many people are first drawn to these styles when pursuing yoga. Then there those individuals who seek out the more dynamic and challenging styles, such as Vinyasa Flow or Hot Yoga. No matter what style a person chooses to start with, he or she has to practice a long time to experience the transformative effects on many levels. In the Yoga Therapy model, these "levels" are referred to as Koshas (energy layers of the body) that define the qualities of the gross to subtle body, from the surface of the skin to the innermost core of our being (Iyengar 2005). I personally feel that practicing yoga not just from a physical level, but with these key factors in mind will allow practitioners to experience the true health benefits of yoga. Yoga can be safe and rewarding if you approach it consciously and mindfully to avoid risks and minimize injuries.

There are hundreds of Hatha yoga poses and categories of poses and movements, such as standing poses, seated poses, backbends, inversions, twists, arm balances, forward bends, and restoratives. Each pose and category of poses has been recognized to have a physical and physiological effect on the body. For example, forward bends typically have a calming effect on the nervous system, twists are good for digestion, and backbends are energizing. B.K.S. Iyengar's book *Light on Yoga* (Iyengar 1979) briefly gives a description of the each asana's unique benefits. This book is an excellent resource to educate teachers and students on the key poses of Hatha yoga. Although some of the poses may look intimidating, there are many variations and modifications available to address the level of the practitioner. An experienced teacher can make the most challenging pose accessible with skillful sequencing, variations, and modifications. A well-rounded yoga class should provide a wide range of postures and movements, yet be adaptable to the level and ability of the participant. This is significant in order for each individual to have a truly rewarding experience with yoga.

I have been practicing yoga consistently for at least twenty years and have experienced profound changes in so many ways. I started with the most basic poses and progressed slowly and mindfully over the years to more advanced postures. Overall, yoga has helped me to straighten my back and minimize pain from scoliosis, alleviate depression, eliminate insomnia, gain confidence, and feel youthful beyond my years. I have been fortunate to have many amazing teachers who have helped me to overcome the obstacles that may appear in the practice of yoga. I've also learned about my body and heightened my awareness of how the body functions in the poses.

LET'S SEE WHAT RESEARCH SAYS . . .

There are many studies that have been done in collaboration with the medical and yoga communities. Some highlights of the research are illuminating and informative, underscoring the vast health benefits of yoga on a range of individuals from children to seniors, breast cancer survivors, and others. Here are some examples:

- "Yoga can improve cardio-respiratory fitness and aerobic capacity as physical exercise intervention in adolescent school children" (Satish et al. 2018).
- "A manualized yoga program for nonspecific chronic low back pain was noninferior to physical therapy for function and pain" (Saper et al. 2017).
- "A relaxation-based yoga programme was found to be feasible and safe for participants with rheumatoid arthritis-related pain and functional disability" (Ward et al. 2017).
- "The identified evidence suggests that combined physical and psychological treatments, medical yoga, information and education

programmes, spinal manipulation and acupuncture are likely to be cost-effective options for low back pain" (Andronis et al. 2016).

- "With few exceptions, previous studies and the recent randomized control trials indicate that yoga can reduce pain and disability, can be practiced safely, and is well received by participants. Some studies also indicate that yoga may improve psychological symptoms, but these effects are currently not as well established" (Chang et al. 2016).
- "Among adults with chronic low back pain, treatment with mindfulness-based stress reduction [training in mindfulness meditation and yoga] . . ., compared with usual care, resulted in greater improvement in back pain and functional limitations at 26 weeks . . . . These findings suggest that mindfulness-based stress reduction may be an effective treatment option for patients with chronic low back pain" (Cherkin et al. 2016).
- "Yoga appears to raise bone mineral density in the spine and the femur safely" (Lu et al. 2016)
- "High-intensity yoga may have positive effects on blood lipids and an anti-inflammatory effect" (Papp et al. 2016).
- While yoga may not alter or undo disc injuries in the back, "within 12 weeks, yoga practice reduced pain and state anxiety" in those who practiced it (Telles et al. 2016).
- "Six weeks of uninterrupted medical yoga therapy is a cost-effective early intervention for non-specific low back pain, when treatment recommendations are adhered to" (Aboagye et al. 2015).
- "Yoga can effectively reduce breast cancer survivors' cognitive complaints and prompt further research on mind-body and physical activity interventions for improving cancer-related cognitive problems" (Derry et al. 2015).
- "Yoga therapy can be safe and beneficial for patients with nonspecific low back pain or sciatica, accompanied by disc extrusions and bulges" (Monro et al. 2015).
- Yoga can lead to possible improvements in psychological health in older adults (Bonura et al. 2014).
- Certain plank exercises performed daily for about 6 months "significantly reduced" unhealthy curvatures of the spine caused by scoliosis (Fishman et al. 2014).
- Yoga may lead to improvements in cognitive function (Gothe et al. 2014; Hariprasad et al. 2013).
- "These results suggest that Iyengar yoga provides better improvement in pain reduction and improvement in health related quality of life in nonspecific chronic back pain than general exercise" (Nambi et al. 2014).
- Yoga, coupled with medical treatments, has been shown to improve quality of life in individuals with bronchial asthma (Sodhi et al. 2014).

- Regardless of race, class, or body mass index, participants in the study found relief from back pain through yoga (Stein et al. 2014).
- Yoga is a useful addition to a school routine to boost social self-esteem (Telles et al. 2013).
- Yoga has a beneficial effect on inflammatory activity and improvement in fatigue among breast-cancer survivors (Bower et al. 2012, 2014).
- Yoga can improve upper-extremity function in individuals with hyper kyphosis, a spine deformity that causes a forward-curved posture of the upper back (Wang et al. 2012) and decreased adult onset kyphosis in seniors (Greendale et al. 2009).
- Yoga helps with stress control (Kiecolt-Glaser et al. 2010).
- Yoga is a helpful way to manage fear of falls and improve balance (Schmidd et al. 2010).
- Yoga can be an effective strategy to help breast-cancer survivors improve quality of life (Speed-Andrews et al. 2010).
- Yoga training in the preseason or as a supplemental activity may lessen the symptoms associated with muscle soreness (Boyle et al. 2004).
- "A yoga-based regimen was more effective than wrist splinting or no treatment in relieving some symptoms and signs of carpal tunnel syndrome" (Garfinkel et al. 1998).

The following yoga sequence was designed by Romy Phillips for you to use in the comfort of your home or at a local park. It is a sample beginner's routine. Although yoga is an excellent form of exercise for many people, not every style or pose is appropriate for certain individuals. Therefore, it is necessary to experiment with different teachers, levels, and styles before committing oneself to the practice, and especially before ruling out yoga altogether. There are a multitude of poses with numerous benefits. I (Romy Phillips) decided to create a sequence that is simple and accessible to many and is ideal for a home practice if you can't make it to a yoga studio.

Despite its benefits, not all yoga poses are safe for individuals with certain conditions.

The author of this book requested I design a very basic yoga sequence for this chapter with an attempt to minimize stress to the lower back. For this reason, I have minimized excess bending and twisting in the sequence I outlined and created a very basic introductory yoga lesson. If you have back pain or any other injury, I highly recommend you work with a qualified medical professional and a yoga instructor to modify this lesson to fit your needs, or learn a different sequence which may be more appropriate for your body.

Individuals who have osteoporosis or someone who underwent back surgery or a total hip replacement will need personalized instruction from a yoga practitioner. For example, people with osteoporosis should typically avoid poses that place them in extreme spinal flexion (forward bending) positions, such as the child's pose, plow pose, seated forward bend pose, and standing forward bend pose. Instead, individuals with osteoporosis may be instructed to focus on neutral spine or spine extension (slight backward arching) positions, such as the bridge pose, mountain pose, chair pose, warrior one pose, warrior two pose, warrior three pose, tree pose, or a plank pose. Also, for further information, you may wish to refer to my book *Yoga Forma: A Visual Resource Guide for the Spine and Lower Back* (Cedar Fort Publishing, 2018).

In this lesson, I will lead you through a series of movements that start you lying down on your back (Part 1) and then get you up to standing (Part 2). Since many people tend to be stiff in the morning, the focus of this short session is to minimize forward bends that may aggravate the lower back. You can always adjust the sequence to fit your time schedule. For example, the first seven postures in the sequence (Part 1) can be a relaxing and gentle practice that minimizes stress to the spine and provides an adequate number of movements to relieve stiffness and let you feel energized and refreshed. In addition, I have provided more detailed instructions that allow you to experience 11 additional postures on a deeper level (Part 2).

Remember that with yoga we are trying to tap into the subtle layers, starting with the outermost layer, the surface of the skin, muscles, and bones and moving inward to connect to what we can't see but feel. Even the simplest postures can have more meaning if you slow down to understand what you're *sensing*. This process allows you to let go of other thoughts and connect to your body. This is really the fundamental concept of the term "mind body." Skillful use of the breath is a subtle way to connect the mind and body. Tremendous healing can begin on this level alone—stress reduction especially because deep breathing, particularly the exhalation, has a calming effect on the nervous system. In my descriptions of the poses (or postures) listed below, I will guide you to direct your focus on certain details of a posture and cue the use of the breath.

You will need the following props for this sequence: two blocks, a strap, blankets, and a bolster (optional). Let's begin your practice by:

PART 1

POSTURE 1: LYING FLAT ON YOUR BACK WITH YOUR KNEES BENT

Place your hands by yours sides or let them rest on your chest and abdomen. The feet can be placed as wide as the mat, inner knees resting together. Breathe evenly through the nose. Notice the gentle rise and fall of your chest as you inhale and exhale. Emphasize lengthening the inhalation by moving the breath slowly from the abdomen to the chest and then pause for a brief moment. Now exhale and slowly release the breath. Repeat this several times, concentrating on the qualities the breath can bring into the body, such as lightness and expansion with each inhale, and releasing tension and stress with each exhale (Figure 6-1).

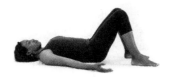

Figure 6-1

POSTURE 2: KNEES-TO-CHEST POSE (APANASANA)

Bring the knees to your chest. Hold on to your shins. If your knees are sensitive, hold on to the back of your thighs. Allow the thighs to softly release toward the torso as you exhale. Focus on releasing tension in the lower back. Keep the back of the head and shoulders resting on the floor. After a few moments, let both feet rest on the floor. The knees are bent (Figure 6-2).

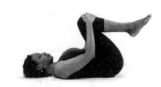

Figure 6-2

POSTURE 3: ONE-KNEE-TO-CHEST POSE (EKA PADA APANASANA)

Hold on to the shin of your left leg and lift it up toward your chest. If your knees are sensitive, you can hold onto the back of your thigh. Straighten the right leg along the floor. If your hamstrings are tight, then keep the right leg bent. Repeat on the right side (Figure 6-3).

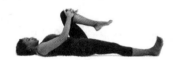

Figure 6-3

POSTURE 4: RECLINING HAND-TO-BIG-TOE POSE (SUPTA PADANGUSTHASANA)

Place both feet on the floor with knees bent. Place a strap on the right foot. Straighten the right leg up toward the ceiling and pause. If your hamstrings are tight, slightly bend the knee and keep the left knee bent as well. If your hamstrings are flexible, straighten both legs. Hold and breathe for 5 breaths. Each inhale and exhale is equal to one breath.

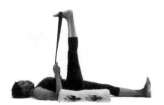

Figure 6-4

The heel and calf of the left leg that is extended along the floor should firmly press against the floor. To avoid hyperextension of the knee, slightly bend the left leg and engage the top of the thigh by firming the quadriceps muscle. Release the inner thigh down toward the floor. Try not to shrug up around the shoulders (Figure 6-4).

Next, place both ends of the strap in the right hand. Lower the right leg and let it rest on a rolled up blanket (Figure 6-5). You should try your best to keep the pelvis and the entire left side of your body balanced. Press the left shoulder, left side of the torso, and left side of the pelvis firmly toward the floor. Imagine that the left hamstring can touch the floor. Pause and hold for a few breaths.

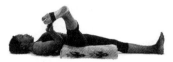

Figure 6-5

Now, bring the leg back up and place both ends of the strap in the left hand. Slowly lower the right leg slightly diagonal across your body (Figure 6-6). Push through the

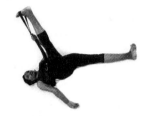

Figure 6-6

heel to lengthen the leg. Turn and look toward your right shoulder. Press the back of the right shoulder toward the floor. Pause here as you reach the foot and hand in the opposite direction. You can go further in the twist if you wish. Slowly release and rest the right leg on the floor. Pause and notice the sensations in your body before repeating the sequence on the left side. Some people feel as if the right leg is slightly longer than the left. What do you feel?

Posture 5: Dynamic Bridge (Setu Bandha Sarvangasana)

Bend your knees and place the feet hip-width apart. The knees should line up directly over the heels. Place your hands down by your sides (Figure 6-7), inhale, and slowly lift the hips and extend your arms overhead (Figure 6-8). Exhale, roll down slowly, and empty out the breath. The hands and pelvis should come to the floor simultaneously. Move very slowly and consciously, noticing any stiffness in the shoulders or spine or tightness in the muscles. Repeat several times.

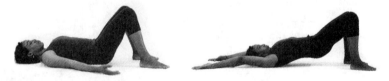

Figure 6-7   Figure 6-8

Posture 6: Knees-to-Chest Pose (Apanasana)

Bring both knees to your chest and hold for a few breaths (See Figure 6-2).

Posture 7: Reclining Mountain Pose (Supta Tadasana)

Inhale, reach the arms overhead, and straighten the legs, lengthening the entire body by reaching out from the fingertips through the heels. Make sure the palms

Figure 6-9

face each other (Figure 6-9). Avoid shrugging up around the neck and shoulders. Soften the front ribs and release the upper back down toward the floor. Release the buttocks toward the heels to lengthen the lower back. Feel the energy moving throughout your entire body. Exhale and release the arms down. Repeat Apanasana again (Figure 6-2).

(Note: You can stop here if you are not getting off the floor. To finish the short version of this sequence, focus on relaxation by continuing to lie on the floor (Savasana) (Figure 6-19). For the Savasana pose, lie on your back, arms down by your sides with your palms facing up. A bolster or blankets can be placed underneath your legs. Lie in the Savasana pose for 5 to 10 minutes.)

If you are continuing, the additional sequences in Part 2 will take you to the standing poses.

PART 2

Posture 8: Downward-Facing Dog (Adho Mukha Svanasana)

Roll to the side and come onto your hands and knees. Make sure your hands are placed shoulder- width apart. Spread the fingers evenly and root down through the palms. Lengthen the spine. Inhale, lift the hips, and move them up and away from the shoulders. If your hamstrings are tight, then bend your knees slightly and place the feet wider at the edges of the mat. Otherwise, the feet are hip-width apart. As you hold the pose for a few moments, try to focus on lifting the tailbone up and away from the upper body. Inhale and lengthen your entire spine, particularly the lower back (lumbar spine). Continue to press down through the width of your palms and firm the outer arms in. Lift the inner arms up toward the ceiling and draw the outer arms down toward the floor (Figure 6-10). Exhale and release into a Child's pose (Figure 6-11).

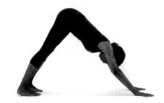

Figure 6-10

POSTURE 9: CHILD'S POSE (BALASANA)

Not only is the Child's pose considered a resting pose, it also prepares parts of the body for other yoga poses. In this case, we are going to focus on the key elements that will release the lower back and open the shoulders (flexion) to prepare for the next Downward-Facing Dog (Adho Mukha Svanasana). Come onto your hands and knees, exhale, and release your hips back toward your heels (Figure 6-11). If your buttocks don't touch the heels, then place a blanket under the pelvis. The forehead can rest lightly on the edge of a

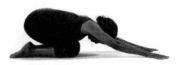

Figure 6-11

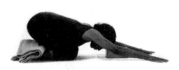

Figure 6-12 (Modified Balasana)

block as well. This encourages length through the entire spine and helps maintain the neutral alignment of the neck (Figure 6-12). The hands are extended forward and placed shoulder- width apart. Spread the fingers and press down through the palms. As you shift back, allow the ribcage to rest on the inner thighs (this protects the lower back). If your forehead doesn't rest on the floor, place a block underneath your forehead. Stay in this supported variation of the Child's pose and breathe for several breaths. Focus on expanding the back as you inhale. Gently release the hips toward your heels as you exhale. Lift the forearms up and away from the floor. Engage the triceps by firming them in. Inhale, press down through your palms, and lengthen the entire body.

POSTURE 10: DOWNWARD-FACING DOG (ADHO MUKHA SVANASANA)

From the Child's pose with your arms engaged, lift the hips up as you exhale (Figure 6-10). Notice the difference in your body as you practice the Downward-Facing Dog pose for a second time. Do you feel more length and opening in the shoulders and back of the legs? Can you straighten the arms even more? Hold the pose and breathe for 5 complete cycles.

POSTURE 11: FORWARD FOLD (UTTANASANA)

From the Downward-Facing Dog pose, walk forward into the Forward Fold pose (Uttanasana) (Figure 6-13). If your hands don't touch the floor, place blocks under the hands or bend your knees. Shift the weight into the center of your feet. The feet can be hip-width apart or placed together evenly. Allow the head to release down toward the floor and

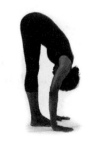

Figure 6-13

feel the tension release in your lower back. If your lower back or hamstrings are tight, bend the knees slightly or place your hands on your shins and extend the spine. Inhale and lengthen the spine to rise up.

POSTURE 12: MOUNTAIN POSE (TADASANA)

The focus here is on strengthening awareness of alignment. Stand with your feet together and your arms down by your sides (your feet should be slightly apart if you are pregnant or having back pain). Align your head over the shoulders. Press down through the feet and spread your toes, lifting the inner arches of the feet. Inhale, firm, and lift the front of your thighs. Lift the front of the hip bones up and release the buttocks down toward the heels. Imagine that you are creating more space between the pelvis and the bottom ribs. Soften the front ribs and widen across the collarbones.

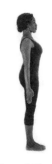

Figure 6-14

The shoulders widen and release away from the ears. Slightly draw the shoulder blades toward each other. Inhale and reach up through the crown of your head. Stand for a while (approximately 5 breaths) working these actions and experience proper alignment and allow this sensation to make an imprint in your mind and body. The Mountain pose (Tadasana) is the root of all standing poses and the key to a healthy spine (Figure 6-14).

POSTURE 13: ONE-HALF SALUTE

Start by standing in the Mountain pose (Tadasana). Next, inhale, lift your arm up, exhale, bow forward, and place your hands on the floor by your feet. If your hamstrings or lower back are tight, place your hands on blocks. Inhale, lengthen your spine, and place the fingertips on the floor or on blocks. Hold this position, placing an emphasis on lengthening your torso by reaching the sternum towards the front of your mat. The knees can also be bent here as well. Exhale and release down into the Forward Fold pose (Uttanasana). Finally, inhale, extend the torso, and rise up to the Mountain pose (Tadasana) (Figure 6-15). Repeat this entire sequence several times.

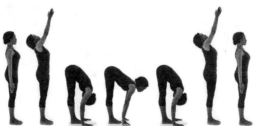

Figure 6-15

Turn to the side and stand in the middle of
your mat in the Mountain pose (Tadasana).

POSTURE 14: TREE POSE (VRKSASANA)

From the Mountain pose (Tadasana), lift your left leg up and place your foot either on your calf or inner thigh. Hands can start out on your hips, then to Anjali Mudra (or the prayer position at the center of the chest) or extended up towards the ceiling (Figure 6-16). The modifications are to use the wall or place your hands on the back of a chair for additional balance. In addition, the heel of the left foot can be placed against the right inner ankle. To work in this pose, I advise that you hold this pose for at least 5 breaths, working up to one minute for a real challenge. As you hold this pose, remember to firm the outer hip in order to avoid the tendency to "sit in the hip" (in other words, make sure you are using muscle effort). Keep lifting up through the sides of your waist and spine and visualize the fundamentals of the Mountain pose (Tadasana).

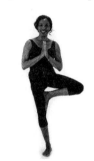

Figure 6-16

POSTURE 15: WARRIOR TWO (VIRABHADRASANA II) (DYNAMIC, THEN HOLD)

From the Mountain pose (Tadasana), spread your feet wide apart. Once again, make sure your feet are parallel to the edges of the mat. Extend the arms out to the sides and align the wrists over the ankles. Bend the right knee and make sure the knee lines up directly over the heel. Inhale, straighten the leg and lift the arms up toward the ceiling, lengthen through both sides of your waist, exhale, lower the arms, and bend the right knee (Figure 6-17). Repeat this several times, making sure the knee is lined up with the toes. Try to bend a little deeper with each repetition. This variation gently opens up the hips. Repeat this sequence on the other side. Do you notice a difference?

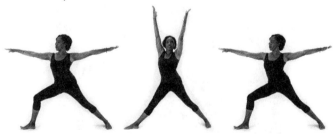

Figure 6-17

POSTURE 16: MOUNTAIN POSE (TADASANA)

Step your feet together and stand in the Mountain pose (Tadasana). Close your eyes. Observe the sensations in the hips, legs, and spine. (Figure 6-14)

Turn toward the top of your mat. From the Mountain pose (Tadasana), perform a One-Half Salute into the Forward Fold pose (Uttanasana). Hold for a moment before coming onto your hands and knees on the floor. Release into the Child's pose (Balasana). Then lie down on your back with your knees bent.

POSTURE 17: SIMPLE TWIST

Bring your knees to your chest (Apanasana) (Figure 6-2). Extend your arms out to your sides and lower the legs toward the floor while exhaling. Turn and look toward your left shoulder. If your legs do not rest easily on the floor, place a blanket under the thighs. This can be done for the back of the left shoulder as well.

For an additional stretch, your right hand can be placed on top of your left thigh and gently applying pressure (Figure 6-18). Hold and breathe, focusing on the gentle rotation of the spine. Repeat on the left side.

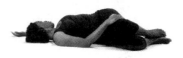

Figure 6-18

POSTURE 18: CORPSE POSE (SAVASANA)

This is your final resting pose. Feel free to prop your legs up on a bolster or two blankets. You may also want to cover yourself with a blanket or place support under your head. Lie down on your back with your palms facing up. Close your eyes (Figure 6-19). Focus on deepening your breath by slowing down each exhalation. Pause for a brief moment at the bottom of each exhale to help release tension in the body. Repeat the flow of the breath to encourage the body to settle against the floor and relax. Rest in this pose for at least 5 minutes and up to 10 minutes.

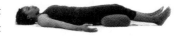

Figure 6-19

This short introduction of a simple home practice is just one of many potential ways to experience yoga—there are infinite possibilities. In fact, this sequence can be adapted to add more postures and can be enhanced or modified for any level of practitioner. For example, for more of a challenge, sun salutations and an inversion can be added. For personalized instruction, I recommend that you study with a certified yoga instructor at a yoga studio in your community. Finally, for an audio-guided instruction to this specific sequence and additional options for sequences, you are welcome to visit my website, yogathology.com, and the Yogathology page on YouTube.

ADDITIONAL RESOURCES

- Certified Ashtanga teachers, Shri K. Patthabi Jois Ashtanga Yoga Institute, kpjayi.org
- Certified Iyengar teachers, Iyengar Yoga National Association of the United States, iynaus.org
- International Association of Yoga Therapists, iayt.org
- MediYoga, en.mediyoga.com
- Yoga Alliance, yogaalliance.org
- Yoga Journal, yogajournal.com
- Yogathology with Romy Phillips, yogathology.com
- YogaWorks, yogaworks.com

REFERENCES

Aboagye E, Karlsson ML, Hagberg J, et al. (2015). Cost-effectiveness of early interventions for non-specific low back pain: A randomized controlled study investigating medical yoga, exercise therapy and self-care advice. *Journal of Rehabilitation Medicine* 47 (2): 167–173.

Andronis L, Kinghorn P, Qiao S, et al. (2017). Cost-effectiveness of non-invasive and non-pharmacological interventions for low back pain: A systematic literature review. *Applied Health Economics and Health Policy* 15 (2): 173-201.

Bonura KB, Tenenbaum G. (2014). Effects of yoga on psychological health in older adults. *Journal of Physical Activity & Health* 11 (7): 1334–1341.

Bower JE, Garet D, Sternlieb B, et al. (2012). Yoga for persistent fatigue in breast cancer survivors: A randomized controlled trial. *Cancer* 118 (15): 3766–3775.

Bower JE, Greendale G, Crosswell AD, et al. (2014). Yoga reduces inflammatory signaling in fatigued breast cancer survivors: A randomized controlled trial. *Psychoneuroendocrinology* 43: 20–29.

Boyle CA, Sayers SP, Jensen BE, et al. (2004). The effects of yoga training and a single bout of yoga on delayed onset muscle soreness in the lower extremity. *Journal of Strength and Conditioning Research* 18 (4): 723–729.

Chang DG, Holt JA, Sklar M, et al. (2016). Yoga as a treatment for chronic low back pain: A systematic review of the literature. *Journal of Orthopedics and Rheumatology* 3 (1): 1–8.

Cherkin DC, Sherman KJ, Balderson BH, et al. (2016). Effect of mindfulness-based stress reduction vs cognitive behavioral therapy or usual care on back pain and functional limitations in adults with chronic low back pain: A randomized clinical trial. *JAMA* 315 (12): 1240–1249.

Derry HM, Jaremka LM, Bennett JM, et al. (2015). Yoga and self-reported cognitive problems in breast cancer survivors: A randomized controlled trial. *Psychooncology* 24 (8): 958–966.

Desikachar TKV. (1995). *The Heart of Yoga: Developing A Personal Practice*. Rochester, VT: Inner Traditions International.

Evans-Wentz WY. (1967). *Tibetan Yoga and Secret Doctrines*. New York, NY: Oxford University Press.

Feuerstein G. (2001). *The Yoga Tradition: Its History, Literature, Philosophy and Practice,* 3rd ed. Prescott, AZ: Hohm Press.

Fishman LM, Groessl EJ, Sherman KJ. (2014). Serial case reporting yoga for idiopathic and degenerative scoliosis. *Global Advances in Health and Medicine* 3 (5): 16–21.

Garfinkel MS, Singhal A, Katz WA, et al. (1998). Yoga-based intervention for carpal tunnel syndrome: A randomized trial. *JAMA* 280 (18): 1601–1603.

Gothe NP, Kramer AF, and McAuley E. (2014). The effects of an 8-week hatha yoga intervention on executive function in older adults. *Journals of Gerontology. Series A, Biological Sciences and Medical Sciences* 69 (9): 1109–1116.

Greendale GA, Huang MH, Karlamangla AS, et al. (2009). Yoga decreases kyphosis in senior women and men with adult-onset hyperkyphosis: Results of a randomized controlled trial. *Journal of the American Geriatrics Society* 57 (9): 1569–1579.

Hariprasad VR, Koparde V, Sivakumar PT, et al. (2013). Randomized clinical trial of yoga-based intervention in residents from elderly homes: Effects on cognitive function. *Indian Journal Psychiatry* 55 (Supplement 3): S357–363.

Iyengar BKS. (1979). *Light on Yoga*. New York, NY: Schocken Books.

Iyengar BKS. (2005). *Light on Life: The Journey to Wholeness, Inner Peace and Ultimate Freedom*. Emmaus, PA: Rodale Books.

Iyengar BKS. (2014). *B.K.S. Iyengar Yoga: The Path to Holistic Health*. New York, NY: DK Publishing.

Kiecolt-Glaser JK, Christian L, Preston H, et al. (2010). Stress, inflammation, and yoga practice. *Psychosomatic Medicine* 72 (2): 113–121.

Lasater JH. (2017). *Restore and Rebalance: Yoga for Deep Relaxation*. Boulder, CO: Shambhala Publications, Inc.

Lu Y-H, Rosner B, Chang G, et al. (2016). Twelve-minute daily yoga regimen reverses osteoporotic bone loss. *Topics in Geriatric Rehabilitation* 32 (2): 81–87.

Monro R, Bhardwaj AK, Gupta RK, et al. (2015). Disc extrusions and bulges in nonspecific low back pain and sciatica: Exploratory randomised controlled trial comparing yoga therapy and normal medical treatment. *Journal of Back and Musculoskeletal Rehabilitation* 28 (2): 383–392.

Nambi GS, Inbasekaran D, Khuman R, et al. (2014). Changes in pain intensity and health related quality of life with iyengar yoga in nonspecific chronic low back pain: A randomized controlled study. *International Journal of Yoga* 7 (1): 48–53.

O'Neill S (ed). (2018). Kuo-Deemer M. Yoga and Qigong. In: *Yoga Teaching Handbook: A Practical Guide for Yoga Teachers and Trainers*. Philadelphia, PA: Singing Dragon.

Papp ME, Lindfors P, Nygren-Bonnier M, et al. (2016). Effects of high-intensity hatha yoga on cardiovascular fitness, adipocytokines, and apolipoproteins in healthy students: A randomized controlled study. *Journal of Alternative and Complementary Medicine* 22 (1): 81–87.

Salem GJ, Yu SS, Wang MY, et al. (2013). Physical demand profiles of Hatha yoga postures performed by older adults. *Evidence-based Complementary and Alternative Medicine* 165763.

Saper RB, Lemaster C, Delitto A, et al. (2017). Yoga, physical therapy, or education for chronic low back pain: A randomized noninferiority trial. *Annals of Internal Medicine* 167 (2): 85–94.

Satish V, Rao RM, Manjunath NK, et al. (2018). Yoga versus physical exercise for cardio-respiratory fitness in adolescent school children: A randomized controlled trial. *International Journal of Adolescent Medicine and Health*. Electronic publication ahead of print.

Schmidd AA, Van Puymbroeck M, and Koceja DM. (2010). Effect of a 12-week yoga intervention on fear of falling and balance in older adults: A pilot study. *Archives of Physical Medicine and Rehabilitation* 91 (4): 576–583.

Sodhi C, Singh S, and Bery A. (2014). Assessment of the quality of life in patients with bronchial asthma, before and after yoga: A randomised trial. *Iranian Journal of Allergy, Asthma, and Immunology* 13 (1): 55–60.

Speed-Andrews AE, Stevinson C, Belanger LJ, et al. (2010). Pilot evaluation of an Iyengar yoga program for breast cancer survivors. *Cancer Nursing* 33 (5): 369–381.

Stein KM, Weinberg J, Sherman KJ, et al. (2014). Participant characteristics associated with symptomatic improvement from yoga for chronic low back pain. *Journal of Yoga and Physical Therapy* 4 (1): 151.

Telles S, Singh N, Bhardwaj AK et al. (2013). Effect of yoga or physical exercise on physical, cognitive and emotional measures in children: A randomized controlled trial. *Child and Adolescent Psychiatry and Mental Health* 7 (1): 37.

Venes D. (Ed.) (2017). *Taber's Cyclopedic Medical Dictionary*, 23rd ed. Philadelphia, PA: FA Davis.

Wang MY, Greendale GA, Kazadi L, et al. (2012). Yoga improves upper-extremity function and scapular posturing in persons with hyperkyphosis. *Journal of Yoga and Physical Therapy* 2 (3): 117.

Wang MY, Yu SS, Hashish R, et al. (2013). The biomechanical demands of standing yoga poses in seniors: The Yoga Empowers Seniors Study (YESS). *BMC Complementary and Alternative Medicine* 13:8.

Ward L, Stebbings S, Athens J, et al. (2017). Yoga for the management of pain and sleep in rheumatoid arthritis: A pilot randomized controlled trial. *Musculoskeletal Care*. Electronic publication ahead of print.

CHAPTER 7

TAI CHI FOR HEALTH

This chapter was completed with the assistance of Derek Plonka, DPT, MTOM, L.Ac, CSCS. Dr. Plonka is a physical therapist and acupuncturist with over 20 years of experience in treating musculoskeletal conditions and movement disorders. As a physical therapist, he has been practicing privately in Santa Monica, California, since 2004 at the Insight Wellness Clinic (www. InsightWellnessClinic.com) and in 2015 he completed his Masters in Traditional Oriental Medicine at Emperor's College of Traditional Oriental Medicine (ECTOM). He remains involved with ECTOM, for which he serves as the Doctoral Program Faculty and CAPSTONE Advisor, helping students mesh together an understanding of Eastern and Western Medicine. It is his multi-faceted approach to patient care which lends a unique perspective to his contributions in this book.

Derek Plonka, DPT, MTOM, L.Ac, CSCS
Doctor of Physical Therapy / Licensed Acupuncturist
Insight Wellness Clinic
Santa Monica, California
www.insightwellnessclinic.com

> *"Empty your mind, be formless, shapeless—like water.*
> *Now you put water in a cup, it becomes the cup;*
> *You put water into a bottle it becomes the bottle;*
> *You put it in a teapot it becomes the teapot.*
> *Now water can flow or it can crash."*
>
> —Bruce Lee

Tai chi is a traditional Chinese martial art in which a series of slow, controlled movements helps improve balance, relaxation, mental concentration, flexibility, and strength (Venes 2017). Tai chi is sometimes considered mind in action or meditation in motion (Chow 1982).

The exact origin of tai chi is unknown. Chinese legend has it that it began about 800 years ago, when a Taoist priest named Zhang Sanfeng witnessed a fight between a bird and a snake. He became fascinated by the fluid motions both animals used in going from offense to defense. Over a period of several years, he experimented with various forms until he developed what is now practiced as tai chi.

Today, there are several styles of tai chi, such as the Yang, Chen, Wu, Hao, and Sun styles, with some forms having more than 100 postures and movements. Traditional styles are associated with family surnames: Chen, Yang (most popular form), Chuan, Wu, and Sun (Kit 2002).

Z Altug's Perspective for Doing Tai Chi

In my clinical practice as a physical therapist, I typically recommend tai chi to patients and clients who need to improve posture and balance, manage stress, and work on mobility. Other general reasons to try tai chi include (Bottomley 2017):

- Relieve stress and tension
- Improve overall health
- Improve flexibility
- Improve breathing
- Improve strength
- Improve endurance
- Improve posture
- Improve balance
- Improve coordination
- Improve circulation
- Help manage pain
- Help prevent falls
- Help manage weight
- Help find inner peace
- Improve socialization (when performed in a group setting)
- Provide a low-cost and low-tech activity

Dr. Derek Plonka's Perspective for Doing Tai Chi

As a physical therapist at heart, my emphasis is to assist with skilled intervention to resolve what a patient can't treat for themselves and progress them toward an independent home exercise program. Most importantly, the patient must be able to comply with the prescribed home program. Many patients have come to me with multiple pages of home exercises, practically the kitchen sink, and are only performing one or two with some regularity. They typically exclude the most important ones because it feels to be too challenging for them. As you have read from the history of tai chi, there are a number of styles and short (24 postures) to long forms (more than 100 postures). For a person just beginning or one with cognitive deficits, even 24 postures can be overwhelming. For this reason, later in this chapter I will outline the Ezy tai chi style.

LET'S SEE WHAT RESEARCH SAYS . . .

- Tai chi may be effective for improving balance, strength, and flexibility while decreasing pain and fatigue in women with fibromyalgia (Wong et al. 2017).
- Tai chi can reduce stress levels in healthy individuals (Zheng et al. 2017).
- Tai chi may be a good way to slow down the age-related decline in muscle strength in a community-dwelling population (Zhou et al. 2016).
- Tai chi can be helpful for improving fitness and arthritis in older adults (Dogra et al. 2015).
- Tai chi and functional balance training benefit older individuals with polyneuropathy (Quigley et al. 2014).
- Tai chi has had modest positive effects on functional status of individuals with Parkinson's disease (Choi et al. 2013; Li et al. 2012).
- Speed and accuracy in math computations has been attributed to the possible relaxed state from a tai chi or yoga class (Field et al. 2010).
- Tai chi can be useful in the treatment of fibromyalgia (Wang et al. 2010).
- Tai chi can improve the quality of life for individuals with chronic obstructive pulmonary disease (COPD) (Yeh et al. 2010).
- Tai chi can lead to balance improvements in people with chronic strokes (Au-Yeung et al. 2009).
- Tai chi improves balance and helps people maintain good postural stability (Li et al. 2008; Mak et al. 2003, Tsang et al. 2004).
- Tai chi can be beneficial for reducing falls (Li et al. 2005; Voukelatos 2007).
- Tai chi can improve sleep quality in older adults (Li et al. 2004).
- Tai chi can improve a person's arthritic symptoms (Song et al. 2003).
- Tai chi can have a positive effect on the immunity that protects against shingles (Irwin et al. 2003).
- Tai chi has been shown to slow the loss of weight-bearing bone in postmenopausal women (Qin et al. 2002; Chan et al. 2004).

🏃 PRACTICAL TAI CHI ROUTINE

The following basic tai chi routine was designed by Dr. Derek Plonka for you to use in the comfort of your home or at a local park.

A number of years ago, I (Derek Plonka) came across what is called the "Ezy tai chi" which consists of only eight postures (Fisher et al. 2004). By implementing this greatly simplified structure to a tai chi routine, I found that tai chi became more "doable" and "digestible" for patients and resulted in an improved patient compliance. The creator of Ezy tai chi, FuZhong Li, Ph.D., is a researcher at the Oregon Research Institute in Eugene, Oregon, and derived the eight-posture series from the simplified form with 24 postures. In a study, he compared patients instructed in Ezy tai chi to a group using a low-stress exercise routine. The results demonstrated that a patient's functional ability, self-assessment health questionnaire, 50-foot walk test, and time to rise from a chair showed significant improvement in the Ezy tai chi group as compared to the low-stress exercise group. The entire eight postures, which consist of a Commencing, Closing, and six transitioning postures, can be completed in approximately three minutes, which allows the entire form to be repeated a number of times. Patients can increase Ezy tai chi's level of difficulty within the established form by varying speed and size of movement, as well as reduce the challenges by using a chair. This establishes Ezy tai chi as an excellent modality for patients with severe balance deficits or in a wheelchair, providing adaptability to a variety of person's physical capabilities. Once you have mastered the Ezy tai chi style, I recommend you consider progressing to the short and long forms of tai chi to enhance your memory, expand your mobility and balance, and improve your endurance. I have revised the concept of a simplified eight-form tai chi practice in my clinical setting and described my adaptation in this chapter.

Principles necessary for the proper practice of tai chi:

1. **Lift in the head:** Allow a lifting or floating feeling to enter your head.
2. **Open the chest and raise the back:** Allow the chest to open to allow the back to lift and follow the head.
3. **Soften in the waist:** Feel the sense of grounded heaviness through your Dan Tian (the area below the navel into the perineum).
4. **Insubstantial versus substantial:** Substantial is when your body is bearing weight through the leg(s) and connecting to the earth. Insubstantial is when a leg or body part is moving freely through space.
5. **Sinking the shoulders and elbows:** Allow the head to float while the arms remain heavier at the shoulder and elbow joints.
6. **Intention in consciousness, not in strength:** Begin all movement with an intention of the mind and allow the body to follow.
7. **Upper and lower follow each other:** As the tail of a kite follows the kite, allow the rest of the body to follow the part that begins the movement.
8. **Internal and external are united:** Be present. The gut, the heart, and the mind should be in concert with each other and the body will happily play together. If the mind wanders away, the heart is held back, or the gut does not know where to go, then the body will be disjointed.

9. **Continuity:** Imagine a silk scarf as it is being pulled through the air. It smoothly floats with direction, following the point it is being tugged at. That is your body doing tai chi.

10. **Tranquility:** If all of the previous principles are in place, then tranquility will be there when you move. Simply draw gentle attention to each principle and ask yourself if you can hold each one in your hands the way one would hold a baby chick. Firm enough to feel safe, and not too tight or loose that the baby chick would squirm away. If a principle squirms away from your hands, gather it up and learn to hold it.

FORM 1: BEGINNING FORM

Beginning Stance: Face forward with feet together, both knees slightly bent, and arms at sides.

1. Gently shift your body weight to the right, with the left foot stepping to the left so that the feet are a full shoulder-width apart and parallel to each other. Allow the arms to hang relaxed at your sides.

2. Raise your arms. *Imagine you have placed your hands onto a bubbling pillar of water.* Your hands will cup the top of the pillar, relaxing at the elbows and allowing the hands to reach the level of your chest (Figure 7-1).

3. Once you have reached chest level for a moment, your hands will return back down and your knees will bend as the hands lower (Figure 7-2).

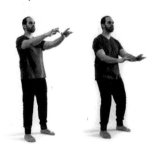

Figure 7-1   Figure 7-2

FORM 2: EAGLE FLAPS ITS WINGS

1. From the previous position, move the right hand down and circle back, eventually raising the hand to shoulder height with the palm rotated upward. At the same time, raise the left arm to chest height and rotate the palm upward. Gently shift your body weight to the right and allow your body to rotate as the arms are moving (Figure 7-3).

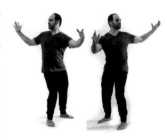

Figure 7-3   Figure 7-4

2. Bring the right hand forward to ball up the energy between both hands, feeling what you have gathered. At the same time, you are returning back to the forward-facing position.

3. Now continue past the front and repeat the same movements to the left. Move the left hand down and circle back, eventually raising the hand to shoulder height with the palm rotated upward. At the same time, raise the right arm to chest height and rotate the palm upward. Gently shift your body weight to the left as the arms are moving (Figure 7-4).

4. Bring the left hand forward to ball up the energy between both hands, feeling what you have gathered. At the same time, you are returning back to the forward-facing position.

Repeat this movement on each side twice.

Form 3: Playing with Silk

This form consists of five parts: (1) Shielding the eyes, (2) Sweeping back, (3) Cover the side, (4) Cover the front, and (5) Push away. *Imagine that you are holding a silk scarf in your hands, playing with it as it frolics through the air, with the silk scarf gently attached to your fingertips.*

1. Shielding the eyes: From the last position and holding the ball of energy in front of you, the left foot steps out to the left side (Figure 7-5) while the upper body rotates 45 degrees to the left. The left hand moves forward, arriving at eye level while pressing the right hand down toward the right hip with the palm facing downward. This is shielding the eyes with silk (Figure 7-6).

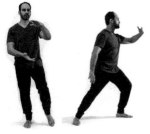

Figure 7-5   Figure 7-6

2. Sweeping back: With the left arm still shielding, bring your right hand up to meet the left hand. Your chest has now also turned to the left and the palms of your hands are now touching, with the left hand turned down and the right hand up (Figure 7-7). *Imagine you are gently holding the silk scarf out to your left, between the palms of your hands.*

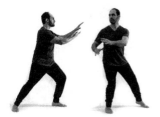

Figure 7-7   Figure 7-8

3. Cover the side: Now rotate the right hand so that the palm is downward and shift the weight of your body to the back right foot. Both hands continue downward to waist height (Figure 7-8). *Imagine you have now covered something in front of you and then behind you with the silk scarf.*

4. Cover the front: *Your body turns back to return the silk scarf.* Turn your body back to the left while shifting your weight back onto the left foot. Once your hands are in front of your body and to the left, with

palms facing down, draw your hands to your waist and press down (Figure 7-9). *Drawing the silk scarf over your left thigh.*

5. Push away: Wrists will tilt up so that your palms will face away from you and your arms will rise up to the level of your chest. Shift your body weight to the left foot and extend the arms to push away (Figure 7-10). *Imagine the silk scarf is being placed on a wall in front of you.*

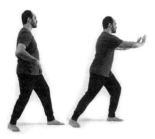

Figure 7-9   Figure 7-10

Repeat this sequence four times to the right.

FORM 4: MOVING HANDS LIKE CLOUDS

Imagine you are standing in a cloud, with cups in each hand, catching the clouds in front of you and dropping them down at your waist.

1. From the previous form's last position, allow the elbows to bend and shift your body weight to the left leg. As your weight is shifting to the left and your body rotates back to the front, the right hand sweeps in front of your face *(catching clouds)* as your left hand sweeps down to your waist *(dropping clouds)* (Figure 7-11).

Figure 7-11   Figure 7-12

2. Both hands continue in circles away from the body. As they simultaneously reach the level of your chest, the left hand turns upward *(catching clouds)* and the right hand turns downward *(dropping clouds)* (Figure 7-12).

3. The right foot now takes a step to be parallel to the left foot. Your feet are now shoulder-width apart. Your hands are now in a position where the right hand is facing upward and the left is facing downward, continuing to *catch clouds* and *drop clouds*.

Repeat this sequence three times only to the left.

Transition Position: Your hands will continue until the left hand is below and the right hand is above, but this time the left hand turns up and the right hand turns down. *Imagine you are now holding a ball of energy supported by the left hand.* This position with the left hand holding the ball completes the sequence and prepares for the next form.

FORM 5: LADY WORKS THE LOOM

1. From the position where the left hand holds the ball, turn your left foot a quarter turn to the left and step out to a comfortable distance (Figure 7-13). As the left foot is stepping out, the left hand rises upward and the right hand pushes forward (Figure 7-14).
2. The right hand then drops downward as your body weight shifts to the left and the right foot does a quarter turn to the right (Figure 7-15). Step out to your right at a comfortable distance. As the right foot is stepping out, the right hand blocks upward and the left hand pushes forward (Figure 7-16).

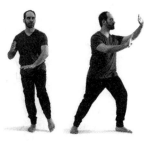

Figure 7-13   Figure 7-14

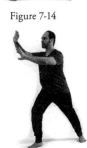

Figure 7-15   Figure 7-16

FORM 6: ROOSTER STANDS ON ONE LEG

1. Shift your body weight back to the left leg, letting the left arm hang down and raising the right arm up with the elbow bent to 90 degrees. Simultaneously lift the right knee to hip height and allow the foot to hang below (Figure 7-17). *Imagine you are standing tall and proud like a rooster waiting for the morning sun.*
2. Lower the right foot to shoulder width and the right hand by your side. Repeat the same position with the left arm and leg (Figure 7-18).

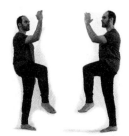

Figure 7-17   Figure 7-18

FORM 7: BRUSH KNEES

1. From the last position, while standing on your right leg, turn your chest to the right as the right hand circles back and up to your head. The elbow is slightly bent and the palm is open to the sky in front of you. The left hand follows the right hand throughout the movement with the left palm facing the right (Figure 7-19). *Your hands are like two birds flying together in unison.*

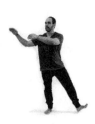

Figure 7-19

2. The left foot steps forward. As the left foot contacts the ground, the left hand drops down to brush past the left knee. The right hand continues past your face and pushes away, with the palm facing forward and the arm extended at chest level (Figure 7-20).

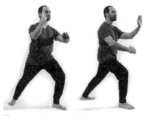

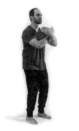

Figure 7-20   Figure 7-21

3. Transition to the left by bringing the right leg forward and balancing on the left leg. Continue by repeating the described sequence to the left side, ending with the right foot in front and the left hand pushing away (Figure 7-21).

FORM 8: ENDING FORM

1. From the previous position, bring the left foot forward to be shoulder-width apart and parallel with the right foot. Both knees are slightly bent. Simultaneously bring the right hand up to cross with the left hand in front of your face. The palms of both hands rotate toward you and lower to the level of your chest (Figure 7-22).

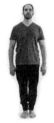

Figure 7-22   Figure 7-23

2. The knees will now straighten, as the hands uncross and allow the arms to rest comfortably at your sides. The eyes will gaze comfortably forward and the body stands tall, restored by the movement of its Qi (in Traditional Chinese Medicine, Qi represents the vital force or the energy of life) (Figure 7-23).

THE PRACTICE

The recommended routine is as follows:

- 10-minute warm-up as a generalized stretching routine to address muscular tightness
- 30 minutes to perform these eight simple tai chi forms, which are intended to be repeated numerous times. Pay attention to the 10 principles to maintain proper form.
- 5-minute cool down to allow a re-integration to regular body movement.
- When performed with a group, socialization is recommended. Speak with friends and smile on the inside as well as the outside, knowing that you have done something good for yourself.

For additional personalized tai chi training, I recommend you visit a martial arts studio or an acupuncture clinic.

ADDITIONAL RESOURCES

- American Tai Chi and Qigong Association, americantaichi.org
- International Sun Tai Chi Association, suntaichi.com
- Tai Chi for Health, taichimania.com

REFERENCES

Au-Yeung SS, Hui-Chan CW, Tang JC. (2009). Short-form tai chi improves standing balance of people with chronic stroke. *Neurorehabilitation and Neural Repair* 23 (5): 515–522.

Bottomley JM. (2017). T'ai Chi: Choreography of body and mind. In: Davis CM. *Integrative Therapies in Rehabilitation: Evidence for Efficacy in Therapy, Prevention and Wellness,* 4th ed. Thorofare, NJ: SLACK.

Chan AW, Lee A, Lee DT, et al. (2013). The sustaining effects of tai chi qigong on physiological health for COPD patients: A randomized controlled trial. *Complementary Therapies in Medicine* 21 (6): 585–594.

Chan K, Qin L, Lau M, et al. (2004). A randomized prospective study of the effects of tai chi chun exercise on bone mineral density in postmenopausal women. *Archives of Physical Medicine and Rehabilitation* 85 (5): 717–722.

Choi HJ, Garber CE, Jun TW, et al. (2013). Therapeutic effects of tai chi in patients with Parkinson's disease. *ISRN Neurology* 548240.

Chow M. (1982). *Classical Yang Style Tai Chi Chuan.* Los Angeles, CA: Wen Lin Associates.

Dogra S, Shah S, Patel M, et al. (2015). Effectiveness of a tai chi intervention for improving functional fitness and general health among ethnically diverse older adults with self-reported arthritis living in low-income neighborhoods: A cohort study. *Journal of Geriatric Physical Therapy* 38 (2): 71–77.

Field T, Diego M, Hernandez-Reif M. (2010). Tai chi/yoga effects on anxiety, heartrate, EEG and math computations. *Complementary Therapies in Clinical Practice* 16 (4): 235–238.

Fisher KJ, Li F, Shirai M. (2004). Ezy Tai Chi: A simpler practice for seniors. *Journal on Active Aging* May/June: 18–26.

Irwin MR, Pike JL, Cole JC, et al. (2003). Effects of a behavioral intervention, Tai Chi Chih, on varicella-zoster virus specific immunity and health functioning in older adults. *Psychosomatic Medicine* 65 (5): 824–830.

Kit WA. (2002). *The Complete Book of Tai Chi Chuan.* Boston, MA: Tuttle Publishing.

Li F, Fisher KJ, Harmer P, et al. (2004). Tai chi and self-rated quality of sleep and daytime sleepiness in older adults: A randomized controlled trial. *Journal of the American Geriatrics Society* 52 (6): 892–900.

Li F, Harmer P, Fisher KJ, et al. (2005). Tai chi and fall reductions in older adults: A randomized controlled trial. *Journals of Gerontology; Series A; Biological Sciences and Medical Sciences* 60 (2): 187–194.

Li F, Harmer P, Fitzgerald K, et al. (2012). Tai chi and postural stability in patients with Parkinson's disease. *New England Journal of Medicine* 366 (6): 511–519.

Li JX, Xu DQ, Hong Y. (2008). Effects of 16-week tai chi intervention on postural stability and proprioception of knee and ankle in older people. *Age and Ageing* 37 (5): 575–578.

Liu J, Wang XQ, Zheng JJ, et al. (2012). Effects of tai chi versus proprioception exercise program on neuromuscular function of the ankle in elderly people: A randomized controlled trial. *Evidence Based Complementary and Alternative Medicine* 265486.

Mak MK, Ng PL. (2003). Mediolateral sway in single-leg stance is the best discriminator of balance performance for tai-chi practitioners. *Archives of Physical Medicine and Rehabilitation* 84 (5): 683–686.

Qin L, Au S, Choy W, et al. (2002). Regular tai chi chuan exercise may retard bone loss in postmenopausal women: A case-control study. *Archives of Physical Medicine and Rehabilitation* 83 (10): 1355–1359.

Quigley PA, Bulat T, Schulz B, et al. (2014). Exercise interventions, gait, and balance in older subjects with distal symmetric polyneuropathy: A three-group randomized clinical trial. *American Journal of Physical Medicine and Rehabilitation* 93 (1): 1–16.

Song R, Lee EO, Lam P, et al. (2003). Effects of tai chi exercise on pain, balance, muscle strength, and perceived difficulties in physical functioning in older women with osteoarthritis: A randomized clinical trial. *Journal of Rheumatology* 30 (9): 2039–2044.

Tsang WW, Hui-Chan CW. (2004). Effects of exercise on joint sense and balance in elderly men: tai chi versus golf. *Medicine & Science in Sports & Exercise* 36 (4): 658–667.

Venes D. (Ed.) (2017). *Taber's Cyclopedic Medical Dictionary*, 23rd ed. Philadelphia, PA: FA Davis.

Voukelatos A, Cumming RG, Lord SR, et al. (2007). A randomized, controlled trial of tai chi for the prevention of falls: the Central Sydney Tai Chi trial. *Journal of the American Geriatrics Society* 55 (8): 1185–1191.

Wang C, Schmid CH, Rones R, et al. (2010). A randomized trial of tai chi for fibromyalgia. *New England Journal of Medicine* 363 (8): 743–754.

Wong A, Figueroa A, Sanchez-Gonzalez MA, et al. (2017). Effectiveness of tai chi on cardiac autonomic function and symptomatology in women with fibromyalgia: A randomized controlled trial. *Journal of Aging and Physical Activity* 1-26.

Yeh GY, Roberts DH, Wayne PM, et al. (2010). Tai chi exercise for patients with chronic obstructive pulmonary disease: a pilot study. *Respiratory Care* 55 (11): 1475–1482.

Zheng S, Kim C, Lal S, et al. (2018). The effects of twelve weeks of tai chi practice on anxiety in stressed but healthy people compared to exercise and wait-list groups-a randomized controlled trial. *Journal of Clinical Psychology* 74 (1): 83–92.

Zhou M, Peng N, Dai Q, et al. (2016). Effect of tai chi on muscle strength of the lower extremities in the elderly. *Chinese Journal of Integrative Medicine* 22 (11): 861–866.

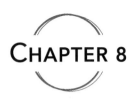

CHAPTER 8

QIGONG FOR HEALTH

This chapter was completed with the assistance of Derek Plonka, DPT, MTOM, L.Ac, CSCS. Dr. Plonka is a physical therapist and acupuncturist with over 20 years of experience in treating musculoskeletal conditions and movement disorders. As a physical therapist, he has been practicing privately in Santa Monica, California since 2004 at the Insight Wellness Clinic (www. InsightWellnessClinic.com) and in 2015 he completed his Masters in Traditional Oriental Medicine at Emperor's College of Traditional Oriental Medicine (ECTOM). He remains involved with ECTOM, for which he serves as the Doctoral Program Faculty and CAPSTONE Advisor, helping students mesh together an understanding of Eastern and Western Medicine. It is his multifaceted approach to patient care which lends a unique perspective to his contributions in this book.

Derek Plonka, DPT, MTOM, L.Ac, CSCS
Doctor of Physical Therapy / Licensed Acupuncturist
Insight Wellness Clinic
Santa Monica, California
www.insightwellnessclinic.com

"Qigong therapy, as well as other branches of Chinese medicine, can be reduced to two simple principles: the cleansing of meridians to achieve harmonious energy flow, and the restoration of yin-yang balance."

—The Art of Chi Kung by Wong Kiew Kit

Qigong (pronounced as "chee-goong") is a traditional Chinese movement therapy (Kerr 2002) and ancient martial art approach to healing that harnesses internal energy through movement (postures involving strength, flexibility, and balance), breathing exercises, relaxation, and meditation. *Qi* (breath, air, spirit) in Chinese stands for "energy of life" and *gong* means "work" or "practice." Thus, *Qi gong* (also known as qigong) means "working with the energy of life" (Johnson 2000; Venes 2017).

The word "qigong" dates back to two published works, in 1915 and 1929, and the therapeutic use of the term dates to 1936. Common use of the term is relatively recent as the practice has been known by many names throughout Chinese history, such as chi kung. There are many forms of qigong, such as Medical qigong, Fragrant qigong, Guo Lin qigong (walking qigong), Five Animals Play qigong, Eight Strands of Brocade qigong (or Eight-Section Brocade), tai chi qigong, and Six Healing Sounds. The term brocade used in this context is to liken qigong movements to a silken and smooth quality.

Also, qigong has several schools with their unique theories, such as Chinese Medical qigong, Daoist qigong, Buddhist qigong, Confucian qigong, and Martial Arts qigong. The earliest qigong-like exercises in China are ritual animal dances and movements. Many qigong postures have names such as Bathing Duck, Leaping Monkey, Turning Tiger, Coiling Snake, Old Bear in the Woods, and Flying Crane (Cohen 1997).

Z ALTUG'S PERSPECTIVE FOR DOING QIGONG

In my clinical practice as a physical therapist, I typically recommend qigong to patients and clients who need to improve posture and balance, manage stress, and work on mobility. In my opinion, individual and small groups of qigong poses tend to be easier to learn than the longer sequences in tai chi. Qigong is a great introduction to some gentle movements used in martial arts. Other general reasons to try qigong include:

- Relieve stress and tension
- Improve overall health
- Improve flexibility
- Improve breathing
- Improve strength
- Improve balance
- Improve posture
- Improve circulation
- Help manage pain
- Help manage weight
- Help find inner peace

DR. DEREK PLONKA'S PERSPECTIVE FOR DOING QIGONG

"The door hinge in an inhabited house will never be insect riddled. Rhythmic movement aids digestion and blood circulation, promoting health."

—Dr. Hua Tou

"Flowing water never freezes and the hinge of a moving door never rusts"

—Unknown

Although the words may differ, the idea is universally understood. The same can be said for qigong (Dao Yin), as there are many different lineages of practice and methods to implement it. What we see is that the door's hinges stay in good working order, but do not always see the door swing and we do not see the inner workings of the hinge. A person may perform the daily movements with their body, but will not see the internal mechanisms that influence how they perform their daily routine. The body may move, but in qigong, the most important movement is the connection inside with the outside. It is your inner mechanism which connects the breath, the mind, and the spirit. Without the connection, a person becomes disjointed and diseases will begin to manifest in the body, the spirit, or the mind.

In my (Derek Plonka) practice, qigong may be used to influence the acupuncture or pressure points of a patient, or I may prescribe a patient the movements (in connection with the breath) to promote Qi (energy) to flow through the channel(s) associated with the organ system(s), which are presenting a disharmony. Deficient conditions would benefit from color visualizations, where an excess condition would benefit from sound resonance. Qigong prescription could be performed while lying on the back, sitting, standing in traditional postures, or walking. The appropriateness of these aspects of qigong needs to be assessed and implemented by an experienced practitioner of Traditional Chinese Medicine (TCM). But for an individual beginning the practice of qigong, the importance is placed on quieting the mind and synchronizing the breath to the body's movements. Staying with a simple and balanced routine, practitioners can promote their own health by performing the Eight-Section Brocade Standing Exercises (also known as **Eight Strands of Brocade Qigong**) presented in this chapter.

LET'S SEE WHAT RESEARCH SAYS . . .

- Guolin-Qigong (or walking qigong) improves quality of life and immunological function during recovery after breast cancer (Liu et al. 2017).
- Qigong exercise involving six healing sounds reduces pro-inflammatory cytokines in people with Parkinson's disease and helps improve sleep quality (Moon et al. 2017).
- Tai chi qigong is useful for improving the quality of sleep in older adults with cognitive impairment (Chan et al. 2016).
- Qigong could be a helpful non-medical method for lessening pain in the chewing muscles, for increasing shoulder mobility, and for lessening sleep problems in survivors of inner nose cancers (Fong et al. 2015).
- There is potential for 'Six Healing Sounds' qigong exercise to improve sleep and other symptoms in breast cancer survivors (Liu et al. 2015).

- Qigong may be effective for reducing fatigue and distress in prostate cancer survivors (Campo et al. 2014).
- Qigong has been shown to be influential to postural stability and to reducing Parkinson's disease-related falls (Loftus 2014).
- Qigong may reduce anxiety and stress in healthy adults (Wand et al. 2014).
- Qigong can improve psychosocial health in individuals with chronic obstructive pulmonary disease (COPD) (Chan et al. 2013).
- Qigong can improve balance in healthy young women (González López-Arza et al. 2013).
- Qigong has been shown to cause short-term improvement of quality of life, pain, and sleep quality in individuals diagnosed with fibromyalgia (Lauche et al. 2013).
- Qigong can reduce chronic neck pain (Rendant et al. 2011).
- Qigong can decrease blood pressure in individuals with essential hypertension, which develops with no apparent cause (Guo et al. 2008).
- Qigong helps elderly individuals with chronic physical and mental illness (Tsang et al. 2003).
- Qigong can help reduce pain and anxiety in individuals with complex regional pain syndrome (Wu et al. 1999).

🏃 PRACTICAL QIGONG ROUTINE

The following basic qigong routine was designed by Dr. Derek Plonka for you to use in the comfort of your home or at a local park.

These qigong exercises have been adapted from various forms of Eight-Section of Brocade qigong (such as the Golden Eight Exercises from Master Hong Liu's book *The Healing Art of Qigong*). Please keep in mind that there are many interpretations to these qigong exercises and this is only one approach. The purpose of this modified Eight-Section Brocade Standing Exercise qigong routine is to help you relax your mind, improve mobility and balance, and improve your overall well-being. There are some precautions to consider before you perform this routine. I recommend you have a sturdy chair nearby for support if you have minor balance difficulties. I also recommend you skip these exercises if you have major balance problems or feel pain in your back, hips, knees, or ankles. Consult with your healthcare provider if you have other concerns or if you need additional ways to modify these exercises for your needs. I recommend you perform the exercises slowly using gentle diaphragmatic breathing or belly breathing (see the index to search for the term if you are unclear). Please keep in mind the benefits for each of the qigong exercises listed are based on the concepts outlined in Traditional Chinese Medicine. You may perform these calming and healing exercises in your living room, backyard, at the park, or any location you feel best.

Starting Position: Quieting the Mind (Opening Position)

Posture: Stand with both feet turned slightly outward and knees straight but relaxed. Relax into the waist and hips. Allow the shoulders to roll forward slightly. Drop the chin and head, but allow the eyes to continue gazing forward and relaxed. Arms hang loosely with fingers naturally turned inward toward each other (Figure 8-1).

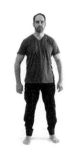

Breath: Mouth hangs open with the tip of the tongue on the palate. Inhale through the nose with a slow, long, even, and deep breath. Exhale through the mouth with a slow, long, even, and deep breath. Apply this practice to all brocades.

Figure 8-1

Purpose: This posture is set at the beginning of the series of eight brocade, in between each of the brocade, and at the end of the series of eight brocade. This position quiets the body, mind, and the breath to provide openness, allowing each brocade's internal action to be fully realized.

Exercise 1: Holding the Sky Up

Brocade: Begin from the Quieting the Mind brocade. Raise your hands to the level of your abdomen and interlace the fingers together. *On the inhale*, allow the interlaced fingers to continue upward, past the chest and over the head, while rotating the palms up to the sky (Figure 8-2). Pause for two seconds. *On the exhale*, release the fingers and allow the arms to lower to your sides.

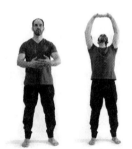

Repeat: Seven times.

Figure 8-2

Internal Action: Moves disease out of the San Jiao (the lymphatic system), lungs, and spleen by releasing tightness in the chest and distended abdomen.

Exercise 2: Drawing the Bow

Brocade: Stand with feet shoulder-width apart, arms hanging by your sides with hands in gentle fists. *On the inhale*, while keeping the torso forward, gently raise both arms to the left while keeping the thumbs pointing up to the sky. When the straight left arm and the right arm aligns with the height of the shoulders, begin raising the left hand's index finger while bending the right arm's elbow (Figure 8-3).

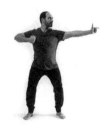

Figure 8-3

The action replicates drawing back the arrow on a bow. Squat and pause for two seconds. *On the exhale*, straighten the legs and allow the arms to return back to the original position.

Repeat: Seven times in each direction.

Internal Action: Treats lung disease and pain in the shoulders and arms.

EXERCISE 3: RAISING AN ARM

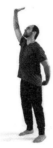

Brocade: Stand relaxed with feet shoulder-width apart and arms hanging by your sides. *On the inhale*, with the palms of your hands facing up, gently raise your hands to a level that is just above the navel. Once there, turn the left palm down and press down behind the buttocks with the finger tips pointing to the right. At the same time, rotate the right hand downward and then up toward the sky with the finger tips pointing to the left. Reach the left palm down and the right palm up, creating space between them (Figure 8-4). Hold for

Figure 8-4

two seconds, with the eyes gazing upward. *On the exhale*, return the hands back to the position just above the navel. Alternate directions of the hands and repeat.

Repeat: Seven times in each direction.

Internal Action: Calms the stomach and spleen for diseases caused by impaired or disorderly flow of qi and, possibly, pain in the shoulders and back.

EXERCISE 4: WISE OWL LOOKS BACK

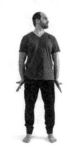

Brocade: Stand relaxed with feet shoulder-width apart and the arms hanging by your sides. *On the inhale*, turn the upper body and then the head as far left as possible while rotating both arms outward so that the palms turn away from the body (Figure 8-5). Pause for two seconds. *On the exhale*, return with the upper body and then the head to the front and allow the arms to return back to their natural resting position. *On the inhale*, turn the upper body and then the head as far right as possible while rotating both arms outward so that the palms turn away from the body. *On the exhale*, return with

Figure 8-5

the upper body and then the head to the front and allow the arms to return back to their natural resting position.

Repeat: Seven times in each direction.

Internal Action: Treats weaknesses of the body and internal damage.

Exercise 5: Shaking the Head and Swaying the Hips

Brocade: Stand relaxed with feet shoulder-width apart and the arms hanging by your sides. Soften the knees, lowering the body into a half-squat, and place your hands on your knees. *On the inhale*, turn the head left and lean over the left knee, while swinging the right hip to the right (Figure 8-6). *On the exhale*, with the body moving first, return back to the forward-facing position. *On the inhale*, turn the head right and lean over the right knee, while swinging the left hip to the left. *On the exhale*, with the body moving first, return back to the forward-facing position. Eyes remain open and follow the movement of the body.

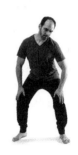

Figure 8-6

Repeat: Seven times in each direction.

Internal Action: Clears internal heat causing mental stress, dark red urine, and pain in the shoulders, waist, and legs.

Exercise 6: Bumping Seven Times

Brocade: Feet are slightly closer than shoulder-width apart. Eyes are gazing forward. Shoulders are slightly shrugged upward. Body remains relaxed. *On the inhale*, raise your body up onto the toes (Figure 8-7). *On the exhale*, drop your heels back to the floor, with the knees bending slightly on the landing.

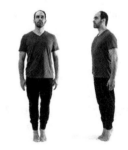

Repeat: Seven times.

Figure 8-7

Internal Action: Treats diseases caused by impaired circulation of qi and blood. Also helps with symptoms of pain one may feel in the neck, waist, knees, ankles, and toes.

Exercise 7: Clenching the Fists with Open Eyes

Brocade: Stand with feet just wider than shoulder-width apart, knees slightly bent, and elbows slightly bent with the palms facing up. Eyes are looking forward with strong intention. *On the exhale*, with both hands clenched in a fist, slowly punch both arms forward while turning the back of the fists upward (Figure 8-8). Pause for two seconds. *On the inhale*, allow the elbows to bend and

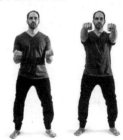

Figure 8-8

draw the fists back to the starting position. *On the exhale*, with a clenched fist slowly punch the right arm to the side with the thumb side of the fist upward. Allow the left elbow to bend and direct the left fist to the right (Figure 8-9). *On the inhale*, allow the elbows to bend and draw the fists back to the starting position. *On the exhale*, with a clenched fist slowly punch the left arm to the side with the thumb side of the fist upward.

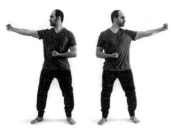

Figure 8-9

Allow the right elbow to bend and direct the right fist to the left. *On the inhale*, allow the elbows to bend and draw the fists back to the starting position.

Repeat: Seven times in each direction.

Internal Action: Strengthens the qi and treats shortness of breath, fatigue, lack of appetite, auto-immune disorders, and upper extremity numbness or pain.

EXERCISE 8: CLASPING THE FEET WITH HANDS

Brocade: Stand comfortably with the feet shoulder-width apart and the arms relaxed at your sides. Reach your arms forward and then directly up to the sky. *On the exhale*, bend forward at the hips and reach down to grasp your feet (only reach as far as you can comfortably) (Figure 8-10). Pause for two seconds. *On the inhale*, with your arms relaxed, gently raise your upper body back to the starting position with the arms relaxed at your sides.

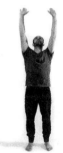
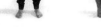

Figure 8-10

Repeat: Seven times.

Internal Action: Strengthens the chest, waist, back, knees, kidneys, and liver to resolve aching of the torso and legs.

ENDING POSITION: QUIETING THE MIND

Posture: Stand with both feet turned slightly outward and knees straight, but relaxed. Relax into the waist and hips. Allow the shoulders to roll forward slightly. Drop the chin and head, but allow the eyes to continue gazing forward and relaxed. Arms hang loosely with fingers naturally turned inward toward each other (Figure 8-11).

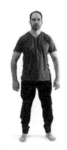

Figure 8-11

Breath: Mouth hangs open with the tip of the tongue on the palate. Inhale through the nose with a slow, long, even, and deep breath. Exhale through the mouth with a slow, long, even, and deep breath. Apply this practice to all brocades.

Repeat: Seven long breaths.

Following the closing position, walk around for a few minutes to reintegrate regular body movements and acclimate to the movement of qi and the awareness that has been brought to your body through this practice. For additional personalized qigong training, I recommend you visit a qigong or martial arts studio or an acupuncture clinic.

ADDITIONAL RESOURCES

- American Tai Chi and Qigong Association, americantaichi.org
- National Qigong Association, nqa.org
- Natural Healing Research Foundation (Grandmaster Hong Liu), naturalhealingresearch.org
- Qigong Institute, qigonginstitute.org
- QiMaster, qimaster.com

REFERENCES

Campo RA, Agarwal N, LaStayo PC, et al. (2014). Levels of fatigue and distress in senior prostate cancer survivors enrolled in a 12-week randomized controlled trial of qigong. *Journal of Cancer Survivorship* 8 (1): 60–69.

Chan AW, Lee A, Lee DT, et al. (2013). Evaluation of the sustaining effects of tai chi qigong in the sixth month in promoting psychosocial health in COPD patients: A single-blind, randomized controlled trial. *Scientific World Journal* 425082.

Chan AW, Yu DS, Choi KC, et al. (2016). Tai chi qigong as a means to improve nighttime sleep quality among older adults with cognitive impairment: A pilot randomized controlled trial. *Clinical Interventions in Aging* 11: 1277–1286.

Cohen KS. (1997). *The Way of Qigong: The Art and Science of Chinese Energy Healing.* New York, NY: Ballantine Books.

Davis CM. (2017). *Integrative Therapies in Rehabilitation: Evidence for Efficacy in Therapy, Prevention and Wellness,* 4th ed. Thorofare, NJ: SLACK.

Fong SS, Ng SS, Lee HW, et al. (2015). The effects of a 6-month tai chi qigong training program on temporomandibular, cervical, and shoulder joint mobility and sleep problems in nasopharyngeal cancer survivors. *Integrative Cancer Therapies* 14 (1): 16–25.

González López-Arza MV, Varela-Donoso E, Montanero-Fernandez J, et al. (2013). Qigong improves balance in young women: A pilot study. *Journal of Integrative Medicine* 11 (4): 241–245.

Guo X, Zhou B, Nishimura T, et al. (2008). Clinical effect of qigong practice on essential hypertension: A meta-analysis of randomized controlled trials. *Journal of Alternative and Complementary Medicine* 14 (1): 27–37.

Jingwei L, Jianping Z. (2014). *An Illustrated Handbook of Chinese Qigong Froms from the Ancient Texts.* London, UK: Singing Dragon.

Johnson JA. (2000). *Chinese Medical Qigong Therapy: A Comprehensive Clinical Text.* International Institute of Medical Qigong. Pacific Grove, CA.

Kerr C. (2002). Translating "mind-in-body": Two models of patient experience underlying a randomized controlled trial of qigong. *Culture, Medicine and Psychiatry* 26 (4): 419–447.

Lauche R, Cramer H, Hauser W. et al. (2013). A systematic review and meta-analysis of qigong for the fibromyalgia syndrome. *Evidence-Based Complementary and Alternative Medicine* 635182.

Liu MH, Perry P. (1997). *The Healing Art of Qigong.* New York, NY: Warner Books.

Liu P, You J, Loo WTY, et al. (2017). The efficacy of Guolin-Qigong on the body-mind health of chinese women with breast cancer: A randomized controlled trial. *Quality of Life Research* 26 (9): 2321–2331.

Liu W, Schaffer L, Herrs N, et al. (2015). Improved sleep after qigong exercise in breast cancer survivors: A pilot study. *Asia Pacific Journal of Oncology Nursing* 2 (4): 232–239.

Loftus S. (2014). Qigong to improve postural stability for Parkinson fall prevention: A neuroplasticity approach. *Topics in Geriatric Rehabilitation* 30 (1): 58–69.

Moon S, Schmidt M, Smirnova IV, et al. (2017). Qigong exercise may reduce serum TNF-alpha levels and improve sleep in people with Parkinson's disease: A pilot study. *Medicines (Basel):* 4 (2).

Rendant D, Pach D, Lüdtke R, et al. (2011). Qigong versus exercise versus no therapy for patients with chronic neck pain: a randomized controlled trial. *Spine (Philadelphia, Pa. 1976)* 36 (6): 419–427.

Tsang HW, Mok CK, Au Yeung YT, et al. (2003). The effect of qigong on general and psychosocial health of elderly with chronic physical illnesses: a randomized clinical trial. *International Journal of Geriatric Psychiatry* 18 (5): 441–449.

Venes D. (Ed.) (2017). *Taber's Cyclopedic Medical Dictionary,* 23rd ed. Philadelphia, PA: FA Davis.

Wang CW, Chan CH, Ho RT, et al. (2014). Managing stress and anxiety through qigong exercise in healthy adults: A systematic review and meta-analysis of randomized controlled trials. *BMC Complementary and Alternative Medicine* 14: 8.

Wu WH, Bandilla E, Ciccone DS, et al. (1999). Effects of qigong on late-stage complex regional pain syndrome. *Alternative Therapies in Health and Medicine* 5 (1): 45–54.

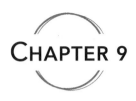

CHAPTER 9

PILATES FOR HEALTH

This chapter was completed with the assistance of Mavis Rode, PT, DPT, CSCS. Dr. Rode developed an interest in functional movement and rehabilitation during her years as a modern dancer. After graduating with a degree in physical therapy, she began her investigation and study of the Pilates method of training for use with her patients. She now maintains a private practice (www.mrodept.com) specializing in orthopedic physical therapy, health and wellness, and dance rehabilitation and injury prevention. Her work with patients, Pilates clients, and fitness clients combines her knowledge and skills as a physical therapist with her experience in Pilates, dance, and other forms of movement re-education.

In addition to her private practice, Dr. Rode is a physical therapist and instructor of kinesiology for the Dance Program at Loyola Marymount University in Los Angeles (2005 to the present).

Dr. Rode earned degrees in biology and in physical therapy from California State University, Northridge, and her Doctor of Physical Therapy degree from Utica College, New York. She is a Certified Sports & Conditioning Specialist (CSCS) with the National Strength and Conditioning Association and an AASDN (American Academy of Sports Dieticians and Nutritionists) Nutrition Specialist.

Mavis Rode, PT, DPT, CSCS
Doctor of Physical Therapy / Pilates Practitioner
Mavis Rode Physical Therapy
Los Angeles, California
www.mrodept.com

> *"Change happens through movement*
> *and movement heals."*
>
> —Joseph Pilates

German-born Joseph H. Pilates (1883–1967) is the creator of the Pilates system, a form of bodywork that uses controlled movements to improve strength, flexibility, balance, and mental concentration. Throughout his career, Pilates developed many original exercise machines (such as the Reformer, Cadillac, Wunda Chair, and Ladder Barrel), created a mat exercise series, wrote two books (Pilates 1934; Pilates et al. 1945), and formulated unique exercise theories.

Z Altug's Perspective for Doing Pilates

In my clinical practice as a physical therapist, I typically recommend Pilates to patients and clients who need to improve core stability and strength and work on posture, balance, and mobility. Other general reasons to try Pilates include:

- Relieve stress and tension
- Improve overall health
- Improve flexibility
- Improve breathing
- Improve circulation
- Help manage weight

Dr. Mavis Rode's Perspective for Doing Pilates

I've been practicing and teaching Pilates for 17 years and I plan to continue until I can't any longer—hopefully, until my last day on this planet. That's how much I love Pilates! Pilates is kind to everybody and I know that you, too, can benefit from Pilates exercises as much as I have and as much as has every one of my patients and clients.

Today there are many variations of the original mat exercises as taught by Joseph Pilates. Exercises can be modified to accommodate those with pain and/or injury and to challenge the most skilled athlete. When using Pilates's apparatus, varying levels of assistance or resistance can be achieved by changing the spring tension and placement. This makes Pilates accessible to people of all ages and fitness levels.

My Pilates patients and clients come to me for all sorts of reasons: examples include dancers who want to improve their performance, who need rehabilitation from an injury, or who want to prevent future injuries; women with osteoporosis who want to stand taller; people with Parkinson's disease who want to improve their ability to walk or climb stairs. With practice, each of these can develop more efficient movement without excess expenditure of energy. This is because Pilates's instruction focuses on postural alignment and balanced use of muscles in a coordinated manner. My greatest joy in teaching Pilates is witnessing the transformation of body and spirit that is possible with committed practice.

Let's See What Research Says . . .

- Pilates exercise "improved postural sway and dynamic balance in young adults with non-specific low back pain" (Lopes et al. 2017).

- Pilates-inspired exercises can improve balance and strength in older women (Vieira et al. 2017).
- Pilates exercise may benefit postmenopausal women with chronic low back pain (Cruz-Diaz et al. 2016).
- Clinical Pilates may improve cognitive functions and quality of life compared with standard exercises in individuals with multiple sclerosis (Kucuk et al. 2016).
- Flexibility and balance can also be improved through Pilates (Valenza et al. 2016), as well as muscular endurance (Kloubec 2010) and abdominal strength and upper-spine posture (Emery et al. 2010).
- Equipment-based Pilates may be superior to mat Pilates for disability and kinesiophobia (fear of movement) in individuals suffering from chronic lower-back pain (da Luz et al. 2014).
- Pilates may lead to decreased fall risk (Stivala et al. 2014).
- Pilates may help improve non-structural scoliosis, and improve flexibility and pain in female college students (Alves de Araújo et al. 2012).
- Pilates can improve abdominal wall muscles (Dorado et al. 2012).
- Pilates can enhance functional capacity in individuals with heart failure when combined with standard medical therapy (Guimarães et al. 2012).
- Pilates can be beneficial for disability, pain, function, and health-related quality of life (Wajswelner et al. 2012).
- Pilates improves mindfulness (changes in mood and perceived stress) (Caldwell et al. 2010).
- Pilates is effective and safe for female breast-cancer patients (Eyigor et al. 2010).
- Pilates is an effective and safe physical activity for individuals with fibromyalgia (Altan et al. 2009).
- Pilates improves thoracic kyphosis (Kuo et al. 2009), or what is commonly known as a hump or a hunchback.
- Pilates improves chronic low back pain in physically active individuals between the ages of 20 and 55 years old (Rydeard et al. 2006).
- Pilates improves the leaping ability of elite rhythmic gymnasts (Hutchinson et al. 1998).

🏃 Practical Pilates Routine

The following basic Pilates routine was designed by Dr. Mavis Rode for you to use in the comfort of your home or at a local park.

A Word before Beginning . . .

Pilates is best with guided instruction from a knowledgeable and skilled instructor. However, the following are beginning versions or preparations for more advanced Pilates mat work and most people can do them safely without formal instruction. I (Mavis Rode) recommend that if you have an injury (especially to any part of the back or neck, shoulders, or hips) that you talk with your physical therapist or medical doctor before trying them on your own.

Don't be too hard on yourself if you find these exercises challenging at first. They will become easier with practice. If you find these exercises aren't challenging enough, congratulate yourself! You are ready to move forward. You might want to look for a qualified instructor who will introduce you to the Pilates equipment.

You'll notice that some of the instructions for starting positions for the exercises are somewhat lengthy. That's because each exercise demands a "whole body" engagement of muscles in an integrated and coordinated fashion. Effective execution of the exercises also requires focused attention to your breath and alignment. The reward of repeated, thoughtful practice of Pilates's exercises is control of movement in a smooth and apparently "effortless" manner.

A word about breath: The focus on your inhalation and exhalation will help keep your mind and body working as an integrated unit. Breathing cues are provided for each exercise, but know that you can try varying your pattern of inhalations and exhalations. Just don't hold your breath.

Finally—no matter your level, from beginning through advanced—there's nothing to gain by "muscling" your way through difficult exercises. Use "just enough" effort to perform the exercise correctly.

SELECTED PILATES EXERCISES

1. THE HUNDRED

Starting Position: Lie on your back with your arms at your sides. Lift one foot at a time until your hips and knees are at 90 degree angles and raise your arms overhead so your fingers are pointing toward the ceiling (Figure 9-1).

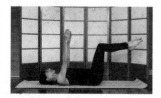

Movement: Inhale, then exhale as you lower your arms, lift your chin toward your chest, and roll your upper body off the mat, keeping the bottom tips of your shoulder blades in contact with the mat. As you roll up, allow the middle and lower parts of your spine to gently round back into to the mat as your chest and belly sink toward your spine. You will feel your lower ribs press into the mat, your abdominal muscles engage, and your lower back flatten. Try to maintain this position throughout the exercise.

Figure 9-1

From this position, pump your arms vigorously as you inhale and exhale (Figure 9-2). Inhale for 5 counts, and then exhale for 5 counts. Breathe deeply, but not forcefully. Keep doing this for a maximum of 100 counts (10 sets).

Purpose: Breathing exercise and warm up preparation.

Helpful Hints: Let your eyes "draw an arc" as you roll up. Keep your arms straight and your shoulders away from your ears.

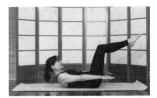

Figure 9-2

Precautions: Avoid if you have osteoporosis. Stop if you're unable to maintain the position or if your neck or back begin to hurt.

2. SINGLE LEG CIRCLES

Starting Position: Lie on your back with both legs straight and allow your spine to sink into the mat. Don't allow your lower back to overly arch. Use your hands to bring your right knee toward your chest and then straighten that knee so your foot is pointing directly toward the ceiling (your hip and trunk at right angles). If you're unable to

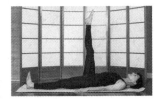

Figure 9-3

do this without the position of your hips or back shifting, it's okay to bend the left knee so that your left foot is flat on the mat. Point the right foot and flex the left foot (unless the left knee is bent). Place your arms by your sides, palms down (Figure 9-3).

Movement: Exhale as you cross your right leg over your body to the left and then circle it back toward the right. Inhale as you continue the circle and raise your right leg back to the starting position (Figure 9-4).

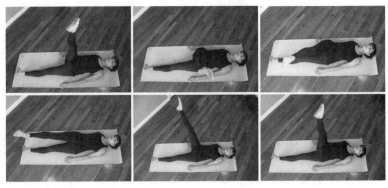

Figure 9-4

Reverse the direction. Exhale as you circle your right leg to the right and down toward the left. Inhale as you continue the circle and lift your right leg back to the starting position. Do 3 to 5 repetitions in each direction and then switch legs. As your leg circles, keep your head, shoulders and upper/mid back stable and flat on the floor. It's okay to allow the hip of the moving leg to lift as that leg crosses over your body, but don't let your back arch. The leg and hip of the non-moving leg should remain anchored in place against the mat without rolling in or out as your other leg circles.

Purpose: To develop control of your trunk position (core); to improve mobility of your hips.

Helpful Hints: Start with small leg circles and progress to larger leg circles as you gain control of the movement. Press your palms into the mat for increased stability while you are learning this exercise. Thinking of pressing your navel into your spine can help maintain stability of your pelvis.

Precautions: If you have hip or lower back pain or injury, try limiting the size of the leg circle and/or positioning the non-circling leg with the knee bent and the foot flat on the mat.

3. SINGLE LEG STRETCH

Starting Position: Sit with your knees bent up and your feet flat on the floor and with your spine curled. Place your left hand on the inside of your right knee and your right hand on the outside of your right ankle (Figure 9-5).

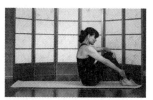

Figure 9-5

Keep your right knee pulled toward your chest as you simultaneously roll your back down toward the mat and straighten your left leg out in front of you. Stop rolling back once the tips of your shoulder blades touch the mat. Your head will be lifted with your chin toward your chest. Lift your left leg only as far as you need to while keeping your back flat. Keep your elbows lifted and to the side (Figure 9-6).

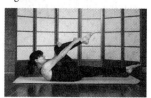

Figure 9-6

Movement: Inhale and allow your abdominals to sink in toward your spine. Exhale as you switch hand and leg positions, then inhale as you again switch hand and leg positions. Switch back and forth 5 times for each leg.

Purpose: Develops core control and abdominal muscle strength.

Helpful Hints: To stay lifted, think of letting your lower ribs sink back into the mat. Pull your abdominal muscles in each time you switch legs. Keep your gaze straight ahead between your knees.

Precautions: Avoid if you have osteoporosis. This exercise can be modified if you have neck or shoulder injuries. A knowledgeable Pilates instructor can help you with this.

4. THE SAW

Starting Position: Sit with your legs straight out in front of you and opened slightly farther than the width of your hips, but no wider than the width of your mat. Flex your ankles so your toes point upward. Sit up tall and reach your arms out to your sides, palms down (Figure 9-7).

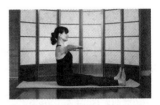

Figure 9-7

Movement: Inhale as you twist from your waist to the left, but keep the right hip firmly pressed into the mat to keep your weight centered over both hips. Exhale as you round forward, stretching your right hand toward the little toe of your left foot and reaching your left arm back as you turn the palm of your left hand up to face the

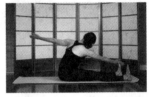

Figure 9-8

ceiling (Figure 9-8). Inhale as you return to the starting position by rolling up through your spine. Your head should come up last. Repeat the movement to the right and do 3 to 4 repetitions to each side.

Purpose: Increases rotation of the spine; helps with posture and sitting up tall; stretches the hamstrings.

Helpful Hints: In your starting position, to keep your shoulder blades wide on your back and to prevent your shoulders from rounding forward, imagine that something is pulling your collar bones and shoulder blades apart at the same time. Reach your arms to touch the walls on either side of you.

Precautions: Bend your knees slightly if you have hip or lower back problems. You could also sit on a rolled up mat or towel. If you have shoulder problems, place your hands on your shoulders or skip this exercise.

5. SINGLE LEG KICK

Starting Position: Lie on your stomach, propped on your forearms with your elbows slightly in front of or directly beneath your shoulders. Make fists with your hands. Your legs and feet should be close together. Press your forearms into the mat to keep your chest lifted away from the mat and your neck in line with your spine. Pull your lower belly (around your navel) up toward your spine and press the front of your hips into the mat to prevent sinking into your lower back. Squeeze your buttocks muscles and press the tops of your feet firmly into the mat (Figure 9-9).

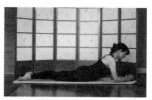
Figure 9-9

Movement: Inhale as you bend one knee and kick toward your buttock with two small pulsing movements. Exhale as you simultaneously lower that leg and kick with the opposite leg (Figure 9-10). Do 6 kicks with each leg. *Challenge: Don't let your foot touch the mat as you straighten your knee.*

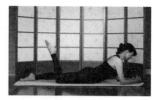
Figure 9-10

Purpose: Strengthens muscles of the shoulders, upper back, buttocks, and back of the thigh; stretches muscles at the front of the thigh.

Helpful Hints: Pick a spot on the floor in front of your hands to look at during the exercise. This will help to keep your neck in alignment with your spine. Imagine your neck and spine are lengthening throughout the exercise.

Precautions: Skip this exercise or lower your upper back and rest your forehead on crossed forearms if you have pinching discomfort in your lower back. If you have knee pain, try limiting how far you bend your knee.

6. SPINE STRETCH FORWARD

Starting Position: Sit with your legs straight out in front of you and opened slightly farther than the width of your hips. Flex your ankles so your toes point upward. Sit up tall and reach your arms in front of you at shoulder height, palms facing each other (Figure 9-11).

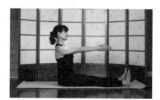
Figure 9-11

Movement: Inhale to begin, sitting up tall. Exhale as you bring your chin to your chest, sink your belly toward your spine to round your back, and reach your arms forward. Remain sitting up tall to keep the front of your hip bones from tipping forward. Stretch as far forward as you can in this position (Figure 9-12). Exhale as you roll up through your spine to the starting position.

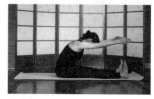
Figure 9-12

Purpose: Helps with posture and sitting up tall; stretches the back of the body; teaches controlled movement through the spine.

Helpful Hints: Imagine you're making a "C" shape with your spine as you round your back. As you roll back up, imagine that you're pressing your back against a wall behind you. You can try switching your breathing pattern, but don't hold your breath.

Precautions: If you have shoulder problems, slide your hands along the floor as you reach forward instead of holding your arms in front of you. Bend your knees slightly if you have hip or lower back problems. Avoid if you have osteoporosis.

7. SIDE KICK (THIS IS ONE OF SEVERAL "SIDE KICK SERIES" EXERCISES)

Starting Position: Lie on your side with the back of your body aligned with one side of your mat. From there, bend both of your legs forward from the hip joint to a 45 degree angle. Rest your head on your outstretched bottom arm and place your top hand, palm down, on the mat in front of your chest. Keep your spine straight and your hips and shoulders stacked one on top of the other. Don't let your waist (mat side) sink into the mat (Figure 9-13).

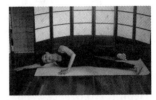

Figure 9-13

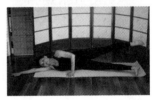

Figure 9-14

Movement: Lift the top leg to hip height. Inhale as you swing the top leg forward with two small pulses (small kicks).

Exhale as you swing the leg behind you with two small pulses without letting your back arch (Figure 9-14).

Repeat each forward and back kick no more than 6 times. Don't allow the alignment of your trunk to change or your body to roll forward or backward during the exercise.

Purpose: Control of trunk position while moving the leg; strengthens hip and trunk muscles.

Helpful Hints: Think of lengthening the top side of your torso as your leg swings. It's not important to swing your leg far in either direction—you can start with small kicks. To prevent the leg from dropping below hip height, think of drawing a line parallel to the floor with your foot. You can bend the bottom knee for more stability.

Precaution: You can use a pillow to support your head and neck to limit stress on your neck.

For personalized Pilates training on a mat, I recommend you visit a Pilates studio in your area. At the Pilates studio, you may also ask about training on various Pilates apparatuses such as the Reformer, Cadillac, Wunda Chair, and Ladder Barrel.

ADDITIONAL RESOURCES

- Balanced Body, www.pilates.com
- BASI Pilates, www.basipilates.com
- Pilates Method Alliance, www.pilatesmethodalliance.org
- Polestar Pilates Education, www.polestarpilates.com
- STOTT Pilates, https://www.merrithew.com/brands/stott-pilates

REFERENCES

Altan L, Korkmaz N, Bingol U, et al. (2009). Effect of Pilates training on people with fibromyalgia syndrome: A pilot study. *Archives of Physical Medicine and Rehabilitation* 90 (12): 1983–1988.

Alves de Araújo ME, Bezerra da Silva E, Bragade Mello D, et al. (2012). The effectiveness of the Pilates method: Reducing the degree of non-structural scoliosis, and improving flexibility and pain in female college students. *Journal of Bodywork and Movement Therapies* 16 (2): 191–198.

Anderson B. (2017). Pilates rehabilitation. In: Davis CM. *Integrative Therapies in Rehabilitation: Evidence for Efficacy in Therapy, Prevention and Wellness*, 4th ed. Thorofare, NJ: SLACK.

Caldwell K, Harrison M, Adams M, et al. (2010). Developing mindfulness in college students through movement-based courses: Effects on self-regulatory self-efficacy, mood, stress, and sleep quality. *Journal of American College Health* 58 (5): 433–442.

Cruz-Diaz D, Martinez-Amat A, Osuna-Perez MC, et al. (2016). Short- and long-term effects of a six-week clinical pilates program in addition to physical therapy on postmenopausal women with chronic low back pain: A randomized controlled trial. *Disability and Rehabilitation* 38 (13): 1300–1308.

da Luz MA., Jr., Costa LO, Fuhro FF, et al. (2014). Effectiveness of mat Pilates or equipment-based Pilates exercises in patients with chronic nonspecific low back pain: A randomized controlled trial. *Physical Therapy* 94 (5): 623–631.

Dorado C, Calbet JAL, Lopez-Gordillo A, et al. (2012). Marked effects of Pilates on the abdominal muscles: A longitudinal magnetic resonance imaging study. *Medicine & Science in Sports & Exercise* 44 (8): 1589–1594.

Emery K, De Serres SJ, McMillan A, et al. (2010). The effects of a Pilates training program on arm-trunk posture and movement. *Clinical Biomechanics* 25 (2): 124–130.

Eyigor S, Karapolat H, Yesil H, et al. (2010). Effects of Pilates exercises on functional capacity, flexibility, fatigue, depression and quality of life in female breast cancer patients: A randomized controlled study. *European Journal of Physical and Rehabilitation Medicine* 46 (4): 481–487.

Guimarães GV, Carvalho VO, Bocchi EA, et al. (2012). Pilates in heart failure patients: A randomized controlled pilot trial. *Cardiovascular Therapeutics* 30 (6): 351–356.

Hutchinson MR, Tremain L, Christiansen J, et al. (1998). Improving leaping ability in elite rhythmic gymnasts. *Medicine and Science in Sports and Exercise* 30 (10): 1543–1547.

Kloubec JA. (2010). Pilates for improvement of muscle endurance, flexibility, balance, and posture. *Journal of Strength and Conditioning Research* 24 (3): 661–667.

Kucuk F, Kara B, Poyraz EC, et al. (2016). Improvements in cognition, quality of life, and physical performance with clinical pilates in multiple sclerosis: A randomized controlled trial. *Journal of Physical Therapy Science* 28 (3): 761–768.

Kuo YL, Tully EA, Galea MP. (2009). Sagittal spinal posture after Pilates-based exercise in healthy older adults. *Spine* 34 (10): 1046–1051.

Lopes S, Correia C, Felix G, et al. (2017). Immediate effects of Pilates based therapeutic exercise on postural control of young individuals with non-specific low back pain: A randomized controlled trial. *Complementary Therapies in Medicine* 34: 104–110.

Pilates JH. (1934). *Your Health: A Corrective System of Exercising that Revolutionizes the Entire Field of Physical Education.* New York, NY: C. J. O'Brien, Inc.

Pilates JH, Miller WJ. (1945). *Return to Life Through Contrology.* New York, NY: J.J. Augustin.

Rydeard R, Leger A, Smith D. (2006). Pilates-based therapeutic exercise: Effect on subjects with nonspecific chronic low back pain and functional disability: A randomized controlled trial. *Jouranl of Orthopaedic and Sports Physical Therapy* 36 (7): 472–484.

Stivala A, Hartley G. (2014). The effects of a Pilates-based exercise rehabilitation program on functional outcome and fall risk reduction in an aging adult status-post traumatic hip fracture due to fall. *Journal of Geriatric Physical Therapy* 37 (3): 136–145.

Valenza MC, Rodriguez-Torres J, Cabrera-Martos I, et al. (2016). Results of a Pilates exercise program in patients with chronic non-specific low back pain: A randomized controlled trial. *Clinical Rehabilitation* 31 (6):753–760.

Vieira ND, Testa D, Ruas PC, et al. (2017). The effects of 12 weeks Pilates-inspired exercise training on functional performance in older women: A randomized clinical trial. *Journal of Bodywork and Movement Therapies* 21 (2): 251–258.

Wajswelner H, Metcalf B, Bennell K. (2012). Clinical Pilates versus general exercise for chronic low back pain: Randomized trial. *Medicine & Science in Sports and Exercise* 44 (7): 1197–1205.

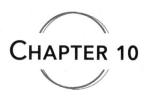

CHAPTER 10

FELDENKRAIS METHOD® FOR HEALTH

This chapter was completed with the assistance of Bridget Quebodeaux, LMFT, GCFP. Bridget is a Guild Certified *Feldenkrais Practitioner*ᶜᵐ with over 20 years of experience. In addition to completing a four-year Professional *Feldenkrais*® training program, Bridget earned an MFA in acting from the California Institute of the Arts in 2000 and a Master's degree in Psychology in 2013. She is a Licensed Marriage and Family Therapist and is on the faculty of the Dynamic Emotion Focused Therapy Institute (DEFTinstitute.com). Bridget has a private Feldenkrais practice (feldenkraiswestla.com) and sees clients at the Center for Physical Health in West Los Angeles (physicalhealth.com).

Bridget's clients come to her for a variety of reasons. She sees people who are recovering from an injury or surgery, managing the symptoms of a chronic illness, suffering with anxiety or depression, and seeking to improve athletic or artistic performance.

For more information about projects Bridget has completed, please refer to the following:
- *Emotion-Focused Workbook: A Guide to Compassionate Self-Reflection* (2015) (amazon.com)
- *Anatomy of Attunement, Feldenkrais Method*® Awareness Through Movement® *audio* lessons for psychotherapists (anatomyofattunement.com)
- *Posture With a Purpose, Feldenkrais Method*® audio recordings (achievingexcellence.com)

"Make the impossible possible, the possible easy, the easy elegant"

—Moshe Feldenkrais

Russian-born engineer, physicist, and judo master, Moshe Feldenkrais (1904-1984), was the creator of the *Feldenkrais Method*®, a system of learning and human improvement. Better posture, improved balance, greater range of motion, pain relief, and stress reduction are commonly reported benefits.

Feldenkrais's own chronic knee injury led to the discovery of ways to tap into the processes through which children learn to move and behave and to use these processes to enhance functioning at any age. He wrote eight books (Feldenkrais 1944, 1949, 1952, 1972, 1977, 1981, 1984, 1985). Over a period of 40 years, Feldenkrais formulated his ideas into an educational method for improving how people move, think, and feel. The method is divided into two parts: *Awareness Through Movement*® (*ATM*®) and *Functional Integration*® (*FI*®).

Awareness Through Movement lessons incorporate verbally directed movements, visualizations, and guided attention for group or individual work. In these lessons participants explore developmental movements, like crawling and rolling, and functions, such as posture and breathing. There are over 1,000 *ATM* lessons, offering an opportunity to develop awareness of habitual movement patterns that contribute to discomfort and limitation and discover easier, more comfortable ways of moving and being.

Functional Integration lessons employ a one-to-one, hands-on approach. During an *FI* lesson the practitioner uses gentle movements and touch to help the client become more aware of how he or she currently holds and organizes his or her body for action and to introduce new, more effective, more pleasurable possibilities.

CASE EXAMPLE
(FROM BRIDGET QUEBODEAUX)

Paula, a 76-year-old woman, came to the *Feldenkrais Method* hoping to get relief from pain and stiffness in her neck. The great difficulty she experienced in turning her head made her afraid to drive and caused her to give up many activities she once enjoyed. Over her lifetime, Paula had developed habitual ways of using her body that put excess strain on certain areas like her neck. In addition to these movement patterns, which included holding her shoulders up and keeping her chest rigid, she had learned attentional patterns, like ignoring her body and pushing through pain.

Paula participated in once-weekly *Functional Integration* sessions during which her practitioner helped her to sense her body more accurately and come to understand how certain habits interfered with easy, coordinated movement. Gradually she was able to retrain her brain to feel and move her body differently. After her third session, Paula sat up with more relaxed shoulders and a more mobile torso. She looked toward the window beside her with a new coordination of previously ignored parts of herself, which now supported the movement of her neck, and she exclaimed, "I can turn my head!" Paula continued weekly sessions for a month and then began *Awareness Through Movement* classes to reinforce her new and improved ways of moving and attending to herself.

Z. ALTUG'S PERSPECTIVE FOR DOING THE FELDENKRAIS METHOD

In my clinical practice as a physical therapist, I typically recommend the *Feldenkrais Method* to patients and clients who need to manage pain and stress, increase mobility, and also improve function in daily activities. Other general reasons to try the *Feldenkrais Method* include:

- Relieve stress and tension
- Improve overall health
- Improve flexibility
- Improve breathing
- Improve posture
- Help manage pain
- Help prevent falls
- Help find inner peace

*"What I'm after is not flexible bodies, but flexible brains . . .
what I'm really after is restoring people to their human dignity."*

—Moshe Feldenkrais

BRIDGET QUEBODEAUX'S PERSPECTIVE FOR DOING THE FELDENKRAIS METHOD

The name of this chapter is *Feldenkrais Method for Health*. Moshe Feldenkrais talked about health not only in terms of avoiding injury or illness, but also in terms of the capacity to recover. Doing this work presupposes the belief that all humans have learning and healing capacity within them. As a *Feldenkrais Practitioner*, I help people tap into that capacity. Sometimes this means that a particular injury or condition will be no more. Sometimes it means that in the face of a diagnosis or structural challenge that cannot be reversed, a person will come to adjust their use of self so that they can live more fully. In my work with clients, I emphasize both awareness and attention to quality of engagement with self. To mindlessly repeat a movement or behavior that is painful or ineffective is to practice the habits that make that movement or behavior problematic. In contrast, to explore what a person does and how he or she does it with compassionate interest is to unlock the human potential to notice, care, learn, and change.

LET'S SEE WHAT RESEARCH SAYS . . .

- The *Feldenkrais Method* could help middle-aged people strengthen their balance, especially for those with certain disabilities (Torres-Unda et al. 2017).
- The *Feldenkrais Method* may offset age-related decline in cognitive function (Ullman et al. 2016).

- "*Feldenkrais Method* is an effective intervention for chronic neck/scapular pain in patients with visual impairment" (Lundqvist et al. 2014)
- The *Feldenkrais Method* positively affects performance of the Four Square Step Test (a test of dynamic balance) and changes in gait in individuals with osteoarthritis (Webb et al. 2013).
- The *Feldenkrais Method* improves balance and mobility (Connors et al. 2010; Ullmann et al. 2010).
- The *Feldenkrais Method* can improve health-related quality of life in individuals with nonspecific musculoskeletal disorders (Malmgren-Olsson et al. 2002).

FELDENKRAIS METHOD AWARENESS THROUGH MOVEMENT LESSON

Hours spent facing forward with eyes locked on a computer screen, the freeway or some other task before us can have detrimental effects on full and comfortable use of the head and neck. The impact can range from nagging discomfort to significant pain and limitation of motion. Many people accept pain and reduced mobility as a sign of aging or they stretch and strain their muscles in an attempt to find relief and regain lost function. This *Feldenkrais Awareness through Movement* lesson offers an alternative.

ATM LESSON: TOWARD TURNING THE HEAD WITH EASE

In this lesson, I (Bridget Quebodeaux) will lead you through a series of movements turning to one side. You may choose to repeat these movements turning to the other side or you may choose to stay with any asymmetry you feel at the end of the lesson. This kind of asymmetry is a novel experience and will invite a heightened state of awareness. Any sense of unevenness you initially notice will dissipate shortly. You may even notice improvement on the side that was not the focus of the lesson.

1. Sit toward the middle or end of a firm chair so that your back is free from the backrest. Allow your hands to hang by your sides or rest them on your legs (Figure 10-1).
2. Moving slowly and without going to a place of stretch or strain, turn and look in one direction and then in the other. Do this a couple of times. In which direction is it easier to turn? Easier may mean that you go further or that there is something about turning in one direction that is just more pleasurable at the moment. Face forward and pause.

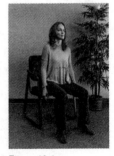

Figure 10-1

Choose one direction you'd like to improve for now—either turning right or turning left. You are only going to turn in this direction for the rest of the lesson.

3. Turn in the direction you have chosen to improve and take note of a spot in the room that marks how far you can see easily when you turn in this direction (Figure 10-2). Once you have identified a spot, face forward once again.

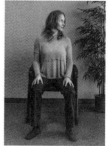

Figure 10-2

4. Lift the shoulder on the side you have chosen to turn toward. Lift it just a little. And then lower it. Do this movement easily and gently 15 to 20 times. If you have chosen to turn to the left for this lesson, you are lifting and lowering the left shoulder (Figure 10-3).

What do you notice as you lift and lower? Go slowly enough to notice the path the shoulder takes. Is it straight up and down? Is there a movement forward or back at the top or bottom of your comfortable range? Sense the shoulder blade sliding along the ribcage as you lift and lower. Rest for a moment.

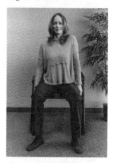

Figure 10-3

5. Now bring your ear in the direction of your shoulder and back to neutral 15 to 20 times. Do only what is easy. Do not stretch or strain the muscles in your neck. If you have chosen to turn to the left, you are taking the left ear toward the left shoulder and away again (Figure 10-4).

Imagine this is the first time you are moving your head and neck in this way and allow yourself to be very curious about how you make this movement. Bring your head back to neutral and rest.

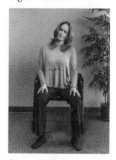

Figure 10-4

6. Put those two movements together. Bring your shoulder toward your ear and your ear toward your shoulder. Repeat 15 to 20 times (Figure 10-5). The shoulder and the ear will each go in the direction of the other, but they don't have to reach each other. It's just a direction, not a destination.

Can you allow this movement to be very easy? We can be so oriented toward doing something big or correct by some external standard. These lessons really are about cultivating and practicing an appreciation of exploration, comfort, and internal ease. Notice if you are tensing the muscles in your face or belly as you bring your ear and shoulder toward and away from each other. Pause with your head and shoulder at neutral.

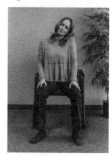

Figure 10-5

7. Turn once or twice in the direction you have chosen and find out if it's a little easier to turn in this direction now. Sit back and rest against the chair.

8. Come back to the middle or front of your chair so you can have your feet on the floor and your back free from the back of the chair. Take the hand that is opposite the side you are turning toward and bring it in front of your face (if you have been turning to the left, put your right hand in front of your face). Bring your elbow out to the side. Keep your shoulder relaxed. Turn your palm toward the ground and let your hand hang limply (Figure 10-6).

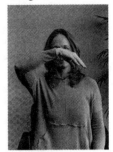

Figure 10-6

9. Turn this whole unit: elbow, shoulder, arm, hand, and head in the direction you have been turning and back to neutral 10 times. Do only what is easy and comfortable (Figure 10-7). Are you moving the arm and hand along the horizon as you turn or does the trajectory curve downward or upward as you progress through the movement? Just notice. As you turn—are you aware of any tension in your face or jaw?

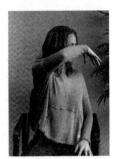

How far through yourself can you feel this movement? Is it a movement that happens only in your head and shoulders? Can you feel your ribs moving as you turn? Are you aware of any holding in your belly or butt? If so, can you let that go? Rest your arm by your side for a moment.

Figure 10-7

10. Return to the previous position (limp hand in front of your face, elbow out to the side, and shoulder relaxed) and return to the movement of turning to the side you have chosen and back to neutral. Do this movement 10 times more. Focus your attention on the movement in your hips.

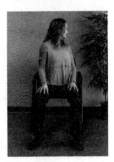

Can you feel that one hip and the corresponding knee move backward as you turn? And the other knee reaches forward? Exaggerate the movement of

Figure 10-8

your hips, accentuating the movement of one hip and knee backward as you turn. Make it a little bigger while staying in a comfortable range (Figure 10-8). How does exaggerating the movement of the hips affect your turning?

11. Turn 5 more times and notice what your eyes do as you turn? Do they move with your head as you turn? Is the movement of the eyes smooth and easy?

   » Turn 5 times taking your eyes opposite your head as you turn. Go easy as this is an unusual use of the eyes and head.

   » Turn once or twice more in the direction you have chosen and take your eyes in the same direction of your head as if there were something you wanted to see in that direction.

Bring your arm down. Face forward and rest against the back of the chair for just a moment.

12. Return to the middle or front of your chair so your feet are on the ground and your back is free from the backrest. Let your hands hang by your sides or place them comfortably in your lap.

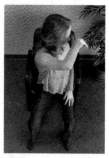

Turn one last time in the direction you've been turning (Figure 10-9). Can you see beyond the spot you identified in the beginning of the lesson? Turn to the other side. Turn one way and then the other way as you did when we started. What has changed? What differences do you notice between turning in one direction and the other? Sit back and rest against the back of the chair.

Figure 10-9

If you can turn further or more easily now than you could when you began, and/ or if you have a greater sense of being supported by your skeleton in sitting, this is largely due to becoming aware of and involving more of yourself in ways that serve your intention (to turn your head). It is also due to eliminating unconscious obstacles to doing what you want.

It might not have happened automatically that you involved your legs, hips, eyes, and chest when you turned from side to side. Perhaps you experienced the involvement of those parts as positively influencing your turning during the lesson. Similarly, you may not have been aware that there was tension in your shoulder, or jaw, or belly, or someplace else that was getting in your way. Bringing obstacles and options to the conscious mind is a big part of this work, and a big part of moving, being, and relating more fully. Moshe Feldenkrais said, "If you know what you are doing, you can do what you want."

Search for a *Feldenkrais Practitioner* or an *Awareness Through Movement* class in your area: www.feldenkrais.com

ADDITIONAL RESOURCES

- Feldenkrais Guild of North America, feldenkrais.com
- Feldenkrais Resources, feldenkraisresources.com
- International Feldenkrais Federation, feldenkrais-method.org (refer to the videos from their archives collection)
- OpenATM.org (free online Feldenkrais Method lessons)
- The Feldenkrais Institute, feldenkraisinstitute.com

References

Connors KA, Galea MP, Said CM. (2010). Feldenkrais Method balance classes are based on principles of motor learning and postural control retraining: A qualitative research study. *Physiotherapy* 96 (4): 324–336.

Connors KA, Pile C, Nichols ME. (2011). Does the Feldenkrais Method make a difference? An investigation into the use of outcome measurement tools for evaluating changes in clients. *Journal of Bodywork & Movement Therapies* 15 (4): 446–52.

Feldenkrais M. (1944). *Judo: The Art of Defense and Attack*. New York, NY: Frederick Warne & Co.

Feldenkrais M. (1949). *Body and Mature Behaviour: A Study of Anxiety, Sex, Gravitation & Learning*. New York, NY: International Universities Press.

Feldenkrais M. (1952). *Higher Judo*. New York, NY: Frederick Warne & Co.

Feldenkrais M. (1972). *Awareness Through Movement: Health Exercises for Personal Growth*. New York, NY: Harper & Row.

Feldenkrais M. (1977). *The Case of Nora: Body Awareness as Healing Therapy*. New York, NY: Harper & Row.

Feldenkrais M. (1981). *The Elusive Obvious or Basic Feldenkrais*. Cupertino, CA: Meta Publications.

Feldenkrais M. (1984). *The Master Moves*. Cupertino, CA: Meta Publications.

Feldenkrais M, Kimmey M. (Ed.). (1985). *The Potent Self: A Guide to Spontaneity*. San Francisco, CA: Harper & Row.

Hillier S, Worley A. (2015). The effectiveness of the Feldenkrais Method: A systematic review of the evidence. *Evidence Based Complementary and Alternative Medicine* 1–12.

Jain S, Janssen K, Decelle S. (2004). Alexander Technique and Feldenkrais Method: A critical overview. *Physical Medicine and Rehabilitation Clinics of North America* 15 (4): 811–825.

Lake B. (1985). Acute back pain. Treatment by the application of Feldenkrais principles. *Australian Family Physician* 14 (11): 1175–1178.

Lundqvist LO, Zetterlund C, Richter HO. (2014). Effects of Feldenkrais Method on chronic neck/scapular pain in people with visual impairment: A randomized controlled trial with one-year follow-up. *Archives of Physical Medicine and Rehabilitation* 95 (9): 1656–1661.

Malmgren-Olsson EB, Branholm IB. (2002). A comparison between three physiotherapy approaches with regard to health-related factors in patients with non-specific musculoskeletal disorders. *Disability and Rehabilitation* 24 (6): 308–317.

Mattes J. (2016). Attentional Focus in Motor Learning, the Feldenkrais Method, and Mindful Movement. *Perceptual and Motor Skills* 123 (1): 258–76.

Myers LK. (2016). Application of neuroplasticity theory through the use of the Feldenkrais Method with a runner with scoliosis and hip and lumbar pain: A case report. *Journal of Bodywork & Movement Therapies*. 20 (2): 300–309.

Ohman A, Astrom L, Malmgren-Olsson EB. (2011). Feldenkrais therapy as group treatment for chronic pain -A qualitative evaluation. *Journal of Bodywork & Movement Therapies* 15 (2): 153–161.

Pugh JD, Williams AM. (2014). Feldenkrais Method empowers adults with chronic back pain. *Holistic Nursing Practice* 28 (3): 171–83.

Reese M. (2002). *Moshe Feldenkrais and his methods: Historical background*. Class notes from Feldenkrais workshop. San Diego, CA: Feldenkrais Southern California Movement Institute. July 12.

Stephens J, Davidson J, Derosa J, et al. (2006). Lengthening the hamstring muscles without stretching using "Awareness Through Movement." *Physical Therapy* 86 (12): 1641–1650.

Stephens J, Miller TM. (2017). Feldenkrais Method in rehabilitation: Using Functional Integration and Awareness Through Movement to explore new movements and solve clinical problems. In: Davis CM. *Integrative Therapies in Rehabilitation: Evidence for Efficacy in Therapy, Prevention and Wellness,* 4th ed. Thorofare, NJ: SLACK.

Teixeira-Machado L, Araújo FM, Cunha FA, et al. (2010). Feldenkrais Method-based exercise improves quality of life in individuals with Parkinson's disease: A controlled, randomized clinical trial. *Alternative Therapies Health Medicine* 21 (1): 8–14.

Torres-Unda J, Polo V, Dunabeitia I, et al. (2017). The Feldenkrais Method improves functioning and body balance in people with intellectual disability in supported employment: A randomized clinical trial. *Research in Developmental Disabilities* 70: 104–112.

Ullmann G, Williams HG. (2016). The Feldenkrais Method can enhance cognitive function in independent living older adults: A case-series. *Journal of Bodywork and Movement Therapies* 20 (3): 512–517.

Ullmann G, Williams HG, Hussey J, et al. (2010). Effects of Feldenkrais exercises on balance, mobility, balance confidence, and gait performance in community-dwelling adults age 65 and older. *Journal of Alternative and Complementary Medicine* 16 (1): 97–105.

Venes D. (Ed.) (2017). Taber's Cyclopedic Medical Dictionary, 23rd ed. Philadelphia, PA: FA Davis.

Verrel J, Almagor E, Schumann F, et al. (2015). Changes in neural resting state activity in primary and higher-order motor areas induced by a short sensorimotor intervention based on the Feldenkrais Method. *Frontiers in Human Neuroscience* 9: 232.

Webb R, Cofre Lizama LE, Galea MP. (2013). Moving with ease: Feldenkrais Method classes for people with osteoarthritis. *Evidence-Based Complementary and Alternative Medicine* 479142.

Zemach-Bersin D, Zemach-Bersin K, Reese M. (1990). *Relaxercise: The Easy New Way to Health and Fitness.* New York, NY: HarperOne.

CHAPTER 11

ALEXANDER TECHNIQUE FOR HEALTH

This chapter was completed with the assistance of Leah Zhang, MFA, AmSAT, CEAS II. Leah Zhang is a nationally-certified teacher of the Alexander Technique with over 1,600 hours of hands-on training. She is a graduate of the Alexander Training Institute-Los Angeles. Leah first learned of the Alexander Technique in 1999 as a young actress in Chicago, and her interests in mind-body unity and an improved posture lead her to train as an Alexander Teacher. In her many years of work with the technique, she has understood how easeful, upright posture brings about more confidence, pain-relief, flexibility, and mind-body awareness. She is passionate about guiding her students toward discovering how to apply this wonderful technique in their everyday lives.

Currently, Leah is the **Movement and Alexander Technique Teacher** at the prestigious **Lee Strasberg Theatre and Film Institute** in West Hollywood, California. She also offers private lessons and group classes in Los Angeles, California. Her students range from actors, singers, and dancers to writers, office workers, and athletes. In addition to her Alexander Technique certification, she is also a certified ergonomics assessment specialist and has helped many office workers learn about proper and easeful positioning and habits while working in front of the computer.

Leah Zhang, MFA, AmSAT, CEAS II
    Alexander Technique Teacher / Ergonomics Specialist
    Leah Zhang Alexander Technique Studio
    Los Angeles, California
    www.leahteachesalexander.com
    https://twitter.com/leahteaches
    www.facebook.com/leahteachesalexander
    www.linkedin.com/in/leahteaches/

> *"Change involves carrying out an activity*
> *against the habit of life."*
>
> —F.M. Alexander

The Alexander Technique is a form of bodywork created by Tasmanian-born Frederick M. Alexander (1869–1955) that promotes postural health (Venes 2017). During his career, Alexander wrote four books (Alexander 1918, 1923, 1932, 1941). Gradually, he developed an educational system that helps reeducate the whole body in proper movement patterns and postural habits. This educational method is known as the Alexander Technique.

Z Altug's Perspective for Doing the Alexander Technique

In my clinical practice as a physical therapist, I typically recommend the Alexander Technique to musicians and individuals who want to improve performance and posture and want to move easier with common daily activities. Other general reasons to try the Alexander Technique include:

- Improve breathing
- Improve walking
- Improve balance
- Improve performance if you are a singer, musician, actor, or dancer

Leah Zhang's Perspective for Doing the Alexander Technique

My students come to me for many different reasons. Some students are performers and would like to gain more control of their physical instrument (their body) without any added or unnecessary tensions during the performance. Other students have experienced years of chronic pain and are searching for a method of moving and being in their bodies that can relieve the pain. I've had other students who are simply curious about themselves and are learning different methods and modalities to add to their self-awareness and self-discovery. For me, even though I have a performance background, I sought out the technique because of my poor posture as a teenager and young adult. During my teenage years I was always told to "sit and stand up straight." I found myself trying to hold the "right" posture for 20 to 30 seconds, but then would collapse into my habitual posture because I felt the "right" one took too much effort. I thought my poor posture was unchangeable and that I had to live with it my whole life. I also didn't realize that my poor posture was contributing to other issues, such as painfully tense shoulders, shallow breathing (not helpful for a young actress working on Shakespeare's plays), lack of confidence, and anxiety.

Fortunately, through the Alexander Technique, I learned that posture is not permanent, and easeful, upright posture is not difficult or exhausting to maintain. I re-learned ways of moving and standing that were hidden under the habits I had developed. In this technique, you will take away a mindset of "to undo." To undo habits, movements, or postures that might be contributing to performance anxiety, excess tension, back pain, shoulder pain, neck pain, difficulty breathing, and/or "poor posture."

- Alexander Technique may serve a role in reducing the negative changes in gait that occur with aging (Hamel et al. 2016).
- Alexander Technique lessons improved posture, mobility, and muscular strength, and led to fewer falls and injuries among those who had previously struggled (Gleeson et al. 2015).
- Alexander Technique lessons and acupuncture both led to significant reductions in neck pain and disability (MacPherson et al. 2015).
- "Alexander Technique sessions may improve performance anxiety in musicians" (Klein et al. 2014).
- "Dynamic modulation of postural tone can be enhanced through long-term training in the Alexander Technique" (Cacciatore et al. 2011).
- The Alexander Technique can significantly improve the posture of surgeons and surgical ergonomics and endurance, and decrease surgical fatigue and incidence of repetitive stress injuries (Reddy et al. 2011).
- "One-to-one lessons in the Alexander technique from registered teachers have long-term benefits [such as decreased back pain and improved quality of life] for patients with chronic back pain. Six lessons followed by exercise prescription were nearly as effective as 24 lessons" (Little et al. 2008).
- "Lessons in the Alexander Technique are likely to lead to sustained benefit [such as less depression and improved activities of daily living] for people with Parkinson's disease" (Stallibrass et al. 2002).
- Alexander Technique instruction may be helpful in improving balance in older women (Dennis 1999).

PRACTICAL ALEXANDER TECHNIQUE LESSON

The following Alexander Technique lesson was designed by Leah Zhang for you to use in the comfort of your home or at a local park.

In this lesson, I (Leah Zhang) will be leading you through an observational experience while standing for you to gain awareness of your balance as you stand and also how to gently undo the tensions and misalignments that might be interfering with you standing in a more balanced and natural way. We'll finish this short lesson by doing a couple of explorations to find balance in your head and neck.

1. Start by standing still somewhere relatively free of visual, audio, and mental distractions. This is a short few minutes where you get to take care of yourself by observing yourself without distractions and judgments.

2. Bring your attention to your feet and notice if you feel an equal amount of weight between your left foot and your right foot. Does one side feel like there's more pressure or weight? How close together are your feet? Are your feet positioned right next to each other or, 2 inches, 6 inches, hip-width, or shoulder-width apart? See if you can shift or gently rock in a way that brings a 50/50 balance of weight to both your right and left feet.

3. Notice the weight on the front of your foot by your toes and the back of your foot by your heels. Is there an equal amount of weight between the front and the heel on both feet? Can you shift or rock in a way that brings 50/50 balance of weight to the front and heel of your feet? After you have shifted to find the 50/50 balance, do you now feel like you are a little more forward than your normal or habitual stance?

4. Move up toward your knees. Do they feel tight or locked? Locked knees means that they are hyperextending or pushing back in space and perhaps causing your calves to be overly arched. Can you gently soften the front and back of your knees so that they no longer feel locked?

5. Move upward toward your hips and pelvis. Do you notice any pressure in your hips? Do the sides feel even with each other? Does the pelvis feel like it's pushing forward in space and is slightly in front of your ankles? Can you shift or gently rock in a way that will align your hips so that they feel like they are directly over your ankles?

6. Move upward toward your shoulders and arms. Does one shoulder or arm feel tighter than the other? Do your arms feel like they are pulling forward and down in space? Does it feel like your arms are pulled back and your shoulders are lifting up in space? Can you think about letting your arms hang lightly at your side without any pulling in any direction? Can you imagine that your arms are like clothes hangers hanging in a closet?

7. Move upward toward your neck and head. Does your neck feel tight? Where? Does your head feel heavy? Does your jaw feel tight? Does it feel like the tightness of your neck is more toward the top of the neck by your jaw or lower in your neck by the shoulders?

Now we will explore the balance of your head. To fully explore the balance of your head, I'd like to give you a mini-anatomy lesson of the head-neck joint. This is a mobile joint that aids in the movement of your head and also helps to prevent unnecessary tightening of the muscles around your neck. In Figure 11-1, you are looking at the atlanto-occipital joint, which is at the top of the spine (your neck). Notice how the joint

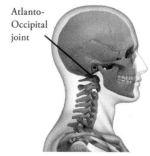

Atlanto-Occipital joint

Figure 11-1

is toward the middle of the neck and underneath the skull. Also notice how high the joint is. It is pretty much at the level in between your ears and very close to the jaw joint.

Experiment 1: Put your fingers on the outside of each ear. Imagine that there is an imaginary stick that goes from finger to finger. The middle point of that finger is where your head balances on the top of your neck/spine at the atlanto-occipital joint.

Experiment 2: I'll now have you experiment with the balance of your head by moving the head from this higher place of balance by your ears. I'd like you to do the following head movements by thinking of allowing the head to move from the atlanto-occipital joint by your ear. You can do these movements with your hands placed in front of your ear if you'd like.

1. Tilt your head back in space and notice if and when it starts to feel heavy (Figure 11-2). Do this about 3 or 4 times to see when you feel the heaviness of the head and when gravity starts to pull it back even further.

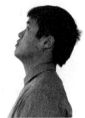

Figure 11-2

2. Tilt your head forward in space so that you are shortening the space in the front of your neck and tucking your chin (Figure 11-3). Notice when your head starts to get heavy as you tilt forward. Notice when you can start to feel the pull of gravity on your head as you move forward. Also do this 3 or 4 times.

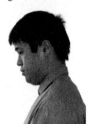

Figure 11-3

3. Now we will explore the lightness and balance of your head. Now that you have a sense of when you feel heaviness by tilting the head forward and back, I'd like you to try to find a middle place between the forward and back. Continue to explore tilting your head backward and when you feel it getting heavy, start to tilt it forward until you find a place when your head feels lighter and more balanced. Also, as you tilt your head forward, you look for the point when you feel heaviness and start to tilt it back until you find a place of lightness and balance (Figure 11-4).

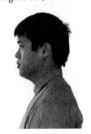

Figure 11-4

This head/neck balance exploration is a great way to experience more awareness in your body design. You are in essence moving your body in a more conscious way. You are attempting to find a position of more balance and ease by exploring the heaviness you feel in the movement of your own head.

EXPERIMENT IN EVERYDAY SITUATIONS

Next time you are sitting at a traffic light, I'd like you to notice your head and if it feels heavy or balanced. Try this same exploration while in your car and notice if your head is tilted forward or back to a position of heaviness. See if you can adjust it by tilting it into a position of lightness and balance (Figure 11-5).

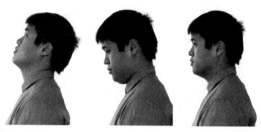

Figure 11-5

Try this at your desk in front of your computer monitor. Do not focus on what you see on your computer screen or on your input devices for 60 seconds. Focus on yourself, or specifically, your head and neck. Notice if your head feels heavy or balanced. Start the exploration of tilting your head to see when it pulls into heaviness and when you are able to find a lighter, more balanced position. Once you've found a more balanced position, bring your focus back to the computer or work at hand.

PRO-TIP

Many of my students tell me they have a difficult time keeping their head and neck balanced while in front of their computers at work. Oftentimes, the work at the computer can be very engaging and causes us to center our attention to the computer and away from an awareness of ourselves. Try the head and neck balance exploration while at your computer. Once you've found a more balanced position of your head and neck, look at the computer and ask yourself if you can still see and read the computer monitor comfortably without moving your head. If the answer is no, then your computer screen is positioned poorly in a way that works against your balanced head and body. If you have to tilt your head backward to see and read the screen, your monitor might be too high. If you have to tilt your head forward to see and read the screen, then your monitor might be too low. Adjust your monitor accordingly. I've included some images below of "poor laptop computer postures" and also some improved versions of these postures. Ideally, your eye level should be at the same level as the top one-third of your monitor while your head is in a balanced position.

1. **Poor Laptop Computer Postures:** Observe how the head and neck are not balanced with the rest of the body and create a heaviness for the worker (Figure 11-6).

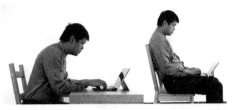

Figure 11-6

2. **Improved Laptop Computer Postures:** Observe the different ways of modifying the laptop setup to create more balance in the head, neck, and body for the worker (Figure 11-7).

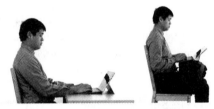

Figure 11-7

Check back in with the head/neck balance exploration often. You can never check in too often, especially at the beginning of your journey with mind-body techniques. The repetition of awareness is how you will begin to build muscle memory at the beginning. The repetition will also strengthen your connection to self-awareness. So often in life we tune out, but this exploration using principles of the Alexander Technique is your opportunity to "tune-in." Only in "tuning-in" can we start to gain control over habits and get out of pain.

In the Alexander Technique, this awakening of our kinesthetic awareness (the ability to perceive extent, direction, or weight of movement) (Venes 2017) is very important to our ability to make change and move out of pain and tension. Oftentimes, tension and pain are results of heaviness and physical collapse. My students often report experiencing a feeling of lightness and ease after an Alexander Technique lesson. This is a result of us bringing the same focus and attention onto different habits and areas of the body during a lesson that we did with the head/neck balance exploration. We not only achieve the immediate benefit of finding release and relief from pain during the lessons, but also gain practical ways in which the student can continue to explore and release during their lives and activities. This awakening of our kinesthetic awareness is how we undo the excess and unnecessary habits. If you are in the Los Angeles area, please feel free to contact me with questions. I wish you the best in your journey of health.

For additional personalized training, I recommend you visit an Alexander Technique studio.

ADDITIONAL RESOURCES

- Alexander Technique International, ati-net.com
- American Society for the Alexander Technique, amsatonline.org
- The Complete Guide to the Alexander Technique, alexandertechnique.com
- UCLA Ergonomics, ergonomics.ucla.edu

REFERENCES

Alexander FM. (1918). *Man's Supreme Inheritance.* New York, NY: E. P. Dutton and Co., Inc.

Alexander FM. (1923). *Constructive Conscious Control of the Individual.* New York, NY: E. P. Dutton and Co., Inc.

Alexander FM. (1932). *The Use of the Self.* New York, NY: E. P. Dutton and Co., Inc.

Alexander FM. (1941). *The Universal Constant in Living.* New York, NY: E. P. Dutton and Co., Inc.

Cacciatore TW, Gurfinkel VS, Horak FB, et al. (2011). Increased dynamic regulation of postural tone through Alexander Technique training. *Human Movement Science* 30 (1): 74–89.

Davis CM. (2017). *Integrative Therapies in Rehabilitation: Evidence for Efficacy in Therapy, Prevention, and Wellness,* 4th ed. Thorofare, NJ: SLACK.

Dawley N, Schapera N, Schapera V. (2010). *Guided Lessons: For Students of the Alexander Technique,* 2nd ed. Cincinnati, OH: FourWinds Press.

Dennis RJ. (1999). Functional reach improvement in normal older women after Alexander Technique instruction. *Journals of Gerontology. Series A, Biological Sciences and Medical Sciences* 54 (1): M8–11.

Gleeson M, Sherrington C, Lo S, et al. (2015). Can the Alexander Technique improve balance and mobility in older adults with visual impairments? A randomized controlled trial. *Clinical Rehabilitation* 29 (3): 244–260.

Hamel KA, Ross C, Schultz B, et al. (2016). Older adult Alexander Technique practitioners walk differently than healthy age-matched controls. *Journal of Bodywork and Movement Therapies* 20 (4): 751–760.

Klein SD, Bayard C, Wolf U. (2014). The Alexander Technique and musicians: A systematic review of controlled trials. *BMC Complementary and Alternative Medicine,* 14: 414.

Little P, Lewith G, Webley F, et al. (2008). Randomised controlled trial of Alexander Technique lessons, exercise, and massage (ATEAM) for chronic and recurrent back pain. *British Journal of Sports Medicine* 42 (12): 965–968.

MacPherson H, Tilbrook H, Richmond S, et al. (2015). Alexander Technique lessons or acupuncture sessions for persons with chronic neck pain: A randomized trial. *Annals of Internal Medicine* 163 (9): 653-662.

Reddy PP, Reddy TP, Roig-Francoli J, et al. (2011). The impact of the Alexander Technique on improving posture and surgical ergonomics during minimally invasive surgery: Pilot study. *Journal of Urology* 186 (Supplement 4): 1658–1662.

Stallibrass C, Sissons P, Chalmers C. (2002). Randomized controlled trial of the Alexander Technique for idiopathic Parkinson's disease. *Clinical Rehabilitation* 16 (7): 695–708.

Venes D. (Ed.) (2017). *Taber's Cyclopedic Medical Dictionary*, 23rd ed. Philadelphia, PA: FA Davis.

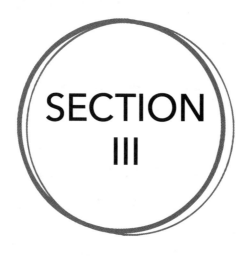

SECTION III

REJUVINATING WESTERN EXERCISE AND MOVEMENT

The purpose of this section is to give you some practical routines to consider and also outline some safe and effective rejuvenating Western exercises you can use in the comfort of your home. I like to think about this part of the book as where the East meets the West.

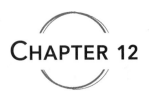

CHAPTER 12

PRACTICAL EXERCISE
PROGRAMS AND ROUTINES

"Life must be lived as play."

—Plato

I'll refer to this chapter as your personal fitness lab. You can experiment with the programs I have provided and eventually create your own variations. I hope these programs will encourage you to train and to move well, but most importantly, to enjoy the process of finding which movements are best suited for your body.

For all the stretches outlined in this chapter, consider doing diaphragmatic breaths instead of just counting. For most individuals, counting 5 to 6 breaths is much more relaxing than counting to 30 or 60 (or watching a clock and letting your mind wander to things like taxes and bills). For example, instead of holding a stretch for 30 seconds, simply do 6 diaphragmatic breaths, or for a 15-second stretch do 3 diaphragmatic breaths. Of course everyone is different, so you can figure out for yourself how many slow diaphragmatic breaths you take in 30 seconds and use that as your guide.

Go ahead and slowly try the following fitness programs to spice up your workouts. Some of the exercises are described in chapter 13. If you come up with new and innovative programs, please feel free to send them to me. Who knows, maybe they will wind up in the next edition of this book!

PROGRAM 1: HOME AEROBIC AND STRENGTH CIRCUIT

Circuit training is a training method that involves moving from one activity or exercise to the other with varying amounts of rest or stretching in between. The advantage of circuit training is that by varying the workouts, you can exercise quickly and efficiently while using many different kinds of equipment. Circuit training may be used to enhance athletic performance, work performance, and activities of daily living (Altug et al. 1990; Morgan et al. 1972). This type of training can be used for general fitness, designed to either emphasize the aerobic, strength, flexibility, or balance components of a workout.

- Start: Warm-up with mobility exercises for 5 minutes.
- Walk in your home for 5 minutes.
- Shortstop Squats for 10 repetitions.
- Walk in your home for 5 minutes.
- Elastic High Rows for 10 repetitions.
- Walk in your home for 5 minutes.
- Supine Bridge for 10 repetitions.
- Walk in your home for 5 minutes.
- Elevated Push-Ups for 10 repetitions.
- Walk in your home for 5 minutes.
- Heel Raises for 10 repetitions.
- Cool down and stretch gently for 5 minutes.
- End: Drink adequate fluids and relax.

🏃 PROGRAM 2: HOME STRENGTH CIRCUIT

- Start: Warm-up with mobility exercises for 5 minutes.
- Slow March in Place for 1 minute.
- Shortstop Squats for 10 repetitions.
- Slow March in Place for 1 minute.
- Heel Raises for 10 repetitions.
- Slow March in Place for 1 minute.
- Tai Chi Steps for 1 minute.
- Slow March in Place for 1 minute.
- Elastic High Rows for 10 repetitions.
- Slow March in Place for 1 minute.
- Elevated Push-ups for 10 repetitions.
- Slow March in Place for 1 minute.
- Supine Bridge for 10 repetitions.
- Slow March in Place for 1 minute.
- Bird Dog pose for 10 repetitions.
- Slow March in Place for 1 minute.
- Cool down and stretch gently for 5 minutes.
- End: Drink adequate fluids and relax.

🏃 PROGRAM 3: TRACK, PARK, OR NEIGHBORHOOD CIRCUIT

- Start: Warm-up with mobility exercises for 5 minutes.

- Walk outdoors for 5 minutes.
- Shortstop Squats for 10 repetitions.
- Walk outdoors for 5 minutes.
- Elevated Push-ups for 10 repetitions.
- Walk outdoors for 5 minutes.
- Tai Chi Steps for 1 minute.
- Walk outdoors for 5 minutes.
- Slow March in Place for 5 repetitions.
- Walk outdoors for 5 minutes.
- Calf Stretch gently for 30 seconds (or for example, 6 diaphragmatic breaths).
- Yawn Stretch gently for 15 seconds.
- Look-Over-Your-Shoulder Stretch gently for 10 seconds.
- End: Drink adequate fluids and relax.

🏃 PROGRAM 4: SENIOR CIRCUIT–HOME

A 70-year-old patient of mine created the following program for herself:

- Start: Outdoor walking warm-up around the house for 5 minutes.
- Walk to the living room and perform Supine Bridging for 10 repetitions.
- Walk to the bedroom and perform Elevated Push-ups from the bed for 10 repetitions.
- Walk to the kitchen and perform Heel Raises while holding on the kitchen counter for 10 repetitions.
- Walk to the front yard and perform Slow March in Place for 10 repetitions.
- Walk to the back yard and perform Shortstop Squats for 10 repetitions . . .
- Walk to the living room and perform Tai Chi Steps for 1 minute.
- Walk outdoors 10 minutes.
- Walk to the living room and perform the Yawn Stretch gently for 15 seconds.
- Stay in the living room and perform the Calf Stretch gently for 30 seconds.
- Stay in the living room and perform the Outer Hip Stretch gently for 30 seconds.
- Stay in the living room and perform the Inner Hip Stretch gently for 30 seconds.
- End: Drink adequate fluids and relax.

🏃 Program 5: Senior Circuit—Mall

An 80-year-old patient of mine created the following program for himself:

- Walk for 5 to 10 minutes around the mall.
- Perform Chair Squats from the mall bench for 10 repetitions.
- Perform Heel Raises while holding onto the back of a bench for 10 repetitions.
- Repeat the first three steps twice.
- Perform the Yawn Stretch gently for 2 sets of 15 seconds.
- Perform the Calf Stretch gently for 2 sets of 30 seconds.
- End: Drink adequate fluids and relax.

🏃 Program 6: Senior Circuit—Fitness Center

Consider the following senior circuit-training program at your local fitness center with your fitness professional nearby for safety:

- Start: Check your blood pressure and heart rate.
- Warm-up on a stationary bike for 5 minutes.
- Shoot some basketballs for 2 minutes.
- Kick a soccer ball for 2 minutes.
- Play a game of table tennis for 2 minutes.
- Perform a few tai chi poses for 2 minutes.
- Perform a few modified yoga poses for 2 minutes.
- Perform a few modified Pilates poses for 2 minutes.
- Perform Shortstop Squats for 10 repetitions.
- Perform Elastic High Rows for 10 repetitions.
- Perform Tai Chi Steps for 1 minute.
- Perform Heel Raises 10 times.
- Perform the Calf Stretch gently for 30 seconds.
- Perform the Yawn Stretch gently for 15 seconds.
- Cool down on a stationary bike for 5 minutes.
- Check your blood pressure and heart rate.
- End: Drink adequate fluids and relax.

🏃 Program 7: Advanced Outdoor Nature Trail Circuit

A fit, 35-year-old client of mine created the following program for himself. Carry a sturdy backpack with water and energy bars, and consider using walking sticks.

- Start: Warm-up with mobility exercises for 5 minutes at the beginning of the trail.
- Walk the trail for 10 minutes.

- Perform Elevated Push-ups from a boulder or log.
- Walk the trail for 5 minutes.
- Perform single-arm rowing movements using a rock (approximately 10 pounds).
- Walk the trail for 5 minutes.
- Perform single-arm overhead lifts using a rock (approximately 10 pounds).
- Walk the trail for 5 minutes.
- Perform a double-arm rock lift, carry a rock (approximately 10 to 25 pounds) for 10 feet, and then lower the rock to the ground, and repeat this sequence 5 times.
- Walk the trail for 5 minutes.
- Perform a slow, double-arm swing (think of the Darth Vader lightsaber swing) using a stick to simulate a battle scene for 1 minute.
- Walk the trail for 10 minutes.
- Perform the Squat Stretch for 15 seconds.
- Perform the Calf Stretch for 30 seconds.
- Perform the Yawn Stretch for 15 seconds.
- Perform the Hands-Behind-the-Back Stretch for 15 seconds.
- Perform the Hands-Behind-the-Neck Stretch for 15 seconds.
- End: Drink adequate fluids and relax.

🏃 PROGRAM 8: FUNCTIONAL CIRCUIT

The following is a quick program that may be applied to movements of daily life (such as getting up and down from the floor) or athletic competition (such as martial arts, wrestling, or gymnastics). You might be surprised at the difficulty of this simple workout. And, like what one of my high school coaches used to say, "Don't drop to the floor like a sack of potatoes."

- Start: Warm-up with mobility exercises for 5 minutes.
- Get-Ups # 1: Start in standing, assume a hands-and knees position, then lie down flat on your stomach, and finally, return to a standing position. Perform the sequence for 5 to 10 repetitions.
- Get-Ups # 2: Start in standing, sit down toward your right side, lie down flat on your *back*, and sit up by partially rolling toward your right and stand up by pushing off the floor from your right side. Once standing, quickly reverse the movements to your left side. Perform the sequence for 5 to 10 repetitions (where a right and left get-up counts as one repetition).
- Get-Ups # 3: Start in standing, sit down toward your right side, lie down on your *stomach*, and roll onto your back toward your right side and stand up by pushing off the floor from your right side. Once standing, quickly reverse the movements to your left side. Perform the

sequence for 5 to 10 repetitions (where a right and left get-up counts as one repetition).

- Cool down and stretch for 5 minutes.
- End: Drink adequate fluids and relax.

🏃 PROGRAM 9: MOTOR CONTROL CIRCUIT

The following program might help train postures and retrain optimal movement patterns (Comerford et al. 2012). These basic movements might be useful for individuals in the early stages of mechanical low-back pain (Aasa et al. 2015) and also help give a person confidence to move with daily activities. See a physical therapist for additional neuromuscular re-education (or motor control) exercise programs for improving stability, coordination, and balance for the neck, shoulder, hand, hip, knee, and foot. Motor control exercises help with purposeful and coordinated movements. The following exercise sequence may be performed up to three times a day to help with back pain:

- Start: Warm-up with walking for 3 to 5 minutes.
- Perform a supine (face up) alternate leg marching where your feet touch the ground for 10 repetitions.
- Perform a prone (face down) alternate leg bending and straightening with your feet in the air for 10 repetitions.
- Perform a gentle quadruped (hands and knees) to a heel sit position for 10 repetitions.
- Perform a seated single-leg straightening and bending for 10 repetitions with each leg.
- Perform the Chair Squats for 10 repetitions.
- Perform the Shortstop Squats for 10 repetitions.
- Perform a deadlift motion using a yardstick or wooden pole for 10 repetitions.
- Perform alternate overhead reaches for 10 repetitions.
- Perform a gentle tennis swing motion on the right and left sides for 10 repetitions.
- Cool down with regular walking for 3 to 5 minutes.
- End: Drink adequate fluids and relax.

🏃 PROGRAM 10: MIND AND BODY FUSION CIRCUIT

The following is a fusion of mind and body movements which might be best suited for a fitness center:

- Start: Warm-up with slow mindful walking (see chapter 1) for 5 minutes.
- Perform a tai chi routine for 5 minutes.

- Perform a qigong routine for 5 minutes.
- Perform a yoga routine for 5 minutes.
- Perform a Pilates mat routine for 5 minutes.
- Perform Feldenkrais Method-based movements for 5 minutes.
- Perform Alexander Technique-based movements for 5 minutes.
- Cool down with mindful walking for 5 minutes.
- End: Drink adequate fluids and relax.

🏃 PROGRAM 11: WEEKLY CROSS-TRAINING

Cross-training has many definitions in the sports world. It refers to applying several sports, activities, or training techniques to improve a person's performance in his or her primary sport or activity (Moran et al. 1997).

In this book, the term "cross-training" indicates a training method in which exercises and activities such as outdoor walking, upper body biking, elliptical training, stair-climbing, tai chi, dancing, tennis, circuit weight-training, aerobic dance, and calisthenics are varied during the month, week, or even in a single workout session. A classic example of cross-training is when triathlon participants train using a combination of running, biking, and swimming.

- Monday: walk or run for 30 to 60 minutes
- Tuesday: weight-training exercises for 30 to 60 minutes
- Wednesday: dance for 30 to 60 minutes
- Thursday: bike for 30 to 60 minutes
- Friday: weight-training exercises for 30 to 60 minutes
- Saturday: tai chi for 30 to 60 minutes
- Sunday: walk or run for 30 to 60 minutes

🏃 PROGRAM 12: SINGLE-SESSION CROSS-TRAINING

Program may range from 30 to 60 minutes

- Start: Warm-up with mobility exercises.
- Walk on an indoor track for 10 to 20 minutes.
- Exercise on an elliptical machine for 10 to 20 minutes.
- Ride a stationary bike for 10 to 20 minutes.
- End: Cool down and stretch.

🏃 PROGRAM 13: WALKING INTERVAL TRAINING

Interval training is a type of training in which periods of high-intensity exercise intervals (such as fast walking, running, fast cycling, fast swimming, or fast rowing) are alternated with low-intensity exercise intervals (such as slow walking, jogging, slow cycling, slow swimming, or slow rowing). Or, it can be thought of as alternating between difficult and easy exercise intervals. This type of training is sometimes also called *fartlek*, which is a Swedish word meaning "speed play."

High-intensity and low-intensity intervals are alternated for a designated amount of cycles and for a specific amount of time. In general, interval-training programs are performed one to two times a week, with the other days of the week focusing on other types of training (Baechle et al. 2008). Interval training can be made less taxing by using fewer high-intensity/low-intensity intervals, reducing the total duration of the workout, reducing the duration of the high-intensity period, or increasing the duration of the low-intensity period. The advantages of interval training are that it can help prevent boredom, potentially reduce overuse injuries by varying the periods of high-intensity exercise and low-intensity exercise, and also help improve physical performance.

Depending on a person's level of conditioning, the fast interval could be as short as 15 seconds or as long as two minutes, and the slow interval can be as short as two minutes or as long as five to 10 minutes. The key is to start slowly and progress gradually.

- Start: Warm-up with mobility exercises.
- Normal-paced walk (typically slow) for 5 to 10 minutes.
- Fast walk (faster than normal pace) for 1 minute.
- Normal-paced walk for 6 minutes.
- Continue with a repetitive cycle of alternating the slow walk (6 minutes) and fast walk (1 minute) for a total of 15 to 45 minutes.
- Cool down and stretch.
- End: Drink adequate fluids and relax.

PROGRAM 14: WALKING/RUNNING INTERVAL TRAINING

- Start: Warm-up with mobility exercises.
- Normal pace or slow walk for 5 to 10 minutes.
- Run or jog for 1 minute.
- Walk for 6 minutes.
- Continue with a repetitive cycle of alternating the walk (6 minutes) and run or jog (1 minute) for a total of 15 to 45 minutes.
- Cool down and stretch.
- End: Drink adequate fluids and relax.

PROGRAM 15: RUNNING OR JOGGING/ SPRINTING INTERVAL TRAINING

- Start: Warm upwith mobility exercises.

- Warm up with normal pace or slow walk for 5 to 10 minutes.
- Run or jog 1 lap around a track.
- Sprint or run fast for 100 yards.
- Continue with a repetitive cycle of alternating the run or jog (1 lap) and a sprint or fast run (100 yards) for a total of 15 to 45 minutes.
- Cool down and stretch.
- End: Drink adequate fluids and relax.

🏃 PROGRAM 16: BIKING INTERVAL TRAINING

- Start: Warm up with mobility exercises.
- Warm up with normal pace or slow biking for 5 to 10 minutes.
- Bike fast for 1 minute.
- Bike slow for 6 minutes.
- Continue with a repetitive cycle of alternating the slow (6 minutes) and fast (1 minute) biking for a total of 15 to 45 minutes.
- Cool down and stretch.
- End: Drink adequate fluids and relax.

🏃 PROGRAM 17: AEROBIC SHORT-BOUT TRAINING

Short-bout training is a type of training in which short-duration periods of exercise are accumulated throughout the day. For some individuals, shorter bouts of training are better suited for their fitness levels (such as deconditioned individuals) or busy lifestyles. Rather than focusing on exercising for one hour continuously, break up activity throughout the day. This removes the burden of having to carve out a big block of time in your schedule, or being physically and mentally overwhelmed by long exercise sessions.

Short-bout exercise (for example, three 10-minute bouts of exercise per day) might fit into your schedule better than one long bout of exercise (one 30-minute workout session per day) (DeBusk et al. 1990). This type of program can keep the body moving throughout the day, as well as prevent stiffness from long work commutes and prolonged sitting.

- Morning: 10- to 15-minute walk (or yoga) before work
- Midday: 10- to 15-minute walk (or yoga) during lunch break
- Evening: 10- to 15-minute walk (or yoga) after work

🏃 PROGRAM 18: STATIC LOADLESS TRAINING

Purpose: This type of training is only a supplement and should not be your sole form of resistance exercise. Try these exercises after recovering from prolonged bed rest, during vacations, or just as a one- to two-week break from your regular strength routines. This routine was inspired by Professor Yuri Verkhoshansky from his book *Supertraining* (Verkhoshansky et al. 2009).

Positions: Standing, sitting, and lying down

Technique:

- *Warm-up*—before starting the program, warm up for at least 5 minutes with walking and mobility exercises for the upper and lower body.
- *Gluteal squeezes*—tense your gluteal muscles while standing or lying supine or prone.
- *Thigh squeezes*—tense your thigh muscles while standing or lying supine.
- *Shoulder blade squeezes*—tense your upper back muscles by squeezing your shoulder blades together while sitting or standing.
- *Biceps squeezes*—tense the front of your arm muscles by bending your elbows 90 degrees while sitting or standing.
- *Triceps squeezes*—tense the back of your arm muscles by straightening your elbow while sitting or standing.
- *Cool-down*—after finishing the program, cool down for at least 5 minutes with walking and mobility exercises for the upper and lower body.

Sets and Reps:

- Perform each exercise by tensing your muscles for 5 to 10 seconds as you count out loud throughout the muscle tension portions. Only tense your muscles hard enough so that you can still count out loud comfortably without experiencing any dizziness or lightheadedness. Apply and release tension slowly to prevent injuries.
- Repeat each exercise 2 to 5 times with at least a 10-second walking rest break after each muscle tension for recovery.
- Perform the exercises 2 to 3 times per week for one to two weeks. During rehabilitation, your physical therapist might advise you to perform these types of exercises more frequently with different sets and reps.

Precautions: Avoid tension exercises if you have high blood pressure; have a history of strokes; have a pacemaker, migraines, or excess eye pressure; underwent eye surgery recently; have a brain or abdominal aneurysm; experience dizziness spells regularly; or think the exercise is painful.

Speak with your healthcare provider if you are in doubt about any other medical conditions. If you are recovering from surgery, do not start any of these exercises until you speak with your physical therapist or physician.

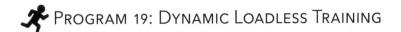

PROGRAM 19: DYNAMIC LOADLESS TRAINING

Purpose: This type of training is only a supplement and should not be your sole form of resistance exercise. Try these exercises after recovering from prolonged bed rest, during vacations, or just as a one- to two-week break from your regular strength routines. This routine was inspired by Professor Yuri Verkhoshansky from his book *Supertraining* (Verkhoshansky et al. 2009).

Position: Standing

Technique:

- *Warm-up*—before starting the program, warm up for at least 5 minutes with walking and mobility exercises for the upper and lower body.
- *Tennis swing*—think tai chi movements (slow motion) as you perform a tennis forehand and backhand swing without a racket. Tense your core, leg, and arm muscles as you slowly go through the tennis swing.
- *Golf swing*—think tai chi movements (slow motion) as you perform a golf swing without a club. Tense your core, leg, and arm muscles as you slowly go through the golf swing.
- *Basketball shot*—think tai chi movements (slow motion) as you perform a basketball shot from the free-throw line without a ball. Tense your core, leg, and arm muscles as you slowly perform the basketball shot.
- *Cool-down*—after finishing the program, cool down for at least five minutes with walking and mobility exercises for the upper and lower body.

Sets and Reps:

- Perform each exercise by tensing your muscles for 5 to 10 seconds as you count out loud throughout the muscle tension portions. Tense your muscles very lightly so that you can still count out loud comfortably without experiencing any dizziness or lightheadedness. Apply and release tension slowly to prevent injuries.
- Repeat each exercise 2 to 5 times with at least a 10-second walking rest break after each muscle tension for recovery.
- Perform the exercises 2 to 3 times per week for one to two weeks.

PROGRAM 20: BASIC POOL CIRCUIT TRAINING

Exercising in a pool or performing aquatic therapy can be beneficial for individuals with pain, and those who are deconditioned or need to recover after injury. Aquatic fitness is a great way to improve cardiovascular fitness, flexibility, and basic strength (Brody et al. 2009).

Purpose: To serve as a basic fitness program

Technique:

- Start: Warm up slowly with walking forward exercises for 5 minutes.
- Walk forward and backward at a challenging pace for 5 minutes.
- Partial squats for 1 minute.
- Push and pull with your hands back and forth in the water while standing for 1 minute.
- Walk forward and backward at a challenging pace for 5 minutes.
- Standing heel raises for 1 minute.
- Standing single-leg balance on each leg for 1 minute.
- "Jog" in the deep end of the pool using a buoyancy belt or vest for 2 minutes.
- Cool down slowly with walking forward exercises for 5 minutes.
- Stretch your calf muscles gently for 30 seconds.
- Stretch your thigh muscles gently for 30 seconds.
- Stretch your hamstring muscles gently for 30 seconds.
- Stretch your chest muscles gently for 30 seconds.
- Stretch your back muscles gently for 30 seconds.
- End: Relax by floating in the water for 1 to 2 minutes.

Duration and Intensity: This program can be performed for 30 to 45 minutes. Use hand webs for extra resistance in the water. Depending on the goals of the pool program, a person may be immersed in the water from waist level to chest level.

Precautions: Wear nonslip footwear for safety around the pool. Work out with a training partner or fitness professional for safety. Also, ideally, have a clear lap lane.

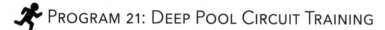

PROGRAM 21: DEEP POOL CIRCUIT TRAINING

Purpose: To serve as a basic fitness program

Equipment: Flotation vest or belt for the first eight exercises

Technique:

- Start: Warm up slowly with walking forward and backward exercises for 5 minutes.
- Perform a slow bicycling motion in the deep end for 5 minutes.
- Perform a running motion in the deep end for 5 minutes.
- Perform a leg open-and-close motion in the deep end for 30 seconds.
- Perform a leg scissor motion in the deep end for 30 seconds.
- Perform a leg open-and-close motion in the deep end for 30 seconds.
- Perform a leg scissor motion in the deep end for 30 seconds.
- Perform a running motion in the deep end for 5 minutes.
- Perform a slow bicycling motion in the deep end for 5 minutes.
- Cool down with walking forward and backward exercises for 5 minutes.
- Stretch your calf muscles gently for 30 seconds.

- Stretch your thigh muscles gently for 30 seconds.
- Stretch your hamstring muscles gently for 30 seconds.
- Stretch your chest muscles gently for 30 seconds.
- Stretch your back muscles gently for 30 seconds.
- End: Relax by floating in the water for 1 minute.

Duration and Intensity: This program can be performed for 30 to 45 minutes. Use hand webs for extra resistance in the water. Depending on the goals of the pool program, a person may be immersed in the water from waist level to chest level.

Precautions: Wear nonslip footwear for safety around the pool. Work out with a training partner or fitness professional for safety. Also, ideally, have a clear lap lane.

Box 9: Holistic Healing

Face Touching and the Flu

To help prevent the flu, minimize the amount you touch your face. Your hands can pick up a virus or other germs when you touch things in your environment (such as doorknobs, shopping cart handles, railings, gas pumps, money, and other people's hands). Therefore, your hands can bring germs directly to your face's critical T-zone, where the "T" is formed by your eyes, nose, and mouth (Bertsch 2010; Elder et al. 2014; Goldmann 2000; Hendley et al. 1973; Nicas et al. 2008; Reed 1975). Not all viruses or bacteria enter the body from this region, but many can and do.

If you must touch your face to scratch an itch, first wash your hands or use a clean tissue. If you can't do either at that moment, gently use your shoulder or the inside of your shirt as a last resort to scratch or wipe your face. This way, you avoid placing your hands—and whatever they've picked up—in your T-zone.

In addition to multiple daily hand washings, frequent facial cleansing should be a key component of daily hygiene. This might be especially true during flu season. Wash your face in the morning and before you go to bed to remove whatever germs have accumulated.

Finally, why should we all cover our mouths when we cough or sneeze or take cover ourselves? Research shows that expelled large droplets may be carried long distances due to sneezing, coughing, and even breathing (Xie et al. 2007, 2009):

- A *sneeze* carries droplets more than six meters (approximately 19 feet) away at approximately 110 mph.
- A *cough* carries droplets more than two meters (approximately six feet) away at approximately 22 mph.
- A normal *breath* carries droplets less than one meter (approximately three feet) away at approximately 2 mph.

ADDITIONAL RESOURCES

- Exercise is Medicine, http://exerciseismedicine.org
- New Interval Training, www.newintervaltraining.com
- For advanced fitness enthusiasts and athletes, look into the Tabata protocol, created by Professor Izumi Tabata at Ritsumeikan University in Japan, using high-intensity interval training (HIIT) with running (outdoors, standard treadmill, or aquatic treadmill) and cycling (Tabata et al. 1996, 1997). A study by Rebold et al. (2013) indicates that the whole Tabata training session is 4 minutes long, where the person altenates between 20 seconds of intense exercise and 10 seconds of rest for total of 8 rounds.

REFERENCES

Aasa B, Berglund L, Michaelson P, et al. (2015). Individualized low-load motor control exercises and education versus a high-load lifting exercise and education to improve activity, pain intensity, and physical performance in patients with low back pain: A randomized controlled trial. *Journal of Orthopaedic and Sports Physical Therapy.* 45 (2): 77–85.

Altug Z, Hoffman JL, Slane SM, et al. (1990). Work-circuit training. *Clinical Management (Magazine of the American Physical Therapy Association)* 10 (5): 41–48.

Baechle TR, Earle RW. (Eds.). (2008). *Essentials of Strength Training and Conditioning,* 3rd ed. Champaign IL: Human Kinetics.

Brody LT, Geigle PR. (2009). *Aquatic Exercise for Rehabilitation and Training.* Champaign, IL: Human Kinetics.

Comerford M, Mottram S. (2012). *Kinetic Control: The Management of Uncontrolled Movement.* Edinburg, United Kingdom: Elsevier Churchill Livingstone.

DeBusk RF, Stenestrand U, Sheehan M, et al. (1990). Training effects of long versus short bouts of exercise in healthy subjects. *American Journal of Cardiology* 65 (15): 1010–1013.

Eguchi M, Ohta M, Yamato H. (2013). The effects of single long and accumulated short bouts of exercise on cardiovascular risks in male Japanese workers: A randomized controlled study. *Industrial Health* 51 (6): 563–571.

Gettman LR, Ayres JJ, Pollock ML, et al. (1978). The effect of circuit weight training on strength, cardiorespiratory function, and body composition of adult men. *Medicine and Science in Sports* 10 (3): 171–176.

Gettman LR, Pollock ML. (1981). Circuit weight training: A critical review of its physiological benefits. *Physician and Sportsmedicine* 9 (1): 44–60.

Jakicic JM, Wing RR, Butler BA, et al. (1995). Prescribing exercise in multiple short bouts versus one continuous bout: Effects on adherence, cardiorespiratory fitness, and weight loss in overweight women. *International Journal of Obesity and Related Metabolic Disorders* 19 (12): 893–901.

Jakicic JM, Winters C, Lang W et al. (1999). Effects of intermittent exercise and use of home exercise equipment on adherence, weight loss, and fitness in overweight women: A randomized trial. *JAMA* 282 (16): 1554–1560.

Kisner C, Colby LA, Borstad J. (2018). *Therapeutic Exercise: Foundations and Techniques,* 7th ed. Philadelphia, PA: FA Davis.

Moran GT, McGlynn GH. (1997). *Cross-Training for Sports*. Champaign, IL: Human Kinetics.

Morgan RE, Adamson GT. (1972). *Circuit Training*, 2nd ed. London, England: G. Bell.

Paoli A, Moro T, Marcolin G, et al. (2012). High-intensity interval resistance training (HIRT) influences resting energy expenditure and respiratory ratio in non-dieting individuals. *Journal of Translational Medicine* 10 (1): 237.

Paoli A, Pacelli QF, Moro T, et al. (2013). Effects of high-intensity circuit training, low-intensity circuit training and endurance training on blood pressure and lipoproteins in middle-aged overweight men. *Lipids in Health and Disease* 12: 131.

Rebold MJ, Kobak MS, Otterstetter R. (2013). The influence of a Tabata interval training program using an aquatic underwater treadmill on various performance variables. *Journal of Strength and Conditioning Research* 27 (12): 3419–3425.

Romero-Arenas S, Blazevich AJ, Martinez-Pascual M, et al. (2013). Effects of high-resistance circuit training in an elderly population. *Experimental Gerontology* 48 (3): 334–340.

Tabata I, Irisawa K, Kouzaki M, et al. (1997). Metabolic profile of high intensity intermittent exercises. *Medicine and Science in Sports and Exercise* 29 (3): 390–395.

Tabata I, Nishimura K, Kouzaki M, et al. (1996). Effects of moderate-intensity endurance and high-intensity intermittent training on anaerobic capacity and VO2max. *Medicine and Science in Sports and Exercise* 28 (10): 1327–1330.

Verkhoshansky Y, and Siff M. (2009). *Supertraining*, 6th ed. Rome, Italy: Verkhoshansky. www.verkhoshansky.com.

HOLISTIC HEALING BOX

Face Touching and the Flu

Bertsch RA. (2010). Avoiding upper respiratory tract infections by not touching the face. *Archives of Internal Medicine* 170 (9): 833–834.

Elder NC, Sawyer W, Pallerla H, et al. (2014). Hand hygiene and face touching in family medicine offices: A Cincinnati area research and improvement group (caring) network study. *Journal of the American Board of Family Medicine* 27 (3): 339–346.

Goldmann DA. (2000). Transmission of viral respiratory infections in the home. *Pediatric Infectious Disease Journal* 19 (Supplement 10): S97–102.

Hendley JO, Wenzel RP, and Gwaltney JM. (1973). Transmission of rhinovirus colds by self-inoculation. *New England Journal of Medicine* 288 (26): 1361–1364.

Nicas M, Best D. (2008). A study quantifying the hand-to-face contact rate and its potential application to predicting respiratory tract infection. *Journal Occupational and Environmental Hygiene* 5 (6): 347–352.

Reed SE. (1975). An investigation of the possible transmission of rhinovirus colds through indirect contact. *Journal of Hygiene (Lond)* 75 (2): 249–258.

Xie X, Li Y, Chwang AT, et al. (2007). How far droplets can move in indoor environments—Revisiting the Wells evaporation-falling curve. *Indoor Air* 17 (3): 211–225.

Xie X, Li Y, Sun H, et al. (2009). Exhaled droplets due to talking and coughing. *Journal of the Royal Society Interface* 6 (Supplement 6): S703–714.

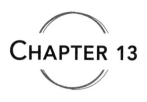

CHAPTER 13

EXERCISE MENU AND HOME PROGRAM GUIDE

"We are what we repeatedly do. Excellence,
then, is not an act, but a habit."

—Aristotle

This chapter focuses more on standard or typical exercises used in Western physical therapy and fitness. However, this does not mean these simple movement patterns and exercises cannot be a part of your home healing program. Many of these exercises have been used successfully in rehabilitation programs and may also be used safely as a part of a fitness program. I talk a little about how to create a healing home gym, which brings some of the concepts from the Eastern world. Finally, I touch a little on feng shui and how to create a home fitness gazebo (which has natural outdoor light, fresh air, and is surrounded by a healing garden).

CREATING A HOME GYM

When creating your home gym, pick a spot where you get outdoor light and fresh air. Now place a few nice plants in your space, hang some inspirational pictures, and set up a good sound system to play your favorite music. These are some potential areas for setting up a gym or fitness center in your home: garage, patio, backyard, living/dining room, spare room, basement, loft, den, sunroom, or a floor-to-ceiling bay window alcove.

HOME EXERCISE EQUIPMENT

Consider purchasing the following equipment for your home gym:

- Quality walking or running shoes for outdoor workouts

- A quality exercise mat (when performing mat or dumbbell exercises in your home, go barefoot or wear flat shoes)
- Dumbbells or kettlebells according to your fitness level (beginner, intermediate, or advanced)
- Elastic resistance bands according to your fitness level (beginner, intermediate, or advanced)
- Stationary bike (unless you plan to walk or hike outdoors)
- Home blood-pressure monitoring unit
- Body-weight scale

Box 10: Holistic Healing

Osteoporosis Information

Osteoporosis: A bone disorder characterized by a reduction in bone density (thickness) accompanied by increasing porosity and brittleness. It is a loss of bone mass that occurs throughout the skeleton, predisposing patients to fractures. According to the World Health Organization, when the bone mineral density exceeds 2.5 standard deviations below normal, it is called osteoporosis (Venes 2017).

When performing any of the following activities, individuals with osteoporosis should use extreme caution or avoid them altogether (Bassey 2001; Beck et al. 2003; Bonner et al. 2003; Katz et al. 1998; Meeks 2008, 2010; Petit et al. 2010; Sinaki 2007; Sinaki et al. 1984):

- Abdominal exercises performed on machines where you sit and bend forward.
- Activities such as golf (Ekin et al. 1993), unloading groceries, or vacuuming, which require leaning and twisting.
- Bending exercises, like standing toe touches or full sit-ups, and stationary rowing machines in which you are seated.
- Yoga poses that focus on extreme bending (Sinaki 2012, 2013). See chapter 6: Yoga for Health for more information.
- Exercises such as jogging, running, aerobics, jump roping, or certain martial arts that involve high-impact kicks, punches, and throws. Although, some individuals may benefit from high-impact exercises.

The following are resources you can use to find more information about osteoporosis treatment and prevention:

- American College of Sports Medicine (search osteoporosis), acsm.org
- International Osteoporosis Foundation, iofbonehealth.org
- International Society for Clinical Densitometry, iscd.org
- National Institutes of Health Osteoporosis and Related Bone Diseases, bones.nih.gov/health-info/bone/osteoporosis
- National Osteoporosis Foundation, nof.org

FENG SHUI FOR FITNESS

Include some feng shui into your home gym or outdoor fitness gazebo to create an energizing, yet calming place for yourself. Feng shui is an ancient Chinese art of interior and architectural design, the objective of which is to create a soothing and healthful living environment that is in accord with the qi (energy or life force) (Venes 2017). Feng shui as used in this book is not about controlling your life, but rather about giving you some guidelines to create a peaceful home-fitness environment and to arrange your furniture and items in a room in a way that brings peace to you. Ultimately, do what makes you happy and what makes sense for your personal needs.

 Consider the following when creating your home gym:

- Ensure area is well lit by natural light and has good air flow
- Install a small ceiling fan for air circulation
- Have an inspiring view (such as your garden, patio, or backyard), along with art and sculptures to help you relax and reflect, as well as plants and flowers to enrich your environment
- Buy a fish tank for relaxation and meditation
- Pick wall and furniture colors for your goals, such as red for energy or blue for relaxation
- Use fabrics made of natural fibers
- Keep clutter to a minimum

ADDITIONAL FENG SHUI RESOURCES
- Association of Feng Shui Consultants, afsc.org.au
- Feng Shui for Real Life, fengshuiforreallife.com
- International Feng Shui Association, intfsa.org
- International Feng Shui Guild, ifsguild.org
- Refer to the book by Nancy SantoPietro *Feng Shui and Health: The Anatomy of A Home: Using Feng Shui to Disarm Illness* (2002).
- Refer to the book by Denise Linn *Feng Shui for the Soul: How to Create a Harmonious Environment That Will Nurture and Sustain You* (1999).

HOME GAZEBO FOR HEALING AND HEALTH

A gazebo in your backyard (or as an extension to your house) provides shade, and it's a great way to entertain friends and family. However, you can also customize your gazebo so that it helps you heal and get fit. One study indicates that outdoor training leads to greater exercise adherence than indoor training in postmenopausal women (Lacharité-Lemieux et al. 2015). So why wait? Go outside and have some fun!

STYLES

- Open gazebo (no windows)—good for warm-weather locations
- Closed gazebo (windows and screens)—good for cold-weather locations

PURPOSE

- Fitness
- Healing
- Meditation
- Relaxation
- Body-based exercise, such as tai chi, qigong, Pilates, or yoga

BENEFITS

- Fresh air
- Natural outdoor light—blue wavelength to help reduce depression
- Some sunshine for vitamin D benefits
- Sustainability—uses very little resources
- Natural aromatherapy from plants
- May use principles of Feng Shui
- Mindfulness training:
  - » Sight—see natural scenery
  - » Sound—hear the birds and wind
  - » Taste—taste the mint or basil plants from your garden around your gazebo
  - » Touch—feel the textures of the herbs and plants around your gazebo

POSSIBLE FEATURES

- Keep a portable massage table in a corner of your fitness gazebo
- Install a pull-up bar to decompress your spine
- Install attachment sites for exercise elastic bands
- Install a wooden rack for dumbbells and kettlebells
- Install hooks for attaching a hammock
- Install a wood floor so you can perform tai chi, qigong, yoga, or Pilates in your private healing gazebo
- Place a rocking chair in the gazebo for sitting while drinking healing green tea
- Create a healing herb garden to surround your fitness gazebo

Exercise Guidelines

Use the following only as a guide to determine how long, how often, and how hard you should perform each type of activity when designing your home routines. Feel free to adjust the *Sample Exercise Prescription Guidelines for Basic Home Fitness* (Table 13-1) to fit your needs and design your own exercise program (Table 13-2). Similar to a well-balanced meal, a proper home fitness program should at minimum have a warm-up routine, aerobic exercises, strength exercises, and flexibility exercises. If you have other specific needs, you may also need some balance, agility, and reaction exercises.

Table 13-1: Home Exercise Prescription Guidelines for Fitness

Type of Activity	Frequency of Activity	Length of Activity	Intensity of Activity
Warm-Up Exercises	Before each aerobic, strength, or balance routine	5–10 minutes	Gentle movements
Aerobic Routine	5+ days per week of moderate aerobic exercise	30–60 minutes of moderate aerobic exercise	Able to talk during the activity ("talk test")
Strength Routine	2–3 days per week	2–4 sets of 8–12 reps for most adults	Able to count reps out loud, with good form and without pain
Flexibility Routine	At least 2–3 days per week but 7 days per week being the most effective	2–4 sets of 10–30 seconds (or 2–6 diaphragmatic breaths) for most adults. Try to accumulate 60 seconds of total stretch for each flexibility exercise	Able to stretch gently without pain (like a yawn)
Balance or Agility Routine (may include tai chi, qigong, or yoga)	At least 2–3 days per week (if needed)	Approximately 20–30 minutes or more may be needed	Able to perform activity safely
Cool-Down Exercises (see warm-up)	After each aerobic, strength or balance routine	5–10 minutes	Gentle movements

Note: Your healthcare provider or fitness professional may need to modify these guidelines for your specific needs.

Adapted from American College of Sports Medicine. (2018). *ACSM's Guidelines for Exercise Testing and Prescription*, 10th ed. Philadelphia, PA: Wolters Kluwer Lippincott Williams & Wilkins.

TABLE 13-2: HOW TO DESIGN YOUR EXERCISE PROGRAM

DESIGN YOUR OWN EXERCISE ROUTINE	SAMPLE EXERCISE ROUTINE
Select Warm-Up Exercises:	**Select Warmup Exercises:**
(Do before your exercise)	(Do before your exercise)
1 Upper Body _____	1 Upper Body _Shoulder March_
1 Lower Body _____	1 Lower Body _Tai Chi Steps_
Select Aerobic Exercises:	**Select Aerobic Exercises:**
(Do at least 5 days per week)	(Do at least 5 days per week)
Outdoor _____	Outdoor _Neighborhood Walk_
Indoor _____	Indoor _Stationary Bike_
Select Srength Exercises:	**Select Srength Exercises:**
(Do at least 2 days per week)	(Do at least 2 days per week)
2 Core _____	2 Core _Get Ups_
_____	_Bird Dog_
2 Upper Body _____	2 Upper Body _Elastic High Rows_
_____	_Elevated Push-Ups_
2 Lower Body _____	2 Lower Body _Shortstop Squats_
_____	_Supine Bridge_
Select Flexibility Exercises:	**Select Flexibility Exercises:**
(Do at least 2 days per week)	(Do at least 2 days per week)
1 Upper Body _____	1 Upper Body _Yawn Stretch_
1 Lower Body _____	1 Lower Body _Calf Stretch_
Select Balance Exercise:	**Select Balance Exercise:**
(Do at least 2 days per week)	(Do at least 2 days per week)
_____	_Heel Raises_
Select Mind Body Exercise:	**Select Mind Body Exercise:**
(Do in place of aerobic or strength day)	(Do in place of aerobic or strength day)
_____	_Yoga Session_

EXERCISE INDEX

Please note that there are many examples of each type of exercise. The exercises used in this index are only examples used in this book. Yes, there are many fancier warm-up, aerobic, strength, flexibility, and balance exercises than what are described in this book, but I have only provided the basics.

WARM-UP EXERCISES

- Shoulder March
- Heel Sits
- Cat/Camel
- March In Place
- Tai Chi Steps

AEROBIC EXERCISES

- Outdoor Walking
- Treadmill Walking
- Stationary Bicycling

STRENGTH EXERCISES

- Get Ups
- Side Leg Lift
- Bird Dog
- Supine Bridge
- Chair Squats
- Shortstop Squats
- Kettlebell Floor Squat
- Elastic High Rows
- Elastic Low Rows
- Elastic Shoulder Blade Squeezes
- Elevated Push-Ups

FLEXIBILITY EXERCISES

- Squat Stretch
- Outer Hip Stretch
- Inner Hip Stretch
- Hamstring Stretch
- Quad Stretch
- Calf Stretch
- Look-Over-Your-Shoulder Stretch
- Hands-Behind-the-Neck Stretch
- Hands-Behind-the-Back Stretch
- Reach-to-the-Sky Stretch
- Yawn Stretch

BALANCE EXERCISES

- Single-Leg Stance (static balance)
- Heel Raises (dynamic balance)

WARM-UP EXERCISES

A warm-up is a low-intensity large-muscle activity, such as walking or light calisthenics, performed *before* a workout for the purpose of easing you into your exercise session.

Warming up before a workout helps prevent injuries and is essential for optimal sports performance (Bishop 2003, 2003). A warm-up should range from five to 10 minutes, or longer, depending on the activity and your medical condition. The following are some facts about the benefits of warm-up exercises:

- Lack of warm-up prevents blood vessels from having adequate time to properly dilate and supply working muscles and the heart with oxygen. This can result in a rapid rise of blood pressure and possibly myocardial ischemia (Abbott 2013; Barnard et al. 1973). Myocardial ischemia is defined as "an inadequate supply of blood and oxygen to meet the metabolic demands of the heart muscle" (Venes 2013).

- The warm-up allows your body to gradually adjust to increasing physiological, biomechanical, and bioenergetic demands placed upon it.

The following are some traditional warm-up exercises you can use in the comfort of your home. Remember, it has been said by many that "motion is lotion." I typically use these simple exercises when designing home exercise programs for my patients and clients since they cover the basic areas in the body. If you are going to participate in an athletic event like a soccer, basketball, or football game, I highly recommend you look into the excellent FIFA 11+ warm-up routine provided by Fédération Internationale de Football Association (http://f-marc.com). Go to FIFA TV (https://www.youtube.com/user/FIFATV/videos) and search for "FIFA 11" for a description of each exercise.

For your home program, you can either select any of the following warm-up exercises (Figures 13-1 to 13-5) for targeting a specific body area, or you could perform them all in a simple circuit fashion before an aerobic, strength, or balance workout. If you are not sure which warm-up exercises to include for your needs, see a physical therapist or a qualified fitness instructor for guidance.

SHOULDER MARCH

Purpose: To warm up and strengthen the shoulder muscles

Position: On hands and knees

Technique:

- Center your hands under your shoulders and your knees under your hips, with hands shoulder-width apart and knees hip-width apart.
- Gently push your left hand into the floor to activate the left shoulder muscles, while raising the right hand off the floor.

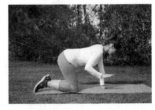
Figure 13-1

- Lower your right hand, and repeat the pushing motion with your right arm.
- Continue slowly marching with your arms—think of a bear lumbering through the woods. It is considered one march when both hands move up and down.
- Do 1 set of 10 repetitions.
- This exercise may be performed daily.

Precautions: Use a soft mat or thick beach towel to cushion your knees. Skip this exercise if it causes pain in your back, neck, shoulders, wrists, or knees. Also, avoid this exercise if you have difficulty or pain getting down to the floor and back up.

Heel Sits

Purpose: To warm up the low back, hips, and knees

Position: On hands and knees

Technique:

- Start with your hands shoulder-width apart and knees hip-width apart, placing your hands slightly in front of your shoulders.
- Slowly bring your hips toward your heels, going only as far as is comfortable without overstretching your knees or lower back.
- Stop the backward movement of the hips toward your heels when you feel a rotation of the pelvis or spine.
- Return to the starting position and repeat.
- Do 1 set of 10 repetitions.
- This exercise may be performed daily.

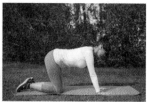
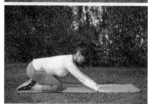

Figure 13-2

Precautions: Use a soft mat or thick beach towel to cushion your knees. Skip this exercise if it causes pain in your back, neck, shoulders, wrist, or knees. Also, avoid this exercise if you have difficulty or pain getting down to the floor and back up. Consult with your healthcare provider or physical therapist before performing this exercise if you've had total hip- or knee-replacement surgery.

Cat/Camel

Purpose: To warm up the core muscles and "lubricate" the spine. Remember, "motion is lotion."

Position: On hands and knees

Technique:

- Center your hands under your shoulders and knees under your hips, with hands shoulder-width apart and knees hip-width apart.
- Gently arch your back toward the ceiling and lower your head slightly.
- Gently lower your abdomen toward the floor as in a scooping motion and lift your head slightly.

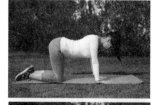
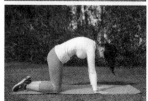

Figure 13-3

- Move your spine between the two midrange positions in a fluid wave-like motion.
- Do 1 set of 10 repetitions.
- This exercise may be performed daily.

Precautions: Use a soft mat or thick beach towel to cushion your knees. Skip this exercise if it causes pain in your back, neck, shoulders, wrist, or knees. Also avoid this exercise if you have difficulty or pain getting down to the floor and back up.

March in Place

Purpose: To warm up the leg muscles and improve coordination and balance

Position: Standing

Technique:

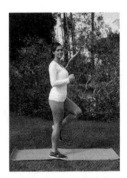

- Start in a standing position with good posture.
- Using an alternate arm and leg motion, march in place.
- Perform 5 normal pace marches, 5 very slow marches, and then 5 fast marches. It is considered one march when both legs move up and down.
- Do 1 set of 10 repetitions, or for 1 minute.
- This exercise may be performed daily.

Figure 13-4

Progression: To increase the difficulty of the exercise, step to the right and then left, forward and then backward, and diagonally forward and then backward as you march.

Precaution: Stand near a solid object for support if you have difficulty with balance or feel unsteady.

Tai Chi Steps

Purpose: To warm up the leg muscles and improve multidirectional coordination and balance

Position: Standing

Technique:

- Standing with good posture, start with your hands on your hips.
- Step straight forward with your right foot (see photo 1), and return to the starting position.
- Step diagonally forward with your right foot (see photo 2), and return to the starting position.

- Step sideways with your right foot (see photo 3), and return to the starting position.
- Repeat the entire 3-step sequence with the left leg. It is considered one set when three steps are completed with the right leg and three steps with the left leg.
- Do 3 sets. No resting between sets.
- This exercise may be performed daily.

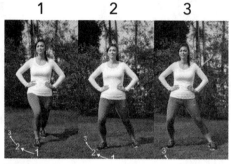

Figure 13-5

Progression: To increase the difficulty of the exercise, move both hands and arms forward (or pushing motion) and backward (or pulling motion) in rhythm (fluid motion like tai chi) with your stepping leg.

Precaution: Stand near a solid object for support if you have difficulty with balance or feel unsteady.

AEROBIC EXERCISES

There are many ways of engaging in aerobic and endurance exercises (also known as cardiorespiratory and cardiovascular fitness) such as walking, hiking, outdoor swimming, outdoor biking, or dancing, plus a variety of sports like tennis, volleyball, soccer, or basketball. Try to perform aerobic exercises at least 3 to 5 times per week. However, a basic low-intensity aerobic program, such as walking, may be performed daily. If you have long work commutes and sit most of the day, an outdoor walk might be your simplest choice for aerobic exercise.

If you are a member of a gym or fitness center, you can choose from an assortment of aerobic training exercises. Try a dance class, elliptical machine, stationary bicycle, recumbent stepper, treadmill, upright bicycle, stair-climber device, ladder-climber device, rowing machine, or an indoor lap pool. Take advantage of all the training tools and expertise a gym or fitness center has to offer. I outline below some common aerobic exercises (Figures 13-6 to 13-8) which may be used as a part of a home program. If going to a gym is not your cup of tea, then spending some money on a quality treadmill or stationary bike for your home may be perfect based on your needs. Look at the descriptions next to each aerobic exercise and decide which one would best fit your home program needs. If you are not sure which aerobic exercises to include for your needs, see a physical therapist or a qualified fitness instructor for guidance.

Outdoor Walking

Benefits of Outdoor Walking:

- Fresh air and sunshine
- Natural bright light for a better mood
- Relaxation by being in nature
- Relief from prolonged sitting positions
- Helps build and maintain bone density for osteoporosis and osteopenia
- Helps relieve back pain for those individuals who find relief with standing and walking

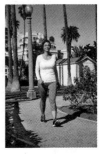

Figure 13-6

Treadmill Walking

Benefits of Treadmill Walking:

- Allows for exercise during cold weather
- Allows for exercise if you have seasonal allergies
- Relief from prolonged sitting positions
- Helps an individual with balance difficulties, especially using a treadmill with two side rails. Once balance is improved, the individual may progress to outdoor walking.
- Helps relieve back pain for those individuals who find relief with standing and walking

Figure 13-7

Stationary Bicycling

Benefits of Stationary Bicycling:

- Allows for exercise during cold weather
- Allows for exercise if you have seasonal allergies
- Relief from prolonged standing positions
- Helps an individual with balance difficulties. Once endurance and lower body strength is improved, the individual may progress to treadmill walking with two side rails or outdoor walking.
- Allows an individual to read and exercise at the same time
- Helps relieve back pain for those individuals who find relief with sitting

Figure 13-8

Strength Exercises

Muscular strength refers to the external force that can be created by a specific muscle or muscle group. *Muscular endurance* is the ability of a muscle group to perform repeated muscle actions over a period of time sufficient to cause muscle fatigue (American College of Sports Medicine 2018).

An article by Vezina et al. (2014) indicates that "strength training by middle-aged and older adults is critical for promoting health, functional fitness, and functional independence." A properly designed strength training program is a safe and effective method for improving muscle strength and reducing weakness in elderly individuals (Aagaard et al. 2010; Coe et al. 2014). The following are practical benefits of strength exercises:

- Greater ability to get in and out of chairs with ease
- Ability to carry groceries and other items without getting injured
- Safer stair climbing
- Greater capacity to do daily chores with more ease
- Increases strength of the bones and muscles for disease prevention (such as osteoporosis and sarcopenia)
- May improve quality of sleep
- May help reduce stress

The following are some traditional strength exercises you can use in the comfort of your home. I typically use these simple exercises when designing home exercise programs for my patients and clients since they cover the basic areas in the body. For your home program, you can either select any of the following strength exercises (Figures 13-9 to 13-19) for targeting a specific body area, or you could perform them all in a simple circuit fashion 2 to 3 times per week for 1 to 2 sets of 10 to 15 repetitions. If you are not sure which strength exercises to include for your needs, see a physical therapist or a qualified fitness instructor for guidance.

Get Ups

Purpose: To strengthen the core. One of the best functional exercises to maintain the ability to get up and down from the floor in a smooth and safe manner. See the study by de Brito et al. (2012) for a practical use of this exercise.

Position: Supine to standing

Technique:

- Start by lying face up on the floor (see photo 1).
- To stand up toward your right side, start by slowly bending your left knee (see photo 2), followed by your right knee to sit down on the floor with your trunk facing to your right (see photo 3).

- Continue pushing off with both hands and placing weight on your feet (see photo 4) as you finally come up to a standing position.
- Now, reverse the sequence by lying down.
- Repeat the sequence of coming up to a standing position toward your left side and then back to lying down. It is considered one repetition when you stand up and then lie back down from both sides.

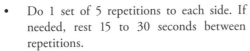

- Do 1 set of 5 repetitions to each side. If needed, rest 15 to 30 seconds between repetitions.
- This exercise may be performed 2 to 3 times per week, every other day. However, it may also be performed daily.

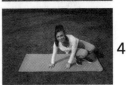

Progression:

- You may also do the exercise while holding a 5- or 10-pound kettlebell in the opposite hand you are using to push off the floor.

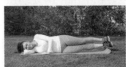

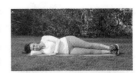

Precautions: Count out loud to promote regular breathing. Skip this exercise if you feel pain in your back, neck, shoulders, elbows, or wrists. Also avoid this exercise if you have difficulty or pain getting down to the floor and back up.

Figure 13-9

SIDE LEG LIFT

Purpose: To strengthen the core (as a modification to a side plank using the arms)

Position: Side-lying

Technique:

- Start by lying on your right side with your right arm under your head for support. Keep your body straight through the shoulder, hip, and knees. Preserve the natural curve in your lower back and neck as you perform this exercise.

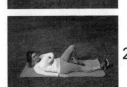

- Place your left hand on the floor in front of your chest for support.

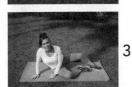

- Slowly lift both legs together so the outside part of your right knee is approximately 1 to 2 inches off the floor.

Figure 13-10

- Hold this position for 3 to 5 seconds, and then relax for 5 to 10 seconds by lowering both legs. It is considered one repetition when both legs are raised and lowered.
- Do 1 to 3 sets of 3 repetitions. Rest 15 to 30 seconds between sets.
- This exercise may be performed 2 to 3 times per week, every other day. However, it may also be performed daily.

Progressions:

- Hold each side leg lift pose for 5 to 10 seconds.
- Do additional sets and repetitions to increase core endurance.
- Other advanced versions of this exercise include side planks. The side plank can be performed by either placing the forearm and knees on the ground, forearm and feet on the ground, or hands and feet on the ground as you lift your hip to form a straight line with your body.

Precautions: Count out loud to promote regular breathing. Use a soft mat or thick beach towel to cushion your hips. Skip this exercise if you feel pain in your back, neck, or shoulders.

Bird Dog

Purpose: To strengthen the core and shoulder muscles

Position: Hands-and-knees

Technique:

- Start in a hands-and-knees position, with your hands shoulder-width and knees hip-width apart. Find the pain-free natural curve in your lower back and neck as you perform this exercise. Stiffen your core muscles just enough to maintain your neck and back curves while still being able to breathe freely.

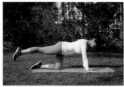
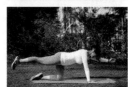

Figure 13-11

- Simultaneously raise your right leg and left arm, thumb pointing to the ceiling and arm approximately 3 to 5 inches away from your head, without losing your spine curve or tilting your hips.
- Slowly return to the starting position, repeating with the opposite leg and arm. It is considered one repetition when both arms and legs are raised and lowered.
- Do 1 to 3 sets of 3 to 5 repetitions. Rest 15 to 30 seconds between sets.
- This exercise may be performed 2 to 3 times per week, every other day. However, it may also be performed daily.

Alternative: This exercise may also be performed with legs or arms only.

Progressions:

- Hold each arm and leg pose for 5 to 10 seconds.
- You may also strap an ankle weight above the knee as extra resistance for strengthening the gluteus maximus muscle (hip and buttocks).

Precautions: Count out loud to promote regular breathing. Use a soft mat or thick beach towel to cushion your knees. Skip this exercise if you feel pain in your back, neck, or shoulders.

SUPINE BRIDGE

Purpose: To strengthen the hips and core

Position: Supine

Technique:

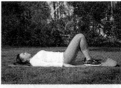

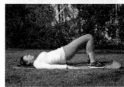

- Lie on your back, with knees bent to 90 degrees.
- Moderately brace or tighten your abdominals and slightly raise your hips while preserving the natural curve in your lower back.
- Return to the starting position.
- Do 1 to 3 sets of 10 repetitions. Rest 15 to 30 seconds between sets.

Figure 13-12

- This exercise may be performed 2 to 3 times per week, every other day. However, it may also be performed daily.

Note: If you feel you are using your hamstrings and not your gluteal muscles, push your feet away from you (but still keeping them on the ground) and tilt your knees slightly outward.

Progressions:

- Hold the bridge pose for 5 to 10 seconds.
- Push your legs outward with elastic bands around your knees.

Precautions: Raising your hips too high might place a strain on your neck. Only raise your hips to where you can slide your forearm under your lower back. Count out loud to promote regular breathing. Skip this exercise if you feel pain in your back, neck, or shoulders.

CHAIR SQUATS

Purpose: To strengthen the legs, hips, and core

Position: Sitting and standing

Technique:

- Push the back of your chair against a wall to keep it from moving away from you as you perform this exercise (or use a sturdy park bench).
- Sit at the edge of the chair with your feet shoulder-width apart and your hands on the top of your thighs.
- Slowly straighten your hips and knees as your trunk leans forward and your knees move slightly in front of your toes as you stand up. Slide both of your hands until your palms are at the front of your hips. Slowly sit back down into the chair as you bend your hips and knees. Think of moving your hips back first and sitting down gently into the chair. Preserve the natural curve in your lower back and neck as you perform this exercise.
- Do 1 to 3 sets of 10 to 15 repetitions. Rest 15 to 30 seconds between sets.
- This exercise may be performed 2 to 3 times per week, every other day. However, it may also be performed daily.

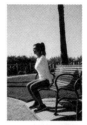
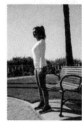

Figure 13-13

Precautions: Count out loud to promote regular breathing. Skip this exercise if you feel pain in your back, hips, or knees.

SHORTSTOP SQUATS

(also called the "ready position" or the "athletic position" in some sports training facilities)

Purpose: To strengthen the legs, hips, and core. May be less painful to the knees than deeper squats

Position: Standing

Technique:

- Stand with your feet shoulder-width apart and hands on the fronts of your thighs.
- Slowly bend your hips and knees as you slide both hands until your fingertips are just above your kneecaps. Be mindful of bringing your hips back and knees at or slightly behind your toes as you squat. Keep your shoulders down and back, and your knees slightly out. Preserve the natural curve in your lower back and neck as you perform this exercise. Do not squat any lower than your ability

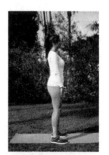
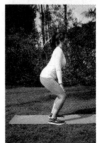

Figure 13-14

to maintain your natural lower back and neck curves. This will vary from person to person.

- Do 1 to 3 sets of 10 to 15 repetitions. Rest 15 to 30 seconds between sets.
- This exercise may be performed 2 to 3 times per week, every other day. However, it may also be performed daily.

Note: To get a little extra power, gently press your feet outward without actually rotating the feet (think of screwing the feet into the ground).

Precautions: Count out loud to promote regular breathing. Skip this exercise if you feel pain in your back, hips, or knees.

KETTLEBELL FLOOR SQUAT

Purpose: To strengthen the legs, hips, and core

Position: Standing

Technique:

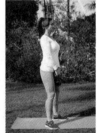

- Choose a weight based on your fitness level (such as 5-, 7-, or 10-pound kettlebells for beginners).
- Stand with your feet shoulder-width apart as you hold a kettlebell close to your body with your arms straight down.
- Slowly bend your hips and knees, keeping the knees at or slightly behind your toes as you bring the kettlebell as close to the floor as possible without losing the natural curve in your lower back. As you squat, keep your shoulders down and back and your knees out. Do not squat any lower than your ability to maintain your natural lower back and neck curves. This will vary from person to person.

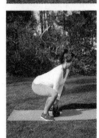

- Do 1 to 3 sets of 10 to 15 repetitions. Rest 15 to 30 seconds between sets.
- This exercise may be performed 2 to 3 times per week, every other day.

Figure 13-15

Alternative: If needed, place a 4-, 6-, or 8-inch block or pad on the floor to stop the kettlebell at a point where your lower back can no longer maintain its natural curve.

Precautions: Stop the squatting motion if you lose the curve in your lower back. Do not force the kettlebell to the floor. Have someone watch your back and give you feedback as you squat. Count out loud to promote regular breathing. Skip this exercise if you feel pain in your back, hips, or knees.

ELASTIC HIGH ROWS

Purpose: To strengthen the shoulders, upper back, and core

Position: Sitting or standing

Technique:

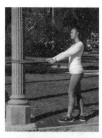

- Start in a sitting or standing position with good posture.
- Place an elastic band around a sturdy object, such as the knob of a securely shut door, a rail, or a post, and step back just enough so the band has some tension.
- Pull or "row" the band from an arms-outstretched position to the elbows-by-your-sides position.
- Do 1 to 3 sets of 10 to 15 repetitions. Rest 15 to 30 seconds between sets.
- This exercise may be performed 2 to 3 times per week, every other day.

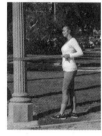

Figure 13-16

Precautions: Count out loud to promote regular breathing. Skip this exercise if you feel pain in your back, neck, shoulders, or arms.

ELASTIC LOW ROWS

Purpose: To strengthen the shoulders, upper back, and core

Position: Sitting or standing

Technique:

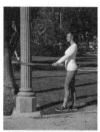

- Start in a sitting or standing position with good posture.
- Place an elastic band around a sturdy object, such as the knob of a securely shut door, a rail, or a post, and step back just enough so the band has some tension.
- Pull the band from an arms-outstretched position to the hands-by-your-hips position.
- Do 1 to 3 sets of 10 to 15 repetitions. Rest 15 to 30 seconds between sets.
- This exercise may be performed 2 to 3 times per week, every other day.

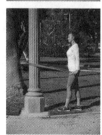

Precautions: Count out loud to promote regular breathing. Skip this exercise if you feel pain in your back, neck, shoulders, or arms.

Figure 13-17

Elastic Shoulder Blade Squeezes

Purpose: To strengthen the shoulders and upper back

Position: Sitting or standing

Technique:

- Start in a sitting or standing position with good posture.
- Place an elastic band in your hands with your palms facing up and your elbows in a bent position.
- Pull the band apart approximately 8 to 10 inches and squeeze your shoulder blades together while keeping your elbows by your sides.
- Do 1 to 3 sets of 10 to 15 repetitions. Rest 15 to 30 seconds between sets.
- This exercise may be performed 2 to 3 times per week, every other day.

Precautions: Count out loud to promote regular breathing. Skip this exercise if you feel pain in your back, neck, shoulders, or arms.

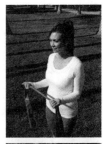
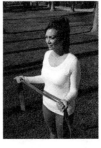

Figure 13-18

Elevated Push-Ups

Purpose: To strengthen the shoulders, chest, arms, and core (front plank)

Position: Standing

Technique:

- Stand and place your hands shoulder-width apart on a bed or other surface that is midthigh to knee height.
- Take several steps backward, placing the fronts of both feet about hip-width apart. Keep your core tight and preserve the natural curve in your lower back and neck as you bend your elbows.
- Stop when your face is approximately 6 inches from the bed, and then push back to the elbows-straight position.
- Do 1 to 3 sets of 10 to 15 repetitions. Rest 15 to 30 seconds between sets.
- This exercise may be performed 2 to 3 times per week, every other day.

Figure 13-19

Precautions: Count out loud to promote regular breathing. Skip this exercise if you feel pain in your back, neck, shoulders, or arms, or have weakness that might lead to injury due to lack of control.

FLEXIBILITY EXERCISES

"*Flexibility* is the ability to move a single joint or series of joints smoothly and easily through an unrestricted, pain-free range of motion" (Kisner et al. 2018). Stretching keeps muscles and joints mobile, and it promotes ease in activities such as bending to tie your shoes or reaching the buttons at the ATM drive-thru. Stretching can be used for relaxing, correcting asymmetries, and increasing range of motion. The following are other practical benefits of stretching and flexibility exercises:

- Reduce muscle tension, pain, and mental stress
- Increase circulation
- Improve posture
- Improve function for daily tasks, such as putting on socks (hip and knee mobility) or removing your coat (shoulder mobility)

Athletes and sports participants should use caution before exercise, activity, and sports, since static stretching has been shown to acutely decrease maximal strength (Fowles et al. 2000; Winchester et al. 2009), strength endurance (Nelson et al. 2005), power (jumping) (Behm et al. 2007), sprint performance (Paradisis et al. 2014; Winchester et al. 2008), performance in short endurance bouts (Lowery et al. 2014), and provides no added benefits to dynamic stretching in terms of injury prevention in high school soccer athletes (Zakaria et al. 2015). Therefore, focusing on dynamic warm-ups before activity or sports participation, and maybe gentle static stretching *after* activity or sports participation might be more beneficial.

The key is to avoid aggressive stretching for general fitness purposes. Keep in mind that you may sometimes need aggressive stretching during certain rehabilitation programs (such as after knee or shoulder surgery). Your physical therapist will guide you in these situations. Remember to stay active throughout the day with a variety of movements (squatting, bending, reaching, and turning) and avoid prolonged sitting or standing positions. This may help minimize or prevent you from getting stiff muscles. As an alternative to stretching, in some cases you could perform tai chi, qigong, yoga, Pilates, and the Feldenkrais Method, which incorporate flexibility and range of motion, into the routines used here.

The following are some traditional flexibility exercises you can use in the comfort of your home. I typically use these simple exercises when designing home exercise programs for my patients and clients since they cover the basic areas in the body. For your home program, you can either select any of the following flexibility exercises (Figures 13-20 to 13-30) for targeting a specific body area, or you could perform them all in a simple circuit fashion after an aerobic, strength, or balance workout. If you are not sure which flexibility exercises to include for your needs, see a physical therapist or a qualified fitness instructor for guidance.

SQUAT STRETCH

Purpose: To stretch the leg and hip muscles
Position: Squatting
Technique:

- Stand with your legs shoulder-width apart.
- Slowly squat down as far as you can go comfortably. Hold the gentle stretch position for 10 to 15 seconds. Stand up and relax for 5 to 10 seconds.
- Do 1 to 3 sets.
- This exercise may be performed daily.

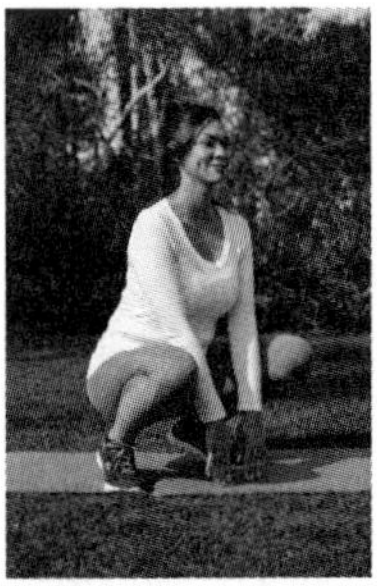

Progression: Try keeping your heels on the ground during the stretch.

Figure 13-20

Precautions: Breathe naturally during the stretch to allow for relaxation. If needed, hold on to a sturdy object for support. Skip this exercise if you feel pain in your back, hips, knees, or ankles. Consult with your healthcare provider or physical therapist before performing this exercise if you've had total hip- or knee-replacement surgery.

OUTER HIP STRETCH

Purpose: To stretch the outer hip muscles

Position: Supine

Technique:

- Lie on your back with both knees bent comfortably.
- Slowly bend your left hip and knee so the outer part of your left foot rests on top of your right thigh.
- Place your right hand on the outer part of your left knee, and very gently apply a force

Figure 13-21

toward you until you feel a stretch in the outer left hip. Hold the gentle stretch position for 10 to 30 seconds. Relax for 5 to 10 seconds.
- Repeat with the other leg.
- Do 1 to 3 sets.
- This exercise may be performed daily.

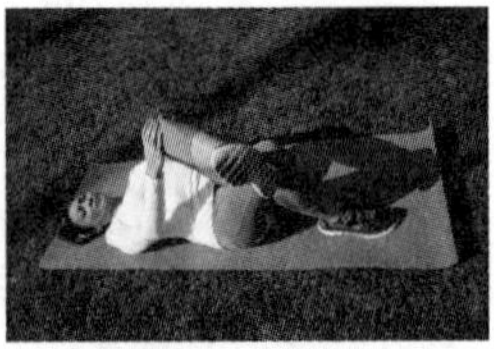

Precautions: Use a small rolled-up towel to support the natural curve in your lower back and a small pillow under your head for support, if needed. Breathe naturally during the stretch to allow for relaxation. Skip this exercise if you feel pain in your back, hips, or knees. Consult with your healthcare provider or physical therapist before performing this exercise if you've had total hip- or knee-replacement surgery.

INNER HIP STRETCH

Purpose: To stretch the inner hip muscles

Position: Supine

Technique:

Figure 13-22

- Lie on your back with both knees bent comfortably.
- Slowly bend your left hip and knee so the outer part of your left foot rests on top of your right thigh.
- Place your left hand on the inner part of your left knee, and very gently apply a force away from you until you feel a stretch in the inner left hip. Hold the gentle stretch position for 10 to 30 seconds. Relax for 5 to 10 seconds.
- Repeat with the other leg.
- Do 1 to 3 sets.
- This exercise may be performed daily.

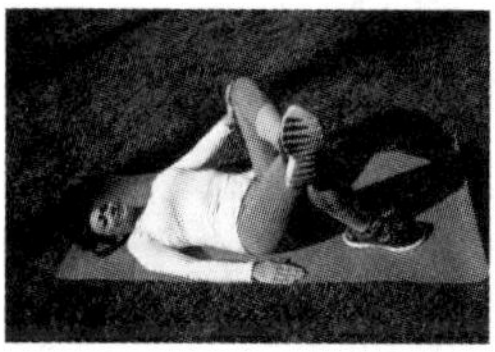

Precautions: Use a small rolled-up towel to support the natural curve in your lower back and a small pillow under your head for support, if needed. Breathe naturally during the stretch to allow for relaxation. Skip this exercise if you feel pain in your back, hips, or knees. Consult with your healthcare provider or physical therapist before performing this exercise if you've had total hip- or knee-replacement surgery.

HAMSTRING STRETCH WITH ANKLE PUMPS

Purpose: To stretch the posterior thigh and calf muscles

Position: Supine

Technique:

- Lie on your back with both knees bent comfortably.
- Place both hands around the back of your upper left leg and bring it toward your chest so it is at arm's length.
- Slowly straighten your left knee until you feel a gentle hamstring stretch.

- Slowly and gently pump your left ankle back and forth, flexing and straightening the foot for 10 repetitions. It is considered one repetition when the foot moves up and down one time.
- Repeat with the other leg.
- Do 1 to 3 sets.
- This exercise may be performed daily.

Alternative: If you are unable to reach the back of your upper leg comfortably, wrap a towel around your upper leg and hold the towel.

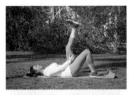

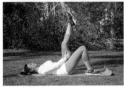

Precautions: Use a small rolled-up towel to support the natural curve in your lower back and a small pillow under your head for support, if needed. Breathe naturally during the stretch to allow for relaxation. Skip this exercise if you feel pain in your back, hips, or knees.

Figure 13-23

QUADRICEPS STRETCH

Purpose: To stretch the anterior thigh muscles

Position: Side-lying

Technique:

- Lie on your left side with both knees bent comfortably. Preserve the natural curve in your lower back and neck as you perform this exercise.
- Using your right hand, grip your right ankle and bring the heel of your right foot toward the back of your hip (or buttocks). Feel the

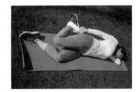

Figure 13-24

 stretch in the front of your right thigh muscles from your knee to the front of your hip. Hold the gentle stretch position for 10 to 30 seconds. Relax for 5 to 10 seconds.
- Repeat with the other leg once you have completed all sets on the right leg.
- Do 1 to 3 sets.
- This exercise may be performed daily.

Alternate: If you have difficulty reaching your ankle, use a towel as an extension (as shown in the photo) to avoid straining your lower back and shoulder.

Precaution: Breathe naturally during the stretch to allow for relaxation. Skip this exercise if you feel pain in your shoulders, neck, back, hips, or knees.

CALF STRETCH

Purpose: To stretch the calf muscles

Position: Standing

Technique:

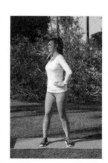

- Stand with your feet hip-width apart. Preserve the natural curve in your lower back and neck as you perform this exercise.
- Place both hands, at about shoulder height, on a wall in front of you.
- Position your right leg in front of you with your right knee slightly bent for support.
- Step back with your left leg, keeping your left knee straight and left foot pointed forward.
- Lean slightly with your hips and torso until you feel a gentle stretch in your left calf, heel cord, and a little in front of your right hip. Hold the gentle stretch position for 10 to 30 seconds. Relax for 5 to 10 seconds.

Figure 13-25

- Repeat with the other leg.
- Do 1 to 3 sets.
- This exercise may be performed daily.

Alternative: For variety, try turning your back foot in or out slightly as you stretch.

Precautions: You might also feel a stretch in the front of the hips, especially if they are tight. Breathe naturally during the stretch to allow for relaxation. Skip this exercise you feel pain in your back, hips, or knees.

LOOK-OVER-YOUR-SHOULDER STRETCH

Purpose: To stretch the chest, shoulders, and back

Position: Standing

Technique:

- Stand erect with good posture and your feet shoulder-width apart.
- Place your hands on your hips.
- Slowly and gently turn your entire trunk and neck so you are looking over your right shoulder for 5 to 10 seconds. Do not force the stretch, and do not bounce.
- Then, slowly and gently turn your trunk and neck so you are looking over your left shoulder for 5 to 10 seconds. Do not force the stretch, and do not bounce.

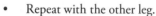

Figure 13-25

- Do 1 to 3 sets.
- This exercise may be performed daily.

Precautions: Breathe naturally during the stretch to allow for relaxation. Skip this exercise if you feel pain in your neck, shoulders, or back. Also, avoid this exercise if you experience dizziness, lightheadedness, or vertigo and report these symptoms to your healthcare provider.

HANDS-BEHIND-THE-BACK STRETCH

Purpose: To stretch the chest, arms, and shoulders

Position: Standing

Technique:

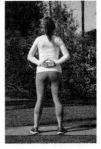

- Stand straight with your feet shoulder-width apart. Preserve the natural curve in your lower back and neck as you perform this exercise.
- Place both hands behind your hips until you feel a light stretching sensation in your shoulders and chest. To increase the stretch, bring your shoulders back. Hold the gentle stretch position for 10 to 30 seconds.
- Do 1 to 3 sets.
- This exercise may be performed daily.

Figure 13-26

Precautions: Breathe naturally during the stretch to allow for relaxation. Skip this exercise if you feel pain in your neck, shoulders, or back.

HAND-BEHIND-THE-NECK STRETCH

Purpose: To stretch the chest, arms, and shoulders
Position: Standing
Technique:

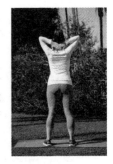

- Stand straight with your feet shoulder-width apart. Preserve the natural curve in your lower back and neck as you perform this exercise.
- Place both hands behind your neck until you feel a light stretching sensation in the back of your arms and shoulders. To increase the stretch, bring your elbows closer to your head. Hold the gentle stretch position for 10 to 30 seconds.
- Do 1 to 3 sets.
- This exercise may be performed daily.

Figure 13-27

Precautions: Breathe naturally during the stretch to allow for relaxation. Skip this exercise if you feel pain in your neck, shoulders, or back.

REACH-TO-THE-SKY STRETCH

Purpose: To stretch the shoulders, arms, and upper back muscles

Position: Standing

Technique:

- Stand with your feet shoulder-width apart, hands by your sides, and thumbs facing forward. Preserve the natural curve in your lower back as you perform this exercise.
- Raise both arms overhead with your palms facing the sky and fingers pointing toward the middle of your body to feel a stretch in your upper back. Finally, yawn as you stretch to relax your facial muscles. Hold the gentle stretch position for 5 seconds.
- Do 1 to 3 sets.
- This exercise may be performed multiple times throughout the day.

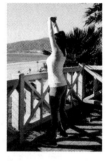

Figure 13-28

Note: Perform the stretch after you have been sitting for prolonged periods, such as after using the computer, watching television, reading a book, sewing or knitting, or driving.

Precautions: Breathe naturally during the stretch to allow for relaxation. Skip this exercise if you feel pain in your neck, shoulders, arms, or back.

YAWN STRETCH

Purpose: To stretch the chest, shoulders, arms, and upper back muscles

Position: Standing

Technique:

- Stand with your feet shoulder-width apart, hands by your sides, and thumbs facing forward. Preserve the natural curve in your lower back as you perform this exercise.
- Rotate your thumbs away from the sides of your body, bend your palms away from the inner part of your wrist, and draw your shoulders slightly back to feel a stretch in your forearms, shoulders, and chest (see photo 1). Hold the gentle stretch position for 5 seconds.
- Bring your arms up to shoulder level, bend your palms away from the inner parts of wrists (palms facing the side walls), and draw your

shoulders slightly back to feel a stretch in your forearms, shoulders, and chest (see photo 2). Hold the gentle stretch position for 5 seconds.

- Raise both arms overhead with your palms facing the ceiling and fingers pointing toward the middle of your body to feel a stretch in your upper back (see photo 3). Finally, yawn as you stretch to relax your facial muscles. Hold the gentle stretch position for 5 seconds.
- Do 1 to 3 sets.
- This exercise may be performed multiple times throughout the day.

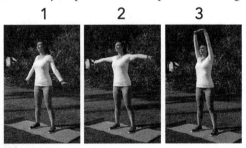

Figure 13-29

Note: Perform the stretch after you have been sitting for prolonged periods, such as after using the computer, watching television, reading a book, sewing or knitting, or driving.

Precautions: Breathe naturally during the stretch to allow for relaxation. Skip this exercise if you feel pain in your neck, shoulders, arms, or back.

BALANCE EXERCISES

Balance, or postural stability, is "the ability to control the center of mass within the boundaries of the base of support" (O'Sullivan 2014). Balance can be either stationary (such as holding a position in standing, sitting, or kneeling) or dynamic (such as with movement during weight shifting from one foot to another, reaching, or stepping). The following are practical areas of improvement from applying balance exercises (Oliveira et al. 2017):

- Walking on uneven surfaces, such as grass, a mountain trail, or old sidewalks
- Going up and down curbs, and climbing stairs without a rail
- Avoiding falls when somebody lightly bumps into you
- Steadily carrying a food plate
- Safely getting in and out of the bathtub
- Reducing injury during sports participation

Balance can be modified by changing feet positions, such as a narrow versus a wide stance, a tandem stance (heel-to-toe position), or a step stance (one foot in front of the other during a normal step), and by keeping your eyes open or closed.

Also, balance exercises can be performed with both legs or using one leg. Finally, try talking during postural stability exercises since it may optimize dynamic control (Massery et al. 2013). As an alternative to traditional balance exercises, in some cases you could perform tai chi, qigong, yoga, Pilates, and the Feldenkrais Method which incorporate balance and agility into the routines used.

Stationary balance exercises can be performed on a stable surface, such as the floor or a low balance beam. Stationary balance exercises can also be performed on an unstable surface, such as a wobble board, hard disc, soft disc, soft stepping pods, foam rubber pad, half foam roll, mini trampoline, or BOSU ball (an exercise tool that has a dome side and platform side, and stands for "both sides up").

The following are types of static and dynamic balance exercises you can use in the comfort of your home. I typically use these simple exercises when designing home exercise programs for my patients and clients. For your home program, you can either select any of the following balance exercises (Figures 13-30 and 13-31) for targeting a specific need, or you could perform both of them as a part of your weekly program. If you are not sure which balance exercises to include for your needs, see a physical therapist or a qualified fitness instructor for guidance.

SINGLE-LEG STANCE

Purpose: To improve static balance

Position: Standing

Technique:

- Stand with your feet hip-width apart near a sturdy object (such as a chair) for support. Keep your eyes open throughout the exercise.
- Slowly lift your right foot off the ground to about midcalf level, without touching your left leg. Hold this position in a safe and steady manner for 1 to 15 seconds, depending on your ability.
- Repeat on the other side.
- Do 3 to 5 sets.
- This exercise may be performed 2 to 3 times per week, every other day. However, it may also be performed daily.

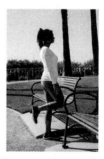

Figure 13-30

Progressions: If you are able to easily stand on each leg for 30 seconds, try the following:

- Slowly swing your arms up and down like you are marching.
- Move your arms across your chest and open them out to the sides.

- Twirl a small towel in your right hand and then your left hand.

Precautions: Breathe naturally during the exercise. Skip this exercise if you experience dizziness, lightheadedness, or vertigo and report these symptoms to your healthcare provider. Also, avoid this exercise if you feel unstable and cannot maintain a safe upright posture. The key is safety and preventing a fall.

HEEL RAISES

Purpose: To strengthen the lower legs and help improve dynamic balance

Position: Standing

Technique:

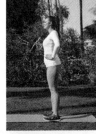

- Stand with your feet hip-width apart and toes pointing straight ahead. Have a sturdy object, such as the back of a chair, to hold on to for safety (only if you have difficulty with balance).
- Slowly raise your heels off the ground as far as is comfortable and return to the starting position.
- Do 1 to 3 sets of 10 to 15 repetitions.
- This exercise may be performed 2 to 3 times per week, every other day. However, it may also be performed daily.

Progressions:

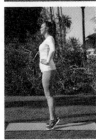

- Perform the exercise without shoes.
- Perform the exercise one leg at a time (with or without holding on for balance).

Precautions: Count out loud to promote regular breathing. Skip this exercise if you feel pain in your back, hips, or knees. Also, avoid this exercise if you feel unstable and cannot maintain a safe upright posture. The key is safety and preventing a fall.

Figure 13-31

BOX 11: HOLISTIC HEALING

FIDGETING AT WORK TO BURN CALORIES AND PREVENT STIFFNESS

A study shows that people who fidget more while standing burned more calories than those who don't fidget as much (Levine et al. 2000). The researchers called it "nonexercise activity thermogenesis" (NEAT, for short). An article by Levine et al. (2006) states that "NEAT is the energy expenditure of all physical activities other than volitional [the act of choosing] sporting-like exercise. NEAT includes all those activities that render us vibrant, unique, and independent beings such as going to work, playing guitar, toe-tapping, and dancing."

You can create your own fidgeting activities and movements such as the following:

- Push up from your chair, and frequently adjust the way you sit. Remember, variable sitting postures are good for preventing stiffness and pressure.
- Change the way you cross your arms and legs, but don't keep your legs crossed too long. It's not the best choice for good circulation.
- Tap your feet while sitting or standing.
- Do the heel-up and toe-up exercise while sitting.
- Turn your feet inward and outward, like windshield wipers, while sitting.
- Bend and straighten your legs one at a time while sitting.
- Wiggle your toes.
- Rise up onto your toes while standing.
- Pinch your shoulder blades together.
- Reach overhead.
- Smile and frown a couple of times to contract and relax your facial muscles.
- Gently turn your head right and left.
- Open and close your hands.
- Stand up and gently shake a leg, like a track athlete before a run.
- Stand up and gently shake your arms, like a swimmer before a race.

Fidgeting not only burns calories, but keeps you from getting stiff and blood flowing freely throughout your body and to your brain. These are all good reasons to keep moving and avoid the "potted plant syndrome."

ADDITIONAL RESOURCES

- International Proprioceptive Neuromuscular Facilitation Association, www.ipnfa.org
- Prague School of Rehabilitation, www.rehabps.com
- PTNow—Rehabilitation Reference Center, www.ptnow.org (this site provides evidence-based exercise prescription for many conditions and diseases).
- Refer to the following books to obtain further information about evidence-based exercises:
  » *ACSM's Guidelines for Exercise Testing and Prescription* (2018)
  » *Therapeutic Exercise: Foundations and Techniques* (2018)
  » *Therapeutic Exercise: Moving Toward Function* (2018)
  » *Essentials of Strength Training and Conditioning* (2016)

REFERENCES

Linn D. (1999). *Feng Shui for the Soul: How to Create a Harmonious Environment That Will Nurture and Sustain You.* Carlsbad, CA: Hay House Inc.

SantoPierto N. (2002). *Feng Shui and Health: The Anatomy of A Home: Using Feng Shui to Disarm Illness, Accelerate Recovery, and Create Optimal Health.* New York, NY: Three Rivers Press.

Venes D. (Ed.) (2017). *Taber's Cyclopedic Medical Dictionary,* 23rd ed. Philadelphia, PA: FA Davis.

Benefits of Warm-Up and Cooldown Exercises

Abbott AA. (2013). Cardiac arrest litigations. *ACSM's Health & Fitness Journal* 17 (1): 31–34.

Allen BA, Hannon JC, Burns RD, et al. (2014). Effect of a core conditioning intervention on tests of trunk muscular endurance in school-aged children. *Journal of Strength and Conditioning Research* 28 (7): 2063–2070.

American College of Sports Medicine. (2014). *ACSM's Resource Manual for Guidelines for Exercise Testing and Prescription,* 7th ed. Philadelphia, PA: Wolters Kluwer Lippincott Williams & Wilkins.

American College of Sports Medicine. (2018). *ACSM's Guidelines for Exercise Testing and Prescription,* 10th ed. Philadelphia, PA: Wolters Kluwer.

Andersen LL, Jay K, Andersen CH, et al. (2013). Acute effects of massage or active exercise in relieving muscle soreness: Randomized controlled trial. *Journal of Strength and Conditioning Research* 27 (12): 3352–3359.

Barnard RJ, Gardner GW, Diaco NV, et al. (1973). Cardiovascular responses to sudden strenuous exercise: Heart rate, blood pressure, and ECG. *Journal of Applied Physiology* 34: 883.

Bishop D. (2003). Warm up I: Potential mechanisms and the effects of passive warm up on exercise performance. *Sports Medicine* 33 (6): 439–454.

Bishop D. (2003). Warm up II: Performance changes following active warm up and how to structure the warm up. *Sports Medicine* 33 (7): 483–498.

Brubaker PH, Kitzman DW. (2011). Chronotropic incompetence: Causes, consequences, and management. *Circulation* 123 (9): 1010–1020.

Dimsdale JE, Hartley LH, Guiney T, et al. (1984). Postexercise peril. Plasma catecholamines and exercise. *JAMA* 251 (5): 630–632.

Haff GG, Triplett NT. (Eds.). (2016). *Essentials of Strength Training and Conditioning,* 4th ed. Champaign IL: Human Kinetics.

Kenney WL, Wilmore JH, Costill DL. (2012). *Physiology of Sport and Exercise,* 5th ed. Champaign, IL: Human Kinetics.

Kisner C, Colby LA, Borstad J. (2018). *Therapeutic Exercise: Foundations and Techniques,* 7th ed. Philadelphia, PA: FA Davis.

Koyama Y, Koike A, Yajima T, et al. (2000). Effects of 'cool-down' during exercise recovery on cardiopulmonary systems in patients with coronary artery disease. *Japanese Circulation Journal* 64 (3): 191–196.

Law RY, Herbert RD. (2007). Warm-up reduces delayed onset muscle soreness but cool-down does not: A randomised controlled trial. *Australian Journal of Physiotherapy* 53 (2): 91–95.

Olsen O, Sjohaug M, van Beekvelt M, et al. (2012). The effect of warm-up and cool-down exercise on delayed onset muscle soreness in the quadriceps muscle: A randomized controlled trial. *Journal of Human Kinetics* 35: 59–68.

Paton CM, Nagelkirk PR, Coughlin AM, et al. (2004). Changes in von Willebrand factor and fibrinolysis following a post-exercise cool-down. *European Journal of Applied Physiology* 92 (3): 328–333.

Spitz MG, Kenefick RW, Mitchell JB. (2013). The effects of elapsed time after warm-up on subsequent exercise performance in a cold environment. *Journal of Strength and Conditioning Research* 28 (5): 1351–1357.

Stickland MK, Rowe BH, Spooner CH, et al. (2012). Effect of warm-up exercise on exercise-induced bronchoconstriction. *Medicine and Science in Sports and Exercise* 44 (3): 383–391.

Takahashi T, Okada A, Hayano J, et al. (2002). Influence of cool-down exercise on autonomic control of heart rate during recovery from dynamic exercise. *Frontiers of Medical and Biological Engineering* 11 (4): 249–259.

Van Gelder LH, Bartz SD. (2011). The effect of acute stretching on agility performance. *Journal of Strength and Conditioning Research* 25 (11): 3014–3021.

Venes D. (Ed.) (2017). *Taber's Cyclopedic Medical Dictionary,* 23rd ed. Philadelphia, PA: FA Davis.

Warm-Up and Mobility Exercises

Andersen CH, Zebis MK, Saervoll, et al. (2012). Scapular muscle activity from selected strengthening exercises performed at low and high intensities. *Journal of Strength and Conditioning Research* 26 (9): 2408–2416.

Brügger A. (2000). *Lehbruch der Funktionellen* Störungen *des Bewegungssystems. [Textbook of the functional disturbances of the movement system].* Zollikon/Benglen, Switzerland: Brügger-Verlag.

Fung V, Ho A, Shaffer J, et al. (2012). Use of Nintendo Wii Fit™ in the rehabilitation of outpatients following total knee replacement: A preliminary randomised controlled trial. *Physiotherapy* 98 (3): 183–188.

Ha SM, Kwon OY, Cynn HS, et al. (2012). Comparison of electromyographic activity of the lower trapezius and serratus anterior muscle in different arm-lifting scapular posterior tilt exercises. *Physical Therapy in Sport* 13 (4): 227–232.

Hardwick DH, Beebe JA, McDonnell MK, et al. (2006). A comparison of serratus anterior muscle activation during a wall slide exercise and other traditional exercises. *Journal of Orthopaedic & Sports Physical Therapy* 36 (12): 903–910.

Janda V, Vávrová M. (1996). Sensory motor stimulation. In: Liebenson C. (Ed.) *Rehabilitation of the Spine: A Practitioner's Manual.* Philadelphia, PA: Lippincott Williams & Wilkins.

Kobesova A, Dzvonik J, Pavel Kolar P, et al. (2015). Effects of shoulder girdle dynamic stabilization exercise on hand muscle strength. *Isokinetics and Exercise Science* 23: 21–32.

Kurokawa D, Sano H, Nagamoto H, et al. (2014). Muscle activity pattern of the shoulder external rotators differs in adduction and abduction: An analysis using positron emission tomography. *Journal of Shoulder and Elbow Surgery* 23 (5): 658–664.

Lee S, Lee D, Park J. (2013). The effect of hand position changes on electromyographic activity of shoulder stabilizers during push-up plus exercise on stable and unstable surfaces. *Journal of Physical Therapy Science* 25 (8): 981–984.

Ludewig PM, Hoff MS, Osowski EE, et al. (2004). Relative balance of serratus anterior and upper trapezius muscle activity during push-up exercises. *American Journal of Sports Medicine* 32 (2): 484–493.

McGill SM. (2016). *Low Back Disorders,* 3rd ed. Champaign IL: Human Kinetics.

McGill SM. (2014). *Building the Ultimate Back: From Rehabilitation to Performance* (course manual). Los Angeles, CA, April 26–27.

Morris CE, Greenman PE, Bullock MI, et al. (2006). Vladimir Janda, MD, DSc: Tribute to a master of rehabilitation. *Spine (Phila Pa 1976)* 31 (9): 1060–1064.

Moseley JB, Jobe FW, Pink M, et al. (1992). EMG analysis of the scapular muscles during a shoulder rehabilitation program. *American Journal of Sports Medicine* 20 (2):128–134.

Preisinger E, Alacamlioglu Y, Pils K, et al. (1996). Exercise therapy for osteoporosis: Results of a randomised controlled trial. *British Journal of Sports Medicine* 30 (3): 209–212.

Sahrmann SA. (2002). *Diagnosis and Treatment of Movement Impairment Syndromes.* St. Louis, MO: Mosby.

Seo SH, Jeon IH, Cho YH, et al. (2013). Surface EMG during the push-up plus exercise on a stable support or Swiss ball: Scapular stabilizer muscle exercise. *Journal of Physical Therapy Science* 25 (7): 833–837.

Shinozaki N, Sano H, Omi R, et al. (2014). Differences in muscle activities during shoulder elevation in patients with symptomatic and asymptomatic rotator cuff tears: Analysis by positron emission tomography. *Journal of Shoulder and Elbow Surgery* 23 (3): e61–67.

Yamada M, Higuchi T, Nishiguchi S, et al. (2013). Multitarget stepping program in combination with a standardized multicomponent exercise program can prevent falls in community-dwelling older adults: A randomized, controlled trial. *Journal of the American Geriatrics Society* 61 (10): 1669–1675.

Yamada M, Tanaka B, Nagai K, et al. (2011). Rhythmic stepping exercise under cognitive conditions improves fall risk factors in community-dwelling older adults: Preliminary results of a cluster-randomized controlled trial. *Aging and Mental Health* 15 (5): 647–653.

Benefits of Aerobic Exercise

American College of Sports Medicine. (2018). *ACSM's Guidelines for Exercise Testing and Prescription,* 10th ed. Philadelphia, PA: Wolters Kluwer Lippincott Williams & Wilkins.

Birnbaum MH. (1984). Nearpoint visual stress: A physiological model. *Journal of the American Optometric Association* 55 (11): 825–835.

Birnbaum MH. (1985). Nearpoint visual stress: Clinical implications. *Journal of the American Optometric Association* 56 (6): 480–490.

Carson SJ. (2013). Effects of emotional exposure on state anxiety after acute exercise. *Medicine & Science in Sports & Exercise* 45 (2): 372–378.

Chapman SB, Aslan S, Spence JS, et al. (2013). Shorter term aerobic exercise improves brain, cognition, and cardiovascular fitness in aging. *Frontiers in Aging Neuroscience* 5: 75.

Earnest CP, Johannsen NM, Swift DL, et al. (2014). Aerobic and strength training in concomitant metabolic syndrome and Type 2 diabetes. *Medicine and Science in Sports and Exercise* 46 (7): 1293–1301.

Erickson KI, Raji CA, Lopez OL, et al. (2010). Physical activity predicts gray matter volume in late adulthood. The Cardiovascular Health Study. *Neurology* 75 (16): 1415–1422.

Pedersen BK, Saltin B. (2006). Evidence for prescribing exercise as therapy in chronic disease. *Scandinavian Journal of Medicine and Science in Sports* 16 (Supplement 1): 3–63.

Aerobic Exercises

Birnbaum MH. (1984). Nearpoint visual stress: A physiological model. *Journal of the American Optometric Association* 55 (11): 825–835.

Birnbaum MH. (1985). Nearpoint visual stress: Clinical implications. *Journal of the American Optometric Association* 56 (6): 480–490.

Buckwalter JA. (2003). Sports, joint injury, and posttraumatic osteoarthritis. *Journal of Orthopaedic & Sports Physical Therapy* 33 (10): 578–588.

Holick MF. (2010). *The Vitamin D Solution: A 3-Step Strategy to Cure Our Most Common Health Problem.* New York, NY: Hudson Street Press.

Kuster MS. (2002). Exercise recommendations after total joint replacement. *Sports Medicine* 32 (7): 433–445.

Turner PL Mainster MA. (2008). Circadian photoreception: Ageing and the eye's important role in systemic health. *British Journal of Ophthalmology* 92 (11): 1439–1444.

Benefits of Strength and Core-Strengthening Exercises

Aagaard P, Suetta C, Caserotti P, et al. (2010). Role of the nervous system in sarcopenia and muscle atrophy with aging: Strength training as a countermeasure. *Scandinavian Journal of Medicine & Sciencein Sports* 20 (1): 49–64.

Akuthota V, Ferreiro A, Moore T. (2008). Core stability exercise principles. *Current Sports Medicine Reports* 7 (1): 39–44.

Alley JR, Mazzochi JW, Smith CJ, et al. (2015). Effects of resistance exercise timing on sleep architecture and nocturnal blood pressure. *Journal of Strength and Conditioning Research* 29 (5): 1378–1385.

American College of Sports Medicine. (2018). *ACSM's Guidelines for Exercise Testing and Prescription,* 10th ed. Philadelphia, PA: Wolters Kluwer Lippincott Williams & Wilkins.

Andersen CH, Zebis MK, Saervoll, et al. (2012). Scapular muscle activity from selected strengthening exercises performed at low and high intensities. *Journal of Strength and Conditioning Research* 26 (9): 2408–2416.

Baechle TR, Earle RW. (Eds.). (2008). *Essentials of Strength Training and Conditioning,* 3rd ed. Champaign IL: Human Kinetics.

Biernat R, Trzaskoma Z, Trzaskoma L, et al. (2014). Rehabilitation protocol for patellar tendinopathy applied among 16- to 19-year old volleyball players. Journal of Strength and Conditioning Research 28 (1): 43–52.

Brody LT, Hall CM. (2018). *Therapeutic Exercise: Moving Toward Function,* 4th ed. Baltimore, MD: Lippincott Williams & Wilkins.

Chinkulprasert C, Vachalathiti R, Powers CM. (2011). Patellofemoral joint forces and stress during forward step-up, lateral step-up, and forward step-down exercises. *Journal of Orthopaedic & Sports Physical Therapy* 41 (4): 241–248.

Cholewicki J, McGill SM, Norman RW. (1991). Lumbar spine loads during the lifting of extremely heavy weights. *Medicine and Science in Sports and Exercise* 23 (10): 1179–1186.

Chung E, Lee BH, Hwang S. (2014). Core stabilization exercise with real-time feedback for chronic hemiparetic stroke: A pilot randomized controlled trials. *Restorative Neurology and Neuroscience* 32 (2): 313–321.

Clemson L, Fiatarone Singh MA, Bundy A, et al. (2012). Integration of balance and strength training into daily life activity to reduce rate of falls in older people (the life study): Randomised parallel trial. *BMJ* 345: e4547.

Coe DP, Fiatarone Singh MA. (2014). Exercise prescription in special populations: Women, pregnancy, children, and older adults. In: Swain DP (Ed.) *ACSM's Resource Manual for Guidelines for Exercise Testing and Prescription,* 7th ed. Philadelphia, PA: Wolters Kluwer-Lippincott Williams & Wilkins.

Cormie P, Pumpa K, Galvao DA, et al. (2013). Is it safe and efficacious for women with lymphedema secondary to breast cancer to lift heavy weights during exercise: A randomised controlled trial. *Journal of Cancer Survivorship* 7 (3): 413–424.

Dusunceli Y, Ozturk C, Atamaz F, et al. (2009). Efficacy of neck stabilization exercises for neck pain: A randomized controlled study. *Journal of Rehabilitation Medicine* 41 (8): 626–631.

Earl JE, Hoch AZ. (2011). A proximal strengthening program improves pain, function, and biomechanics in women with patellofemoral pain syndrome. *American Journal of Sports Medicine* 39 (1): 154–163.

Ekstrom RA, Donatelli RA, Carp KC. (2007). Electromyographic analysis of core trunk, hip, and thigh muscles during 9 rehabilitation exercises. *Journal of Orthopaedic & Sports Physical Therapy* 37 (12): 754–762.

Escamilla RF, Lewis C, Bell D, et al. (2010). Core muscle activation during Swiss ball and traditional abdominal exercises. *Journal of Orthopaedic & Sports Physical Therapy* 40 (5): 265–276.

Fiatarone MA, Marks EC, Ryan ND, et al. (1990). High-intensity strength training in nonagenarians. Effects on skeletal muscle. *JAMA* 263 (22): 3029–3034.

Fiatarone MA, O'Neill EF, Ryan ND, et al. (1994). Exercise training and nutritional supplementation for physical frailty in very elderly people. *New England Journal of Medicine* 330 (25): 1769–1775.

Figuers CC. (2010). Physical therapy management of pelvic floor dysfunction. In: Irion JM, and Irion GL. *Women's Health in Physical Therapy*. Philadelphia, PA: Wolters Kluwer Lippincott Williams & Wilkins.

Guo LY, Wang YL, Huang YH, et al. (2012). Comparison of the electromyographic activation level and unilateral selectivity of erector spinae during different selected movements. *International Journal of Rehabilitation Research* 35 (4): 345–351.

Ha SM, Kwon OY, Cynn HS, et al. (2012). Comparison of electromyographic activity of the lower trapezius and serratus anterior muscle in different arm-lifting scapular posterior tilt exercises. *Physical Therapy in Sport* 13 (4): 227–232.

Hardwick DH, Beebe JA, McDonnell MK, et al. (2006). A comparison of serratus anterior muscle activation during a wall slide exercise and other traditional exercises. *Journal of Orthopaedic & Sports Physical Therapy* 36 (12): 903–910.

Hulme JA. (2002). *Pelvic Pain and Low Back Pain: A Handbook for Self-Care & Treatment*. Missoula, MT: Phoenix Publishing. http://phoenixcoresolutions.com.

Idland G, Sylliaas H, Mengshoel AM, et al. (2014). Progressive resistance training for community-dwelling women aged 90 or older: A single-subject experimental design. *Disability and Rehabilitation* 36 (15): 1240–1248.

Jang EM, Kim MH, Oh JS. (2013). Effects of a bridging exercise with hip adduction on the EMG activities of the abdominal and hip extensor muscles in females. *Journal of Physical Therapy Science* 25 (9): 1147–1149.

Kahle N, Tevald MA. (2014). Core muscle strengthening's improvement of balance performance in community-dwelling older adults: A pilot study. *Journal of Aging and Physical Activity* 22 (1): 65–73.

Kim MH, Kwon OY, Kim SH, et al. (2013). Comparison of muscle activities of abductor hallucis and adductor hallucis between the short foot and toe-spread-out exercises in subjects with mild hallux valgus. *Journal of Back and Musculoskeletal Rehabilitation* 26 (2): 163–168.

Kisner C, Colby LA, Borstad J. (2018). *Therapeutic Exercise: Foundations and Techniques*, 7th ed. Philadelphia, PA: FA Davis.

Lee BC, McGill SM. (2015). Effect of long-term isometric training on core/torso stiffness. *Journal of Strength and Conditioning Research*. 29 (6): 1515–1526.

Lee IH, Park SY. (2013). Balance improvement by strength training for the elderly. *Journal of Physical Therapy Science* 25 (12): 1591–1593.

Leetun DT, Ireland ML, Willson JD, et al. (2004). Core stability measures as risk factors for lower extremity injury in athletes. *Medicine and Science in Sports and Exercise* 36 (6): 926–934.

Liebenson C. (2007). *Rehabilitation of the Spine: A Practitioner's Manual*, 2nd ed. Philadelphia, PA: Lippincott Williams & Wilkins.

Ludewig PM, Hoff MS, Osowski EE, et al. (2004). Relative balance of serratus anterior and upper trapezius muscle activity during push-up exercises. *American Journal of Sports Medicine* 32 (2): 484–493.

Lynn SK, Padilla RA, Tsang KK. (2012). Differences in static- and dynamic-balance task performance after 4 weeks of intrinsic-foot-muscle training: The short-foot exercise versus the towel-curl exercise. *Journal Sport Rehabilitation* 21 (4): 327–333.

Mavros Y, Kay S, Anderberg KA, et al. (2013). Changes in insulin resistance and hba1c are related to exercise-mediated changes in body composition in older adults with Type 2 diabetes: Interim outcomes from the GREAT2DO trial. *Diabetes Care* 36 (8): 2372–2379.

McGill SM. (2010). Core training: Evidence translating to better performance and injury prevention. *Strength and Conditioning Journal* 32 (3): 33–46.

McGill SM. (2014). *Ultimate Back Fitness and Performance*, 5th ed. Waterloo, Ontario, Canada: Backfitpro Inc. (formerly Wabuno Publishers).

McGill SM. (2016). *Low Back Disorders*, 3rd ed. Champaign IL: Human Kinetics.

McGill SM, Karpowicz A, Fenwick C. (2009). Ballistic abdominal exercises: Muscle activation patterns during three activities along the stability/mobility continuum. *Journal of Strength and Conditioning Research* 23 (3): 898–905.

McGill SM, Karpowicz A, Fenwick C. (2009). Exercises for the torso performed in a standing posture: Motion and motor patterns. *Journal of Strength and Conditioning Research* 23 (2): 455–464.

McGill SM, McDermott A, Fenwick C. (2009). Comparison of different strongman events: Trunk muscle activation and lumbar spine motion, load, and stiffness. *Journal of Strength and Conditioning Research* 23 (4): 1148–1161.

Meinhardt U, Witassek F, Petro R, et al. (2013). Strength training and physical activity in boys: A randomized trial. *Pediatrics* 132 (6): 1105–1111.

Myers TW. (2014). *Anatomy Trains: Myofascial Meridians for Manual and Movement Therapists*, 3rd ed. London, England: Churchill Livingstone Elsevier.

Nachemson AL. (1975). Toward a better understanding of low-back pain: A review of the mechanics of the lumbar disc. *Rheumatology and Rehabilitation* 14 (3): 129–143.

Nachemson AL. (1976). The lumbar spine: An orthopaedic challenge. *Spine* 1 (1): 59–71.

Nachemson AL. (1981). Disc pressure measurements. *Spine (Phila Pa 1976)* 6 (1): 93–97.

National Academy of Sports Medicine. (2010). *NASM Essentials of Corrective Exercise Training*. Baltimore, MD: Lippincott Williams & Wilkins.

National Academy of Sports Medicine. (2011). *NASM Essentials of Personal Fitness Training*, 4th ed. *Baltimore*, MD: Lippincott Williams & Wilkins.

National Strength and Conditioning Association. (2008). *Exercise Technique Manual for Resistance Training*, 2nd ed. Champaign, IL: Human Kinetics.

Page P, Frank CC, Lardner R. (2010). *Assessment and Treatment of Muscle Imbalance: The Janda Approach*. Champaign IL: Human Kinetics.

Richardson C, Hodges P, Hides J. (2004). *Therapeutic Exercise for Lumbopelvic Stabilization: A Motor Control Approach for the Treatment and Prevention of Low Back Pain*, 2nd ed. New York, NY: Churchill Livingstone.

Salo P, Ylonen-Kayra N, Hakkinen A, et al. (2012). Effects of long-term home-based exercise on health-related quality of life in patients with chronic neck pain: A randomized study with a 1-year follow-up. *Disability and Rehabilitation* 34 (23): 1971–1977.

Seo SH, Jeon IH, Cho YH, et al. (2013). Surface EMG during the push-up plus exercise on a stable support or Swiss ball: Scapular stabilizer muscle exercise. *Journal of Physical Therapy Science* 25 (7): 833–837.

Sharma A, Geovinson SG, Singh Sandhu J. (2012). Effects of a nine-week core strengthening exercise program on vertical jump performances and static balance in volleyball players with trunk instability. *Journal of Sports Medicine and Physical Fitness* 52 (6): 606–615.

Sinaki M, Brey RH, Hughes CA, et al. (2005). Significant reduction in risk of falls and back pain in osteoporotic-kyphotic women through a spinal proprioceptive extension exercise dynamic (speed) program. *Mayo Clinic Proceedings* 80 (7): 849–855.

Tarnanen SP, Siekkinen KM, Hakkinen AH, et al. (2012). Core muscle activation during dynamic upper limb exercises in women. *Journal of Strength and Conditioning Research* 26 (12): 3217–3224.

Verkhoshansky Y, Siff M. (2009). *Supertraining,* 6th ed. Rome, Italy: Verkhoshansky. www.verkhoshansky.com.

Vezina JW, Der Ananian CA, Greenberg E, et al. (2014). Sociodemographic correlates of meeting US Department of Health and Human Services muscle strengthening recommendations in middle-aged and older adults. *Preventing Chronic Disease* 11: E162.

Voight ML, Hoogenboom BJ, Prentice WE. (2007). *Musculoskeletal Interventions: Techniques for Therapeutic Exercise.* New York, NY: McGraw Hill Medical.

Ylinen J, Takala EP, Nykanen M, et al. (2003). Active neck muscle training in the treatment of chronic neck pain in women: A randomized controlled trial. *JAMA* 289 (19): 2509–2516.

Yu W, An C, Kang H. (2013). Effects of resistance exercise using Thera-band on balance of elderly adults: A randomized controlled trial. *Journal of Physical Therapy Science* 25 (11): 1471–1473.

Strength Exercises

Ahlund S, Nordgren B, Wilander EL, et al. (2013). Is home-based pelvic floor muscle training effective in treatment of urinary incontinence after birth in primiparous women? A randomized controlled trial. *Acta Obstetricia et Gynecologica Scandinavica* 92 (8): 909–915.

Altug Z. (2016). *Sustainable Fitness: A Practical Guide to Health, Healing, and Wellness.* North Charleston, SC: CreateSpace.

Altug Z, Hoffman JL, Martin JL. (Ed.) (1993). *Manual of Clinical Exercise Testing, Prescription, and Rehabilitation.* Norwalk, CT: Appleton & Lange.

Altug Z, Altug T, Altug A. (1987). A test selection guide for assessing and evaluating athletes. *National Strength & Conditioning Association Journal* 9 (3): 62–66.

Badiuk BW, Andersen JT, McGill SM. (2014). Exercises to activate the deeper abdominal wall muscles: The Lewit: A preliminary study. *Journal of Strength and Conditioning Research* 28 (3): 856–860.

Barton CJ, Kennedy A, Twycross-Lewis R, et al. (2014). Gluteal muscle activation during the isometric phase of squatting exercises with and without a Swiss ball. *Physical Therapy in Sport* 15 (1): 39–46.

Berry JW, Lee TS, Foley HD, et al. (2015). Resisted side-stepping: The effect of posture on hip abductor muscle activation. *Journal of Orthopaedic and Sports Physical Therapy* 45 (9):675–682.

Bo K. (2006). Pelvic floor muscle training. In: Chapple CR, Zimmern PE, Brubaker, L, et al. (Eds.). *Multidisciplinary Management of Female Pelvic Floor Disorders.* Philadelphia, PA: Churchill Livingstone Elsevier.

Bo K, Berghmans B, Morkved S, et al. (2007). *Evidence-Based Physical Therapy for the Pelvic Floor: Bridging Science and Clinical Practice.* New York, NY: Churchill Livingstone Elsevier.

Bo K, Talseth T, Holme I. (1999). Single blind, randomised controlled trial of pelvic floor exercises, electrical stimulation, vaginal cones, and no treatment in management of genuine stress incontinence in women. *British Medical Journal* 318 (7182): 487–493.

Boren K, Conrey C, Le Coguic J, et al. (2011). Electromyographic analysis of gluteus medius and gluteus maximus during rehabilitation exercises. *International Journal of Sports Physical Therapy* 6 (3): 206–223.

Braekken IH, Majida M, Engh ME, et al. (2010). Can pelvic floor muscle training reverse pelvic organ prolapse and reduce prolapse symptoms? An assessor-blinded, randomized, controlled trial. *American Journal of Obstetrics and Gynecology* 203 (2): 170.e171–177.

Buatois S, Miljkovic D, Manckoundia P, et al. (2008). Five times sit to stand test is a predictor of recurrent falls in healthy community living subjects aged 65 and older. *Journal of American Geriatrics Society* 56 (8): 1575–1577.

Cambridge ED, Sidorkewicz N, Ikeda DM, et al. (2012). Progressive hip rehabilitation: The effects of resistance band placement on gluteal activation during two common exercises. *Clinical Biomechanics (Bristol, Avon)* 27 (7): 719–724.

Carriere B. (2002). *Fitness for the Pelvic Floor.* New York, NY: Georg Thieme Verlag.

Carriere B, Feldt CM. (2006). *The Pelvic Floor.* New York, NY: Georg Thieme Verlag.

de Brito LB, Ricardo DR, de Araujo DS, et al. (2012). Ability to sit and rise from the floor as a predictor of all-cause mortality. *European Journal of Preventive Cardiology* 21 (7): 892–898.

Distefano LJ, Blackburn JT, Marshall SW, et al. (2009). Gluteal muscle activation during common therapeutic exercises. *Journal of Orthopaedic & Sports Physical Therapy* 39 (7): 532–540.

Edwards PK, Ebert JR, Littlewood C, et al. (2017). A systematic review of electromyography studies in normal shoulders to inform postoperative rehabilitation following rotator cuff repair. *Journal of Orthopaedic and Sports Physical Therapy* 47 (12): 931-944.

Fenwick, C, Brown SH, McGill SM. (2009). Comparison of different rowing exercises: Trunk muscle activation and lumbar spine motion, load, and stiffness. *Journal of Strength and Conditioning Research* 23 (5): 1408–1417.

Flanagan S, Salem GJ, Wang MY, et al. (2003). Squatting exercises in older adults: Kinematic and kinetic comparisons. *Medicine and Science in Sports and Exercise* 35 (4): 635–643.

Flanagan SP, Song JE, Wang MY, et al. (2005). Biomechanics of the heel-raise exercise. *Journal of Aging Physical Activity* 13 (2): 160–171.

Garcia-Vaquero MP, Moreside JM, Brontons-Gil E, et al. (2012). Trunk muscle activation during stabilization exercises with single and double leg support. *Journal of Electromyography and Kinesiology* 22 (3): 398–406.

Guo LY, Wang YL, Huang YH, et al. (2012). Comparison of the electromyographic activation level and unilateral selectivity of erector spinae during different selected movements. *International Journal of Rehabilitation Research* 35 (4): 345–351.

Heron SR, Woby SR, Thompson DP. (2017). Comparison of three types of exercise in the treatment of rotator cuff tendinopathy/shoulder impingement syndrome: A randomized controlled trial. *Physiotherapy* 103 (2): 167-173.

Holmberg D, Grantz H, Michaelson. (2012). Treating persistent low back pain with deadlift training: A single subject experimental design with a 15-month follow-up. *Advances in Physiotherapy* 14: 61–70.

Jang EM, Kim MH, Oh JS. (2013). Effects of a bridging exercise with hip adduction on the EMG activities of the abdominal and hip extensor muscles in females. *Journal of Physical Therapy Science* 25 (9): 1147–1149.

Janssen WG, Bussmann HB, and Stam, H. J. (2002). Determinants of the sit-to-stand movement: A review. *Physical Therapy* 82 (9): 866–879.

John D. (2009). *Never Let Go: A Philosophy of Lifting, Living and Learning.* Aptos, CA: On Target Publications.

John D. (2013). *Intervention: Course Corrections for the Athlete and Trainer.* Aptos, CA: On Target Publications.

Jones CJ, Rikli RE, Beam WC. (1999). A 30-s chair stand test as a measure of lower body strength in community residing older adults. *Research Quarterly for Exercise and Sport* 70 (2): 113–119.

Jung DY, Koh EK, Kwon OY. (2011). Effect of foot orthoses and short-foot exercise on the cross-sectional area of the abductor hallucis muscle in subjects with pes planus: A randomized controlled trial. *Journal of Back and Musculoskeletal Rehabilitation* 24 (4): 225–231.

Kegel A. (1948). Progressive resistance exercises in the functional restoration of the perineal muscles. *American Journal of Obstetrics and Gynecology* 56: 238–249.

Kegel A. (1951). Physiologic therapy for urinary incontinence. *JAMA* 146: 915–917.

Kegel A. (1952). Sexual function of the pubococcygeus muscle. *Western Journal of Surgery Obstetrics and Gynecology* 10: 521.

Kegel A. (1956). Stress incontinence of urine in women: Physiologic treatment. *Journal of the International College of Surgeons* 25: 487–499.

Kushner AM, Brent JL, Schoenfeld BJ, et al. (2015). The back squat: Targeted training techniques to correct functional deficits and technical factors that limit performance. *Strength and Conditioning Journal* 37 (2): 13–60.

Liebenson C, Shaughness G. (2011). The Turkish get-up. *Journal of Bodywork and Movement Therapies* 15 (1): 125–127.

MacAskill MJ, Durant TJS, Wallace DA. (2014). Gluteal muscle activity during weightbearing and non-weightbearing exercise. *International Journal of Sports Physical Therapy* 9 (7): 907–914.

McBeth JM, Earl-Boehm JE., Cobb SC, et al. (2012). Hip muscle activity during 3 side-lying hip-strengthening exercises in distance runners. *Journal of Athletic Training* 47 (1): 15–23.

McGill SM. (2016). *Low Back Disorders*, 3rd ed. Champaign IL: Human Kinetics.

McGill SM, Marshall LW. (2012). Kettlebell swing, snatch, and bottoms-up carry: Back and hip muscle activation, motion, and low back loads. *Journal of Strength and Conditioning Research* 26 (1): 16–27.

Moeller CR, Bliven KC, Valier AR. (2014). Scapular muscle-activation ratios in patients with shoulder injuries during functional shoulder exercises. *Journal of Athletic Training* 49 (3): 345–355.

Moon DC, Kim K Lee SK. (2014). Immediate effect of short-foot exercise on dynamic balance of subjects with excessively pronated feet. *Journal of Physical Therapy Science* 26 (1): 117–119.

Myer GD, Ford KR, Hewett TE. (2004). Rationale and clinical techniques for anterior cruciate ligament injury prevention among female athletes. *Journal of Athletic Training* 39 (4): 352–364.

Noble E. (2003). *Essential Exercises for the Childbearing Year*, 4th ed. Harwich, MA: New Life Images.

Nuzik S, Lamb R, VanSant A, et al. (1986). Sit-to-stand movement pattern. A kinematic study. *Physical Therapy* 66 (11): 1708–1713.

Pelaez M, Gonzalez-Cerron S., Montejo R, et al. (2014). Pelvic floor muscle training included in a pregnancy exercise program is effective in primary prevention of urinary incontinence: A randomized controlled trial. *Neurourology and Urodynamics* 33 (1): 67–71.

Schenkman M, Berger RA, Riley PO, et al. (1990). Whole-body movements during rising to standing from sitting. *Physical Therapy* 70 (10): 638–648

Selkowitz DM, Beneck GJ, Powers CM. (2013). Which exercises target the gluteal muscles while minimizing activation of the tensor fascia lata? Electromyographic assessment using fine-wire electrodes. *Journal of Orthopaedic & Sports Physical Therapy* 43 (2): 54–64.

Sharma G, Lobo T, Keller L. (2014). Postnatal exercise can reverse diastasis recti. *Obstetrics and Gynecology* 123 (Supplement 1): 171s.

Sidorkewicz N, Cambridge ED, McGill SM. (2014). Examining the effects of altering hip orientation on gluteus medius and tensor fascae latae interplay during common non-weight-bearing hip rehabilitation exercises. *Clinical Biomechanics (Bristol, Avon)* 29 (9): 971–976.

Silva P, Franco J, Gusmao A, et al. (2015). Trunk strength is associated with sit-to-stand performance in both stroke and healthy subjects. *European Journal of Physical and Rehabilitation Medicine* 51 (6): 717–724.

Souza GM, Baker LL, Powers CM. (2001). Electromyographic activity of selected trunk muscles during dynamic spine stabilization exercises. *Archives of Physical Medicine and Rehabilitation* 82 (11): 1551–1557.

Swinton PA, Lloyd R, Keogh JW, et al. (2012). A biomechanical comparison of the traditional squat, powerlifting squat, and box squat. *Journal of Strength and Conditioning Research* 26 (7): 1805–1816.

Tarnanen SP, Siekkinen KM, Hakkinen AH, et al. (2012). Core muscle activation during dynamic upper limb exercises in women. *Journal of Strength and Conditioning Research* 26 (12): 3217–3224.

Thigpen CA, Shaffer MA, Gaunt BW, et al. (2016). The American Society of Shoulder and Elbow Therapists' consensus statement on rehabilitation following arthroscopic rotator cuff repair. *Journal of Shoulder and Elbow Surgery* 25 (4): 521-535.

Uhl TL, Carver TJ, Mattacola CG, et al. (2003). Shoulder musculature activation during upper extremity weight-bearing exercise. *Journal of Orthopaedic and Sports Physical Therapy* 33 (3): 109-117.

Webster KA, Gribble PA. (2013). A comparison of electromyography of gluteus medius and maximus in subjects with and without chronic ankle instability during two functional exercises. *Physical Therapy in Sport* 14 (1): 17–22.

Benefits of Stretching Exercises

American College of Sports Medicine. (2018). *ACSM's Guidelines for Exercise Testing and Prescription*, 10th ed. Philadelphia, PA: Wolters Kluwer Lippincott Williams & Wilkins.

Avolio AP, Deng FQ, Li, WQ, et al. (1985). Effects of aging on arterial distensibility in populations with high and low prevalence of hypertension: Comparison between urban and rural communities in china. *Circulation* 71 (2): 202–210.

Behm DG, Kibele A. (2007). Effects of differing intensities of static stretching on jump performance. *European Journal of Applied Physiology* 101 (5): 587–594.

Cortez-Cooper MY, Anton MM, Devan AE, et al. (2008). The effects of strength training on central arterial compliance in middle-aged and older adults. *European Journal of Cardiovascular Prevention and Rehabilitation* 15 (2): 149–155.

Cristopoliski F, Barela JA, Leite N, et al. (2009). Stretching exercise program improves gait in the elderly. *Gerontology* 55 (6): 614–620.

Fowles JR, Sale DG, MacDougall JD. (2000). Reduced strength after passive stretch of the human plantar flexors. *Journal of Applied Physiology (1985)* 89 (3): 1179–1188.

Kokkonen J, Nelson AG, Tarawhiti T, et al. (2010). Early-phase resistance training strength gains in novice lifters are enhanced by doing static stretching. *Journal of Strength and Conditioning Research* 24 (2): 502–506.

Lowery RP, Joy JM, Brown, LE, et al. (2014). Effects of static stretching on 1-mile uphill run performance. *Journal of Strength and Conditioning Research* 28 (1): 161–167.

Nelson AG, Kokkonen J, Arnall DA. (2005). Acute muscle stretching inhibits muscle strength endurance performance. *Journal of Strength and Conditioning Research* 19 (2): 338–343.

Nelson AG, Kokkonen J, Winchester JB, et al. (2012). 10-week stretching program increases strength in the contralateral muscle. *Journal of Strength and Conditioning Research* 26 (3): 832–836.

Paradisis GP, Pappas PT, Theodorou AS, et al. (2014). Effects of static and dynamic stretching on sprint and jump performance in boys and girls. *Journal of Strength and Conditioning Research* 28 (1): 154–160.

Winchester JB, Nelson AG, Kokkonen J. (2009). A single 30-s stretch is sufficient to inhibit maximal voluntary strength. *Research Quarterly for Exercise and Sport* 80 (2): 257–261.

Winchester JB, Nelson AG, Landin D, et al. (2008). Static stretching impairs sprint performance in collegiate track and field athletes. *Journal of Strength and Conditioning Research* 22 (1): 13–19.

Wong A, Figueroa A. (2014). Eight weeks of stretching training reduces aortic wave reflection magnitude and blood pressure in obese postmenopausal women. *Journal of Human Hypertension* 28 (4): 246–250.

Yamamoto K, Kawano H, Gando Y, et al. (2009). Poor trunk flexibility is associated with arterial stiffening. *American Journal of Physiology. Heart and Circulatory Physiology* 297 (4): H1314–1318.

Zakaria AA, Kiningham RB, and Sen A. (2015). The effects of static and dynamic stretching on injury prevention in high school soccer athletes. A randomized trial. *Journal of Sport Rehabilitation* 24 (3):229–235.

Stretching Exercises

American College of Sports Medicine. (2018). *ACSM's Guidelines for Exercise Testing and Prescription*, 10th ed. Philadelphia, PA: Wolters Kluwer Lippincott Williams & Wilkins.

Hartmann H, Wirth K, Klusemann M. (2013). Analysis of the load on the knee joint and vertebral column with changes in squatting depth and weight load. *Sports Medicine* 43 (10): 993–1008.

Lamontagne M, Kennedy MJ, Beaule PE. (2009). The effect of cam FAI on hip and pelvic motion during maximum squat. *Clinical Orthopaedics and Related Research* 467 (3): 645–650.

Winters MV, Blake CG, Trost JS et al. (2004). Passive versus active stretching of hip flexor muscles in subjects with limited hip extension: A randomized clinical trial. *Physical Therapy* 84 (9): 800–807.

Benefits of Balance Exercises

Bieryla KA, Dold NM. (2013). Feasibility of Wii Fit training to improve clinical measures of balance in older adults. *Clinical Interventions in Aging* 8: 775–781.

Furman JM, Cass SP, Whitney SL. (2010). *Vestibular Disorders: A Case Study Approach to Diagnosis and Treatment*, 3rd ed. New York, NY: Oxford University Press.

Herdman SJ. (2007). *Vestibular Rehabilitation*, 3rd ed. Philadelphia, PA: FA Davis.

Hirase T, Inokuchi S, Matsusaka N, et al. (2015). Effects of a balance training program using a foam rubber pad in community-based older adults: A randomized controlled trial. *Journal of Geriatric Physical Therapy* 38 (2): 62–70.

Lee S, Park J, Lee D. (2013). Effects of an exercise program using aero-step equipment on the balance ability of normal adults. *Journal of Physical Therapy Science* 25 (8): 937–940.

Liao CD, Liou TH, Huang YY, et al. (2013). Effects of balance training on functional outcome after total knee replacement in patients with knee osteoarthritis: A randomized controlled trial. *Clinical Rehabilitation* 27 (8): 697–709.

Madureira MM, Takayama L, Gallinaro AL, et al. (2007). Balance training program is highly effective in improving functional status and reducing the risk of falls in elderly women with osteoporosis: A randomized controlled trial. *Osteoporosis International* 18 (4): 419–425.

Massery M, Hagins M, Stafford R, et al. (2013). Effect of airway control by glottal structures on postural stability. *Journal of Applied Physiology (1985)* 115 (4): 483–490. www. masserypt.com.

Ogaya S, Ikezoe T, Soda N, et al. (2011). Effects of balance training using wobble boards in the elderly. *Journal of Strength and Conditioning Research* 25 (9): 2616–2622.

Oliveira AS, de Brito Silva P, Lund ME, et al. (2017). Balance training enhances motor coordination during a perturbed side-step cutting task. *Journal of Orthopaedic and Sports Physical Therapy* 47 (11): 853–862.

O'Sullivan SB, Schmitz TJ, Fulk GD. (2014). *Physical Rehabilitation,* 6th ed. Philadelphia, PA: FA Davis Company.

Holistic Healing Boxes

Osteoporosis Information

Bassey EJ. (2001). Exercise for prevention of osteoporotic fracture. *Age and Ageing* 30 (Supplement 4): 29–31.

Beck BR, Snow CM. (2003). Bone health across the lifespan—Exercising our option. *Exercise and Sport Sciences Reviews* 31 (3): 117–122.

Bonner FJ, Sinaki M, Grabois M, et al. (2003). Health professional's guide to rehabilitation of the patient with osteoporosis. *Osteoporosis International* 14 (Supplement 2): S1–S22.

Ekin JA, Sinaki M. (1993). Vertebral compression fractures sustained during golfing: Report of three cases. *Mayo Clinic Proceedings* 68: 566–570.

Katz WA, Sherman. (1998). Exercise for osteoporosis. *Physician and Sportsmedicine* 26 (2): 43.

Meeks SM. (2008). *The Physical Therapy Management of Bone Health: A Clinician's Guide,* 2nd ed. Minneapolis, MN: Orthopedic Physical Therapy Products.

Meeks SM. (2010). *Walk Tall! An Exercise Program for the Prevention and Treatment of Back Pain, Osteoporosis and the Postural Changes of Aging,* 2nd ed. Gainesville, FL: Triad Publishing Company.

Petit MA, Hughes JM, Warpeha JM. (2010). Exercise prescription for people with osteoporosis. In: American College of Sports Medicine. *ACSM'S Resource Manual for Guidelines for Exercise Testing and Prescription,* 6th ed. Philadelphia, PA: Wolters Kluwer Lippincott Williams & Wilkins.

Sinaki M. (2007). The role of physical activity in bone health: A new hypothesis to reduce risk of vertebral fracture. *Physical Medicine and Rehabilitation Clinics of North America* 18 (3): 593–608.

Sinaki M. (2012). Exercise for patients with osteoporosis: Management of vertebral compression fractures and trunk strengthening for fall prevention. *PM & R* 4 (11): 882–888.

Sinaki M. (2013). Yoga spinal flexion positions and vertebral compression fracture in osteopenia or osteoporosis of spine: Case series. *Pain Practice* 13 (1): 68–75.

Sinaki M, Brey RH, Hughes CA, et al. (2005). Significant reduction in risk of falls and back pain in osteoporotic-kyphotic women through a spinal proprioceptive extension exercise dynamic (speed) program. *Mayo Clinic Proceedings* 80 (7): 849–855.

Sinaki M, Canvin JC, Phillips BE, et al. (2004). Site specificity of regular health club exercise on muscle strength, fitness, and bone density in women aged 29 to 45 years. *Mayo Clinic Proceedings* 79 (5): 639–644.

Sinaki M, Itoi E, Wahner HW, et al. (2002). Stronger back muscles reduce the incidence of vertebral fractures: A prospective 10 year follow-up of postmenopausal women. *Bone* 30 (6): 836–841.

Sinaki M, Khosla S, Limburg PJ, et al. (1993). Muscle strength in osteoporotic versus normal women. *Osteoporosis International* 3 (1): 8–12.

Sinaki M, Mikkelsen BA. (1984). Postmenopausal spinal osteoporosis: Flexion versus extension exercises. *Archives of Physical Medicine and Rehabilitation* 65 (10): 593–596.

Sinaki M, Pfeifer M, Preisinger E, et al. (2010). The role of exercise in the treatment of osteoporosis. *Current Osteoporosis Reports* 8 (3): 138–44.

Venes D. (Ed.) (2017). *Taber's Cyclopedic Medical Dictionary*, 23rd ed. Philadelphia, PA: FA Davis.

Fidgeting at Work to Burn Calories and Prevent Stiffness

Levine JA. (2014). *Get Up! Why Your Chair is Killing You and What You Can Do About It.* New York, NY: Palgrave Macmillan.

Levine JA, Schleusner SJ, and Jensen MD. (2000). Energy expenditure of nonexercise activity. *American Journal of Clinical Nutrition* 72 (6): 1451–1454.

Levine JA, Vander Weg MW, Hill JO, et al. (2006). Non-exercise activity thermogenesis: The crouching tiger hidden dragon of societal weight gain. *Arteriosclerosis, Thrombosis and Vascular Biology* 26 (4): 729–736.

Levine JA, Yeager S. (2009). *Move a Little, Lose a Lot: Use N.E.A.T.* Science to: Burn 2,100 Calories a Week at the Office, Be Smarter in as Little as 3 Hours, Reduce Fatigue by 65%, Extend Your Lifespan by 4 Years.* New York, NY: Three Rivers Press.

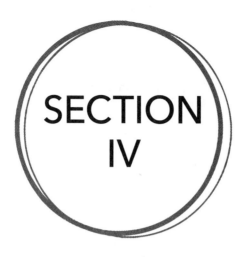

SECTION IV

SELF-CARE STRATEGIES

This section outlines some strategies you can use to understand your body reactions better and also track your progress. I use these strategies with many of my patients. Also, I compiled some simple weight management tips for you to consider since this is one of the key areas I frequently get asked in the clinic. Finally, I outlined some key self-management strategies you can use as a part of your home healing program. I routinely incorporate these strategies into the therapy programs for my patients and clients.

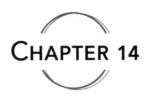

CHAPTER 14

TRACKING YOUR PROGRESS

"The unexamined life is not worth living."

—Socrates

Have you ever wondered, "Why do I hurt all over today?" or "Why don't I have any energy this week?" or "How come I haven't lost this extra weight?" It all goes back to what my Dad said about how we feel is rarely a random event. Again, it is mainly our habits, choices, and environment which influence our health. We really shouldn't blame genetics for everything.

A practical way to establish daily focus on good health, before tackling any other tasks, is to ask yourself these five questions first thing every morning:

- "What will I eat today for meals and snacks?"
- "What type of physical exercise am I going to do?"
- "What am I going to do for fun?"
- "What are my personal goals for today?"
- "What time am I going to sleep tonight?"

A personal diary is an important tool you can use to track habits and goals. As I mentioned in the Introduction section of this book, I have used a daily journal and diary for many years to help me understand my mind and body so I can make appropriate adjustments. Your diary can help guide you as you lose and maintain weight, get in shape, monitor and figure out dietary intake and chronic pain (if pain is present), and also log sleep patterns. Once you know which habits are beneficial to you, you'll be able to better incorporate them into your lifestyle. A diary also encourages you to develop discipline and make the most of each day. Write in a small journal book (Altug 2011), on a paper calendar (Altug 2011), electronic calendar (such as one on a computer, smartphone, or tablet) (Hutchesson et al. 2015), or a personal blog. Use your personal diary to track any of the following:

Workouts

Track strength, aerobics, and flexibility.

Sample entry: "Exercise—Monday, walk x 60 minutes"

Daily Diet

Keep track of all foods to encourage healthfully balanced eating and prevent overeating. You can also use your journal to note any food sensitivities or allergies.

Sample entry: "Breakfast—two eggs, two slices of bread with honey, one orange, water—8:00 a.m."

Daily Supplements

Keeping track of the brands, amounts, and times of any supplements you take can help you and your physician figure out if they are effective, causing you discomfort, or interfering with other medications. For instance, calcium supplements should *not* be taken with thyroid medications (such as Synthroid) because they affect the absorption of your medication, making it less effective.

Sample entry: "Supplement—calcium 500 mg—12:30 p.m."

Weight Loss

Track weekly weight loss, taking note of how certain activities and habits coincide with changes in your body weight.

Sample entry: "Weight—135 pounds—Sunday, two pounds lost since last weighed on Thursday"

Sleep Pattern

Keep a log of sleep patterns and compare to certain foods and activities noted in your journal. For example, perhaps you'll notice that you experienced insomnia the same night you swigged an after-dinner double cappuccino.

Sample entry: "Sleep—10:00 p.m.–6:00 a.m. = eight hours uninterrupted"

Stress Level

Record daily stress levels to pinpoint triggers. Use a numeric scale of zero to ten for gauging stress: zero represents no stress, five is moderate stress, and ten is the worst possible stress. For example, a high level of stress right around rush hour could mean it's time to find a solution to your long, hectic commute. Change your route, or join a vanpool.

Sample entry: "Stress level—eight out of 10—5:00 p.m."

Pain Level

Make note of pain and symptoms related to headaches, fibromyalgia, neck pain, and back pain. By tracking your pain along with your diet, exercise, sleep, and stress levels, you might notice patterns. For example, if you're regularly waking up in the morning with pain, it might be time to get a new mattress. It also helps you better describe symptoms to your physician. Incorporate a pain scale, similar to the stress scale noted above, with zero being no pain, five as being moderate pain, and ten the worst possible pain.

Sample entry: "Lower-back pain—six out of ten—5:00 a.m."

Blood Sugar

Keep track of your blood sugar if you are diabetic. Again, watch for patterns. For example, take notice if your blood sugar is off-kilter before breakfast.

Sample entry: "Sugar—105 mg/dL—7:30 a.m."

Blood Pressure

Keep track of your blood pressure if you have hypertension.

Sample entry: "Blood Pressure—130/80—7:30 a.m."

Medications

Keep track of your medications. Many medications need to be taken consistently at the same time so they are effective.

Sample entry: "Medication—Synthroid, 50 mcg—6:00 a.m."

Home Rehabilitation

Track the progress of your physical therapy (PT) or home rehabilitation exercise program.

Sample entry: "PT—10 minutes—10:00 a.m."

Personal Thoughts

Keep track of any personal thoughts, dreams, and goals to make them real. Each day matters. Or keep track of your emotions and frustrations as a way to release and relieve stress.

Sample entry: "Tomorrow I ask for a raise" or "Today I got my raise!" or "First day of my European vacation" or "I will reassess my skill set to see what I can improve upon for a future job opportunity."

Sample Wellness Journal Format

The following sample daily wellness journal (Table 14-1) shows an example of a diary format you can create either in a paper journal or on an electronic blog:

Table 14-1: Sample Daily Wellness Journal

Date: July 1, 2018

Exercise:
Morning Yoga x 15 minutes
Evening Walk x 30 minutes

Meditation:
Morning Self-Hypnosis / Meditation x 5 minutes

Nutrition:
Breakfast—bowl of gluten-free oatmeal with blueberries, avocado, walnuts, and honey, one cup almond yogurt, one cup tea
Lunch—turkey-and-vegetable sandwich (gluten-free), mixed salad with olive oil, one banana, one cup yogurt, two cups water
Dinner—salmon steak, mixed salad with olive oil, one pear, two cups water
Snacks—water throughout day, nuts, fruits

Diary:
I had a great day today. My project got accepted! Tonight, I'm going dancing with my friends to celebrate.

(Note: For the nutrition section, the portion sizes and type of foods need to be adjusted for the person's needs and preferences.)

Sample Wellness Calendar Format

Track your home fitness program, body weight, and goals by using the following calendar samples. The first outline is a suggested way for you to fill in the various spaces (Table 14-2).

The second is blank so you can copy or scan for personal use (Table 14-3). Write in the month and corresponding days, and then complete the body weight, exercises, and goals sections as you progress with your fitness program.

TABLE 14-2: SAMPLE WELLNESS CALENDAR

JUNE 2018

SUN	MON	TUES	WED	THURS	FRI	SAT
					1 a.m. Walk x 30 min p.m. Walk x 30 min	2 Weights x 30 min
Diary: My goal for this week is to add some weight training.						
3 Tai Chi x 30 min BW: 140	4 a.m. Walk x 30 min p.m. Walk x 30 min	5 Walk x 30 min	6 Weights x 30 min	7 Yoga x 30 min	8 a.m. Walk x 30 min p.m. Walk x 30 min	9 Weights x 30 min
Diary: I lost two pounds this week by exercising and by consuming no soft drinks.						
10 Tai Chi x 30 min BW: 138	11 a.m. Walk x 30 min p.m. Walk x 30 min	12 a.m. Walk x 30 min	13 Weights x 30 min	14 Yoga x 30 min	15 a.m. Walk x 30 min p.m. Walk x 30 min	16 Weights x 30 min
Diary: My energy level was excellent.						
17 Tai Chi x 30 min BW: 136	18 a.m. Walk x 30 min p.m. Walk x 30 min	19 a.m. Walk x 30 min	20 Weights x 30 min	21 Yoga x 30 min	22 a.m. Walk x 30 min p.m. Walk x 30 min	23 Weights x 30 min
Diary: My goal for this week is to drink more water.						
24 Tai Chi x 30 min BW: 134	25 a.m. Walk x 30 min p.m. Walk x 30 min	26 a.m. Walk x 30 min	27 Weights x 30 min	28 Yoga x 30 min	29 a.m. Walk x 30 min p.m. Walk x 30 min	30 Weights x 30 min
Diary: This month I lost six pounds!						

BW = body weight in pounds
(Note: Modify the program for your needs and replace activities based on your interests.)

TABLE 14-3: WELLNESS CALENDAR

SUN	MON	TUES	WED	THURS	FRI	SAT
BW:						
Diary:						
BW:						
Diary:						
BW:						
Diary:						
BW:						
Diary:						
BW:						
Diary:						

BW = body weight in pounds

Sample Lifestyle Assessment

Identify specific things you need to improve or modify in each category (Table 14-4).

Table 14-4: Your Lifestyle Assessment

MEDICAL CONDITIONS	
FOOD INTOLERANCES	
ALLERGIES	
VEGETABLES	
FRUITS	
MEATS	
DAIRY	
GRAINS	
OILS	
BEVERAGES	
SUPPLEMENTS	

FOODS IN GENERAL	
SLEEP	
STRESS MANAGEMENT	
EXERCISES	
CHEMICAL PRECAUTIONS	

BOX 12: HOLISTIC HEALING

TOP 10 HEALTH PRODUCTS

The following are products which most likely won't trend up or down considerably, but are important for your well-being:

- Good bed and pillow along with comfortable sheets
- Good toothbrush, floss, and a gum massager
- Comfortable walking and dress shoes
- Self-massage devices for the neck, back, and foot
- Good dumbbells and kettlebells
- Sturdy exercise elastic bands
- Comfortable exercise mat
- Quality cookware
- Quality kitchen drinking water filter and shower filter
- Quality lunchbox for nutritious meals and snacks

What's on your list?

ADDITIONAL RESOURCES

- Habit Nest (The Morning Sidekick Journal), habitnest.com
- Intelligent Change, Inc. (The Five Minute Journal), intelligentchange. com. Also, check out their app on iTunes.
- Moleskine, us.moleskine.com/en
- SuperTracker, supertracker.usda.gov

References

Altug Z. (2011). *2012 Healthy Lifestyle Engagement Calendar.* Indianapolis, IN: TF Publishing.

Altug Z. (2011). *2012 Healthy Lifestyle Wall Calendar.* Indianapolis, IN: TF Publishing.

Anderson CM, MacCurdy MM. (1999). *Writing and Healing: Toward an Informed Practice.* Urbana, IL: National Council of Teachers of English.

Bassett D. (2010). Assessment of physical activity. In: *ACSM's Resource Manual for Guidelines for Exercise Testing and Prescription,* 6th ed. American College of Sports Medicine. Philadelphia, PA: Wolters Kluwer Lippincott Williams & Wilkins.

DeSalvo L. (1999). *Writing as a Way of Healing: How Telling Our Stories Transforms Our Lives.* Boston, MA: Beacon Press.

Hollis JF, Gullion CM, Stevens VJ, et al. (2008). Weight loss during the intensive intervention phase of the weight-loss maintenance trial. *American Journal of Preventive Medicine* 35 (2): 118–126.

Hutcheson MJ, Rollo ME, Callister R, et al. (2015). Self-monitoring of dietary intake by young women: Online food records completed on computer or smartphone are as accurate as paper-based food records but more acceptable. *Journal of the Academy of Nutrition and Dietetics* 115 (1): 87–94.

Pennebaker JW. (2004). *Writing to Heal: A Guided Journal for Recovering from Trauma & Emotional Upheaval.* Oakland, CA: New Harbinger Publications, Inc.

Petrie KJ, Fontanilla I, Thomas MG, et al. (2004). Effect of written emotional expression on immune function in patients with human immunodeficiency virus infection: A randomized trial. *Psychosomatic Medicine* 66 (2): 272–275.

Schaefer EM. (2008). *Writing through the Darkness: Easing Your Depression with Paper and Pen.* Berkeley, CA: Celestial Arts.

Shay LE, Seibert D, Watts D, et al. (2009). Adherence and weight loss outcomes associated with food-exercise diary preference in a military weight management program. *Eating Behaviors* 10 (4): 220–227.

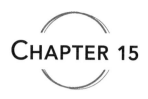

CHAPTER 15

HEALING FASTER

"The symptoms or the sufferings generally considered to be inevitable and incident to the disease are very often not symptoms of the disease at all, but of something quite different—of the want of fresh air, or of light, or of warmth, or of quiet, or of cleanliness, or of punctuality and care in the administration of diet, of each or of all of these."

—Florence Nightingale

One of the key questions I frequently get asked in physical therapy is "What can I do to heal faster?" Over the years I have accumulated lots of tips and research on this topic. Read through the following tips and see which ones make the most sense to you. If you are not sure, ask your healthcare provider for some guidance. I wish you all the best in your healing and recovery journey. Please keep in mind that some of the sections outlined in this chapter are not evidence-based (such as Biological Grounding or Earthing and the table outlining the Six Healing Sounds). However, these sections are presented as theories and potential areas researchers may explore in the near future.

The rate and the quality of healing in the body is affected by many factors such as a person's age, illness, medical conditions (such as diabetes, hypertension, obesity, high cholesterol, or osteoporosis), lifestyle habits (such as smoking or inappropriate alcohol consumption), type and severity of injury (such as mild, moderate, or severe), type of tissue affected (such as tendon, muscle, ligament, bone, or cartilage), sleep, psychological stress, nutrition, and exercise (Abe et al. 2018; Abtahi et al. 2015; Avishai et al. 2017; Berman et al. 2017; Sandrey 2003; Tashjian et al. 2010; Taylor et al. 2017; Thorud et al. 2017; Toyoda et al. 2018). This chapter will provide some basic resources for you to consider for helping you optimize your healing and recovery.

SEE YOUR PRIMARY PHYSICIAN

Speak with your physician about medications and other recommended strategies for speeding up the healing process. For example, ask your physician about platelet-rich plasma (PRP) to improve early tendon healing and repair (Lamplot et al. 2014).

SEE A PHYSICAL REHABILITATION SPECIALIST

A specialist, such as a physical therapist, occupational therapist, speech therapist, acupuncturist, or chiropractor, might provide appropriate healing techniques and strategies, so ask your physician about a possible referral. See a physical therapist or occupational therapist about unloading tissues by utilizing techniques such as joint protection guidelines (Table 15-1), proper body mechanics guidelines for daily tasks (Table 15-2), energy conservation guidelines (Table 15-3), and fall prevention guidelines (Table 15-4), which can all help with the healing process. See the tables below for some examples of how your rehabilitation specialist may help you with personalized instructions:

TABLE 15-1: JOINT PROTECTION GUIDELINES

Use this sample checklist to protect your neck:

- Avoid prolonged sitting positions (generally no more than 30 minutes). Set a quiet food timer or other soft alarm next to your computer as a reminder to get up.
- Avoid lying on a sofa with your head propped too far forward.
- Avoid prolonged sleeping on your stomach.
- Avoid clenching your jaw at rest.
- Sleep on your side or back with arms below chest level.
- Store household items at levels that are not too high or too low.
- Avoid squeezing the phone between your ear and shoulder.
- Avoid prolonged bending of the neck during tasks such as texting (also known as "text neck"), reading, laptop use, sewing, writing, or any activity involving detailed work with the hands.

Use this sample checklist to protect your lower back:

- Avoid prolonged sitting. Follow the 30-30 guideline, by getting up and moving around for at least 30 seconds after 30 minutes of sitting.
- If you already have lower back and leg pain, consider limiting prolonged standing to no longer than 40 minutes.
- Avoid twisting at the waist when holding a heavy object.
- When lifting heavy items, bend at the hips and knees, not at the waist. For lifting a heavy object, first tighten (or "lock") the abdominal muscles and then lift the item. Just remember, "Lock and lift."

When sneezing or coughing, bend your knees slightly and place one hand behind your back or on your hip, or hold on to a solid object for support to avoid a sudden forward bend.

(Adapted from Altug 2010; Coenen et al. 2017; McGill 2016; Sheon 1985; Sheon et al. 1996; Thosar et al. 2015.)

TABLE 15-2: PROPER BODY MECHANICS GUIDELINES

Use this sample checklist to lift and carry items safely:

- First, plan your lift. Remove obstructions along your path ahead of time. Decide how you are going to hold and move the object. Get help if the object is too heavy for you.
- Get a firm hold on the object so it won't slip.
- Lift the object with control and avoid jerky motions.
- Plant your feet firmly on the ground for a solid base when lifting.
- Bend your knees and hips, not your back.
- Keep objects you are lifting or carrying close to your body.
- Minimize or avoid twisting your spine when lifting or carrying objects. Adjust your feet instead of twisting excessively at the trunk. A simple rule to remember is this: "Your nose should follow your toes."
- Maintain the normal arch in your lower back as you lift and carry. As the saying goes, "Preserve the curve."
- Use tools such as hoists, lifts, and dollies to avoid unnecessary lifting and carrying.
- Remember to "tighten and lift." When lifting a moderate to heavy object, brace the abdominal muscles or stiffen your midsection just enough to support your back before you lift.

(Adapted from Aleksiev 2014; Delitto et al. 1992; McGill 2016; Vera-Garcia et al. 2007.)

TABLE 15-3: ENERGY CONSERVATION GUIDELINES

Knowing how to use your energy wisely as a part of your daily activities may be an essential part of your recovery process and preventing injury. Personal energy conservation involves finding ways to reduce the amount of effort and energy needed to accomplish tasks to help you experience less fatigue and pain.

Use this sample checklist to help you conserve energy with your daily tasks:

- Determine which activities trigger discomfort or pain, and plan how to modify them.
- Figure out what is the easiest and safest way to perform a task. For instance, is it easier to clean your bathroom by using tools with longer handles?
- Do the most strenuous daily tasks when you have the most energy.
- Alternate difficult tasks with easy tasks to prevent overloading the muscles and joints.
- Take brief rest periods for recovery during your daily chores and activities.
- Pace yourself. Exhausting all of your energy at the beginning of the day can leave you feeling run-down later.
- Change the location of household equipment and supplies for easier access.
- Minimize excess stair-climbing, frequent bending and squatting, and heavy lifting and carrying.
- Take advantage of labor-saving devices (such as a dishwasher) and tools (such as a power screwdriver).
- Avoid unnecessary trips to the store by planning ahead with shopping lists.
- Partner with gravity. Slide, push, or pull instead of lifting an object.
- Use assistive devices (such as a cane or walker), braces, and splints as needed.
- Ask for help, or delegate tasks and chores when needed.

(Adapted from Altug 2011; Gerber et al. 1987; Iversen et al. 2014; Mathiowetz et al. 2005; Young 1991.)

Table 15-4: Fall Prevention Guidelines

Use this sample checklist to help you prevent falls in your home and in the community:

- Widen pathways in your home by rearranging furniture and removing clutter.
- Hold on to sturdy handrails when going up and down stairs.
- Check that there is adequate lighting in the stairwell area.
- Keep stairs free of clutter.
- Provide adequate lighting throughout your house.
- Space your home furniture to allow comfortable maneuvering.
- Remove throw rugs that might cause you to slip or trip.
- Remove electrical cords that extend across the floor.
- Keep a flashlight in every room and near your bed for emergencies.
- Avoid highly polished floors.
- Don't walk around your house in socks, especially on hardwood or tile floors.
- Avoid climbing ladders if you are unsteady.
- Be careful when carrying large items, like laundry baskets, that prevent you from seeing your walking path.
- Be careful when wearing long coats, dresses, night garments, or pants.
- Avoid rushing to the phone to answer calls. Have phones throughout the house or a cellular phone you can carry with you.

(Adapted from the Academy of Geriatric Physical Therapy [2018].)

See a Mental Health Professional

Consider a consultation with a psychologist, counselor, or psychiatrist for treatments such as talk therapy, counseling, cognitive behavioral therapy (CBT), and possibly medications as prescribed by a psychiatrist.

Ask Your Doctor about Preoperative Training

There is some evidence that getting in shape before surgery can help you recover faster and reduce complications after surgery (dos Santos Alves et al. 2014; Humphrey et al. 2015). Consider this as the "better in, better out" approach (Hoogeboom et al. 2014). Ask your doctor if you would benefit from preoperative physical therapy and fitness training. Before your surgery is also a good time to quit smoking, limit alcohol, improve your diet, establish better sleep patterns, and learn to control your stress levels. If you do smoke, talk to your doctor for more information on quitting smoking.

You can also have a discussion with your healthcare provider about how you can prepare your home for after surgery, such as installing grab bars in the shower or purchasing a raised toilet seat or safety rails around the toilet for assistance in sitting and standing.

Ask Your Doctor or
Therapist about BEMER

BEMER (Bio-Electro-Magnetic-Energy-Regulation) is a medical device which increases microcirculation and helps reduce pain and support the body's own self-healing and regeneration processes. For more information about BEMER, refer to the BEMER group website www.bemergroup.com.

A study by Gyulai et al. (2015) shows that "BEMER physical vascular therapy reduced pain and fatigue in the short term in patients with chronic low back pain, while long-term therapy appears to be beneficial in patients with osteoarthritis of knee." Another study by Piatkowski et al. (2009) shows "a beneficial effect of BEMER intervention on multiple sclerosis (MS) fatigue."

Go for a Nature Walk
and Get Green Exercise

Here is what a study by Li et al. (2016) says about forest bathing. "The forest environment has long been enjoyed for its quiet atmosphere, beautiful scenery, calm climate, pleasant aromas, and clean fresh air. Researchers in Japan have tried to find preventive effects against lifestyle-related diseases from forests and have proposed a new concept called 'forest bathing.' What is forest bathing? In Japan, a forest bathing is a short leisurely visit to a forest, called '*Shinrin-yoku*' in Japanese, which is similar in effect to natural aromatherapy, for the purpose of relaxation. '*Shinrin*' means forest and '*yoku*' means bathing in Japanese."

Another study by Barton et al. (2010) indicates that green exercise is where you are exercising in nature. The researchers found that green exercise improved both self-esteem and mood, especially in the presence of water. For further information, refer to the Green Exercise website www.greenexercise.org and MovNat (Natural Movement Fitness) website www.movnat.com.

Brighten Your Home

Pull back the curtains, and open the shades. Bring more natural outdoor light into your home during the day to help you heal (Beauchemin et al. 1996, 1998).

Create a Healing Garden

Being exposed to nature can help reduce psychological stress and allow you to heal by promoting relaxation (Mitrione 2008). A garden inspires you to be outside in the fresh air and sunshine, and among serene wildlife, such as butterflies and hummingbirds.

Use your senses to heal your mind and body in your home garden:

- **Touch** various textures of plants, and put your hands in the soil
- **See** an array of colors
- **Listen** to the birds or a backyard waterfall
- **Smell** a variety of plants such as mint, rosemary, and basil
- **Taste** an assortment of teas brewed from garden herbs

Try growing the following in your backyard or greenhouse or in pots on your porch, balcony, patio, or windowsill:

- *Fruits*—apples, berries, grapes, plums
- *Healing plants*—aloe vera (Moriyama et al. 2016), lavender (Sasannejad et al. 2012)
- *Herbs*—basil, mint, parsley, rosemary
- *Vegetables*—cucumbers, tomatoes

You might also consider caring for a bonsai tree. Caroll Hermann states in her doctoral thesis that "There is an ancient Japanese saying that 'tears are dried, pain disappears and heartaches mended when one is pulling weeds or watering a flower'. In ancient Japanese culture, the spiritual rebirth by Nature is contained in the peaceful cultivation of Bonsai" (Hermann 2015).

GET ADEQUATE VITAMIN D

See your physician to get your vitamin D level checked. Vitamin D might help optimize recovery after injury since it is reduced after inflammatory insult (such as knee replacement surgery) and is essential for optimal bone health and muscle function (Bogunovic et al. 2010; Reid et al. 2011; Stratos et al. 2013). An article by Pludowski et al. (2013) states that "adequate vitamin D status seems to be protective against musculoskeletal disorders (muscle weakness, falls, fractures), infectious diseases, autoimmune diseases, cardiovascular disease, type 1 and type 2 diabetes mellitus, several types of cancer, neurocognitive dysfunction and mental illness, and other diseases."

GET ENOUGH SLEEP

The body's tissue healing mechanisms are altered from sleep deprivation (Siengsukon et al. 2017). An article by Patel et al. (2008) indicates that "immune system dysfunction, impaired wound healing, and changes in behavior are all observed in patients who are sleep-deprived."

Get Social Support and Have Hope

A study indicates that "hope and social support are psychological strengths that may be beneficial to an injured athlete's rehabilitation and subjective well-being" (Lu et al. 2013).

Give a Hug

A simple hug can help heal illness, depression, and anxiety. A study by Matsunaga et al. (2009) suggests that "psychological stress may be reduced and we may feel happiness when we kiss and hug a romantic partner." So go for a single hug, group hug, pet hug, or even hug that tree. Just give a hug. For more information, refer to the Touch Research Institute website www6.miami.edu/touch-research.

Go on a Spiritual Retreat

A study shows spiritual retreats that "included guided imagery, meditation, drumming, journal writing, and nature-based activities" increased hope while reducing depression in individuals with acute coronary syndrome (Warber et al. 2011).

Box 13: Holistic Healing

Women's Health Highlights

This section highlights some issues related to women's health.

Let's See What Research Says . . .

- "Supervised physical exercise during pregnancy reduces the level of depression and its incidence in pregnant women" (Perales et al. 2015).
- High-heeled shoes can exacerbate muscle overuse and lead to lower-back problems (Mika et al. 2012).
- "Acupuncture in an integrated system that includes therapeutic techniques such as diet therapy and Tuina self-massage [a traditional method of Chinese massage where the body is lifted, squeezed, and pushed to improve circulation] can be used to treat hot flushes [also known as hot flashes] and selected symptoms in postmenopausal women" (Baccetti et al. 2014; Venes 2017).
- According to the American Congress of Obstetricians and Gynecologists (www.acog.org) educational pamphlet *Premenstrual Syndrome*, "for many women, regular aerobic exercise lessens premenstrual syndrome (PMS) symptoms."

- A good-fitting bra is not only important for comfort and health, but also might encourage women to be more physically active without exercise-related breast discomfort (Bowles et al. 2013; Brown et al. 2014; McGhee 2009).
- "Fatigue may interfere with breastfeeding, so interventions minimizing fatigue are important" (Milligan et al. 1996). The authors continued by saying that mothers reported significantly less fatigue when nursing in the side-lying versus the sitting position.

The following are some resources for women's health:

- American Congress of Obstetricians, www.acog.org and search for the educational pamphlet titled *Breastfeeding Your Baby*
- American Congress of Obstetricians, www.acog.org and search for the educational pamphlet titled *Exercise During Pregnancy*
- American Physical Therapy Association—Section on Women's Health, www.womenshealthapta.org
- Breast Research Australia, www.facebook.com/BreastResearchAustralia
- Lady-Comp Fertility Monitors, www.lady-comp.com
- Office on Women's Health, http://womenshealth.gov
- Sports Bra App available on iTunes at www.bra.edu.au. This app was created by sports physiotherapist Dr. Deirdre McGhee, who is a researcher for Breast Research Australia, and a senior lecturer in the School of Medicine at the University of Wollongong. Also, refer to the YouTube video at www.youtube.com/watch?v=eY_ybnXFDFc.
- Sports Medicine Australia, http://sma.org.au and search for Exercise and Breast Support
- The North American Menopause Society, www.menopause.org
- Refer to the book *Essential Exercises for the Childbearing Year* (Noble 2003) by physical therapist Elizabeth Noble, PT, for further self-help techniques during and after pregnancy.
- Refer to the book *Women's Health in Physical Therapy* (Irion et al. 2010).
- Refer to the book *Your Best Pregnancy: The Ultimate Guide to Easing the Aches, Pains, and Uncomfortable Side Effects During Each Stage of Your Pregnancy* (Hoefs et al. 2014).
- Refer to the article by Litos (2014) titled "Progressive Therapeutic Exercise Program for Successful Treatment of a Postpartum Woman With a Severe Diastasis Recti Abdominis."

TAKE A VACATION

Consider taking a vacation at a mind body healing resort or holistic retreat center to recover and recuperate. It could be a great experience for the entire family to learn about various self-healing techniques such as massage, aromatherapy, music therapy, yoga, tai chi, qigong, meditation, cooking, and exercise. A study by Mills et al. (2016) concludes that "a short-term intensive program providing holistic instruction and experience in mind-body healing practices can lead to significant and sustained increases in perceived well-being." Refer to the following for a relaxing and healthy vacation:

- CanyonRanch, canyonranch.com
- Eastover, eastover.com
- Esalen, esalen.org
- Hollyhock, hollyhock.ca

INTERACT WITH A PET

It's no secret that dogs are humans' best friends and we are cats' best friends. Pets can serve as important sources of social support (McConnell et al. 2011), enhance daily living of older individuals (Raina et al. 1999), and help people heal. So, give your huggable pet a big squeeze.

KEEP A JOURNAL OR DIARY

The authors of one study (Koschwanez et al. 2013) state that "expressive writing can improve wound healing in older adults and women. Future research is needed to better understand the underlying cognitive, psychosocial, and biological mechanisms contributing to improved wound healing from these simple, yet effective, writing exercises." Another study by Burton et al. (2004) indicates that "writing about intensely positive experiences was also associated with significantly fewer health center visits for illness."

Why not try a little journal right now and see how that makes you feel. Just enter whatever thoughts you have or perhaps something you are grateful for this past week. Go ahead and write in the book below (unless it's a library book or your friend's copy!) (Figure 15-1).

🧘 YOUR PERSONAL DIARY

DATE:

_____

_____

_____

_____

Figure 15-1

Keep on the Sunny Side

Wadey et al. (2013) indicates that "as optimism increased, the likelihood of injury occurrence decreased." Also, optimism can be important for cardiovascular health (Roy et al. 2010).

Let Go of Stress

Studies have shown that controlling acute and chronic stress can have a positive effect on healing (Altemus et al. 2001; Glaser et al. 1999; Kiecolt-Glaser et al. 1995; Stults-Kolehmainen et al. 2014). To relax and reduce stress, simply smile, laugh, whistle, sing, hum, play a fun game, read some comics, or watch a funny movie. If these simple techniques do not work, then consider seeing your doctor for additional medical care.

Let Music Mend Your Mind and Body

Music therapy might help reduce pain and anxiety, which can promote speedy healing (Bradt et al. 2013; Meghani et al. 2017; Nilsson 2008). Music can help heal the mind and body. Studies have shown that music can decrease pain in an intensive care unit (ICU) setting (Chiasson et al. 2013) and anxiety after heart surgery (Nilsson 2009). A study by Lubetzky et al. (2010) indicates that "exposure to Mozart music significantly lowers resting energy expenditure in healthy preterm infants. We speculate that this effect of music on resting energy expenditure might explain, in part, the improved weight gain that results from this 'Mozart effect.'" Refer to the Music Mends Minds, Inc. website www.musicmendsminds.org to learn more about the therapeutic benefits of music.

Of course, everyone has his or her own tastes and preferences for music. Consider including some of my personal favorites on your healing playlist (Table 15-5):

Table 15-5: Music for Your Heart and Soul

Bach, Johann Sebastian	**Brahms, Johannes**
"Air on the G String"	"Wiegenlied, Op. 49, No. 4 (Lullaby)"
"Brandenburg Concertos"	
"Goldberg Variations"	**Chopin, Frédéric François**
"Suite for Solo Cello No. 1 in G major"	"Nocturne in E-flat major, Op. 9, No. 2"
	"Waltz in A minor"
Beethoven, Ludwig van	"Waltz in C-sharp minor, Op. 64, No. 2"
"Bagatelle No. 25 in A minor (Für Elise)"	
"Ode to Joy"	**Grieg, Edvard**
	"Morning Mood, Peer Gynt, Op. 23"

Handel, George Frideric
"Water Music"

Liszt, Franz
"Consolations, No. 3"

Massenet, Jules
"Méditation (Thaïs)"

Mozart, Wolfgang Amadeus
"Piano Concerto No. 21 in C major, K. 467: II. Andante"
"Violin Concerto No. 3 in G major, K. 216, II. Adagio"
"Violin Concerto No. 5 in A major, K. 219, II. Adagio"

Pachelbel, Johann
"Canon in D major"

Puccini, Giacomo
"O mio babbino caro"

Rodrigo, Joaquín
"Concierto de Aranjuez—Adagio"

Saint-Saëns, Camille
"The Swan–Carnival of the Animals"

Strauss II, Johann
"The Blue Danube Waltz"

Tchaikovsky, Pyotr Ilyich
"Dance of the Sugar Plum Fairy"
"Piano Concerto No. 1 in B-flat minor, Op. 23"

Vivaldi, Antonio
"The Four Seasons"

SIX HEALING SOUNDS

According to Traditional Chinese Medicine (TCM) beliefs, healing "sounds should actually physically vibrate the targeted organ like an inner-massage" (Moon et al. 2017; Voigt 2010-2011). Also see chapter 8: Qigong for Health for more research on healing sounds. To the best of my knowledge, the effects of making healing sounds have not been proven in Western medicine, but healing sounds may be used as a part of some Eastern approaches to healing.

For more information about the Six Healing Sounds (Table 15-6) see the Wikipedia website en.wikipedia.org/wiki/Liu_Zi_Jue. See a TCM practitioner to learn how, in a safe manner, to make your own vocal healing sounds such as these:

TABLE 15-6: SIX HEALING SOUNDS

XU	pronounced like "shoe"	for Liver Qi
HE	pronounced like "her"	for Heart Qi
HU	pronounced like "who"	for Spleen/Pancreas Qi
SI	pronounced like "sir"	for Lung Qi
CHUI	pronounced "chway" or "chwee"	for Kidney Qi
XI	pronounced like "she"	for Triple Burner Qi

You can also create healing sounds with the following tools (Goldsby et al. 2017), but I recommend you consult with a TCM practitioner to determine the best options for your needs:

- Baoding balls (Chinese exercise balls for the hands)
- Bells and Dorges (or Dorje)
- Chimes
- Crystal bowls
- Drums
- Flutes
- Gongs
- Tibetan singing bowls (singing bowl meditation)
- Ting-shas (tiny cymbals)

For additional information about singing bowls, refer to the Himalayan Bowls website (himalayanbowls.com) or the Best Singing Bowls website (bestsingingbowls.com).

Finally, did you know that cats may purr as a form of self-healing (Lyons 2006)? I personally find it very relaxing when my cats are purring while I'm writing or reading.

SINGING, WHISTLING, AND HUMMING

A study by Pongan et al. (2017) concludes that "singing and painting interventions may reduce pain and improve mood, quality of life, and cognition in patients with mild Alzheimer's disease." Another review article by Kang et al. (2017) states that "singing can also cause changes in neurotransmitters and hormones, including the upregulation of oxytocin, immunoglobulin A, and endorphins, which improves immune function and increases feelings of happiness."

What about whistling and humming. To the best of my knowledge, people rarely whistle or hum while they are sad. Most people tend to whistle or hum when they are happy, content, or perhaps trying to blow off some stress. I periodically catch myself whistling or humming the melody *Beautiful Dreamer* from Stephen Foster (1826-1864). Do I have a study to cite here about the benefits of whistling or humming? No, but if you do, please send it to me! For additional information, refer to the books *Healing Sounds: The Power of Harmonics* (2002) and *The Humming Effect: Sound Healing for Health and Happiness* (2017) by Jonathan Goldman. Also refer to his *Humming Effect* Instructional Audio Tracks at audio.innertraditions.com/humeff.

So, go ahead and sing, whistle, or hum your favorite tune right now. Or better yet, make up your own melody. See how you feel with each one.

BIOLOGICAL GROUNDING OR EARTHING

"Grounding or earthing refers to direct skin contact with the surface of the Earth, such as with bare feet [such as walking on the beach or grass] or hands [such as working in the garden], or with various grounding systems [such as commercial wrist band and mat products]. Subjective reports that walking barefoot on the Earth enhances health and provides feelings of well-being can be found in the literature and practices of diverse cultures from around the world" (Oschman et al. 2015). This proposed theory suggests that earthing or grounding has the potential to be a simple, natural, and accessible strategy for degenerative and inflammatory-related diseases" (Sinatra et al. 2017). For additional information about the proposed benefits of earthing, refer to the Earthing Center website http://earthingcenter.org and the Earthing website www.earthing.com.

LET YOUR MIND HEAL YOUR BODY

Sometimes our thoughts and approaches to life get in the way of healing and health. By freeing the mind of clutter, the body can focus its energy on healing and well-being. Practice the following (Kross et al. 2014; Rein et al. 1995):

- Nix the negative self-talk
- Resist the urge to judge
- Walk away from arguments that serve little purpose
- Lose the stubbornness
- Let go of anger
- Be more tolerant
- Always show respect
- Act more pleasant and kind

MANAGE ANGER

A study by Gouin et al. (2008) indicates that "the impact of anger control on wound healing has clinical relevance. Individuals with low control over the expression of their anger were 4.2 times more likely to take more than four days to heal, compared to those with higher levels of anger control." The authors conclude that "these findings suggest that the ability to regulate the expression of one's anger has a clinically relevant impact on wound healing." I recall Dad telling me that "anger was usually a journey with no destination" when I was being an unruly teenager. That statement always made me stop and think. Perhaps the stopping to think about what that actually meant was what made my teen angst go away for the moment.

Pray and Meditate

Practicing your personal spiritual beliefs, including engaging in prayer and meditation, can help you cope with illness (Brown et al. 2009; Crane 2009).

Quit Smoking

A study shows that smokers had less improvement than nonsmokers after lumbar stenosis surgery (Sanden et al. 2011). If this applies to back surgery, it most likely applies to other types of surgery as well as for injuries. See chapter 3: Getting Enough Sleep for more information on quitting smoking.

Read or Write a Poem

Let the creation and expression through poetry be your guide for healing (Carroll 2005). Also, refer to the National Association for Poetry Therapy website www .poetrytherapy.org.

See a Manual Therapy Specialist

Manual therapy, massage, and bodywork can help a person heal. The following list outlines just a few forms (Kassolik et al. 2015; Kumar et al. 2017) and styles of manual therapy and bodywork used for healing, recovery, and relaxation:

- Active Release Technique (ART), activerelease.com
- Acupressure, exploreim.ucla.edu (search for acupressure)
- Aston Kinetics (bodywork, movement, ergonomics, fitness), astonkinetics .com
- Ayurvedic massage, theayurvedaexperience.com
- BodyTalk, bodytalksystem.com
- Chakra stones (such as the 7 main Chakras used as a part of some bodywork), chakras.info, chopra.com
- Craniosacral therapy, upledger.com
- Cupping, cuppingtherapy.org
- Dry needling, aaaomonline.org (search for dry needling)
- Graston (instrument-assisted soft tissue mobilization), grastontechnique .com
- Gua Sha (instrument-assisted soft tissue mobilization), guasha.com
- Hellerwork, hellerwork.com
- Hot stones (used in massage), amtamassage.org
- Jin Shin Do (acupressure), jinshindo.org
- Joint manipulation (also known as spinal manipulation), aaompt.org (search for joint manipulation)

- Joint mobilization, aaompt.org (search for joint manipulation)
- Manual lymph drainage (also referred to as complete decongestive therapy), vodderschool.com
- Moxibustion (form of heat therapy that stimulates acupuncture points in the body), nih.gov (search for moxibustion)
- Muscle energy techniques, leonchaitow.com (search for muscle energy)
- Myofascial Release, myofascialrelease.com
- Reflexology, reflexology-usa.org
- Reiki (also known as energy medicine or biofield therapy), reiki.org
- Rolfing, rolf.org
- Shiatsu, shiatsusociety.org
- Sports massage, amtamassage.org (search for sports massage)
- Swedish massage (also known as traditional massage), amtamassage.org (search for Swedish massage)
- Tensegrity (also known as biotensegrity), anatomytrains.com, biotensegrity.com
- Thai massage, thaimassageassociation.com
- Therapeutic touch, therapeutictouch.org
- Trager Approach, trager.com
- Trigger point therapy, myofascialtherapy.org
- Tuina (also Tui-na), acupuncturetoday.com (search for tuina)
- Visceral manipulation, barralinstitute.com

SHELF THE ALCOHOL

Alcohol delays the healing of bone and soft tissues such as tendons and muscles (Jung et al. 2011). It's best to wait until you are completely healed after surgery or injury before consuming alcohol even in moderation.

TRY LABYRINTH WALKING

Refer to the Labyrinth Walking Program in chapter 1.

TRY TAI CHI

This gentle martial arts practice might help boost your immune system (Burke et al. 2007).

TRY VISUALIZATION, RELAXATION, AND GUIDED IMAGERY

These methods before and after surgery promote faster healing and also reduce pain and anxiety (Huddleston 2012). A study by Broadbent et al. (2012)

indicates that relaxation and guided imagery prior to surgery "can reduce stress and improve the wound healing response in surgical patients." A study by Maddison et al. (2012) indicates that guided "imagery intervention improved knee laxity [slackness or looseness] and healing-related neurobiological factors." Also, a study by Cupal et al. (2001) shows that individuals who underwent a guided imagery intervention had "greater knee strength and significantly less reinjury anxiety" after anterior cruciate ligament reconstruction.

TRY A ROCKING CHAIR

Rocking chairs are relaxing and comfortable, and might be better than static seating. Rocking causes the feet and ankles to pump blood back to the heart and brain, thus preventing overall stiffness. A rocking chair can help manage pain from trigger points in the gluteus medius, piriformis, gastrocnemius, and soleus muscles (Travell et al. 1992). So, why sit in a standard chair while watching television or reading when you could be rocking away comfortably in a rocking chair, especially if the seat is padded? Also, check out hammocks and porch swings for relaxation. We definitely need to reduce sitting time in our culture, but rocking chairs are good alternatives for the times we do sit. Rock on!

USE HEALING RECIPES

A well-balanced diet *before* and *after* surgery (or injury) is crucial for optimal healing (Kratzing 2011). Micronutrients most important for wound healing include vitamin A, vitamin C, and zinc (Hwang et al. 2012). Vitamin K (good sources are green, leafy vegetables) assists in proper blood clotting, healing of fractures, and protecting against inflammation (Bitensky et al. 1988; Shea 2008). Consult with a dietitian about providing healing recipes for your needs. Refer to the Academy of Nutrition and Dietetics website www.eatright.org. For information about finding a dietitian specializing in your needs near your home, click the Find an Expert (Registered Dietitian Nutritionist) link.

HEAL WITH AROMATHERAPY

Aromatherapy is the "therapeutic use of essential oils distilled from plants in baths, as inhalants, or during massage to treat skin conditions, anxiety and stress, headaches, and depression" (Venes 2017). I was introduced to aromatherapy through my parents without even knowing it. When I was in high school, I asked Mom why my pillowcase smelled like lavender and she answered "It helps keep the wolves away so the sheep can sleep." I guess I was a restless sleeper, and she was trying to help. I also remember Dad, an internal medicine physician as you may recall, having me smell fresh-cut lemons to help me feel better when I had the flu or felt nauseated. Both of these strategies worked for me and they may do the same for you. Consider giving it a try.

For safe and effective use of all essential oils, consult with a professional experienced in aromatherapy. The following are examples of oil scents that can have surprising health benefits:

- **Bergamot** might be useful in reducing preoperative anxiety (Ni et al. 2013).
- **Lavender** can be an essential part of the multidisciplinary treatment for pain after a cesarean section (Olapour et al. 2013), might decrease the number of required analgesics following pediatric tonsillectomy (Soltani et al. 2013), and could help alleviate premenstrual emotional symptoms (Matsumoto et al. 2013).
- **Lemon** can be effective in reducing nausea and vomiting during pregnancy (Yavari et al. 2014).
- **Orange** might reduce salivary cortisol and pulse rate due to anxiety during a child's dental treatment (Jafarzadeh et al. 2013).
- **Peppermint** is effective in relieving postoperative nausea or vomiting when used in conjunction with controlled breathing (Sites et al. 2014). Also, local use of peppermint oil may help relieve a tension headache (Kligler et al. 2007).

Other essential oils to consider include basil, cinnamon, clove, cypress, eucalyptus, myrtle, nutmeg, oregano, rosemary, sage, spearmint, and wintergreen. I recommend consulting with the following resources to learn more about the uses and effects of essential oils:

- Alliance of International Aromatherapists, alliance-aromatherapists .org
- Aromatherapy Registration Council, aromatherapycouncil.org
- International Federation of Aromatherapists, ifaroma.org
- MSDS Solutions Center, msds.com (material safety data sheets)
- National Association for Holistic Aromatherapy, naha.org
- Refer to the book *Clinical Aromatherapy: Essential Oils in Healthcare* (Buckle 2014).
- Refer to the book, *Essential Oil Safety: A Guide for Health Care Professionals* (Tisserand et al. 2014), roberttisserand.com.

HEAL WITH COLOR

An article by Azeemi et al. (2005) hypothesizes that various colors have different healing characteristics. Unfortunately, very few reliable scientific studies show the effectiveness of chromotherapy for treating a variety of medical conditions. For example, pink light is proposed to having a tranquilizing and calming effect.

Further research is needed in this area. However, for the purpose of this book, consider using color generically and according to your personal preferences for enhancing your mood. For example, red, yellow, and orange can be thought of for stimulation and excitement, and blue, green, and violet for relaxation. Pink, on the other hand, is thought to reduce aggression (Schauss 1979, 1985). So the next time you are angry or agitated, think pink.

HEAL WITH VISUAL ARTS

Art can be used as a tool for healing (Bozcuk et al. 2017; Rollins 2005; Svensk et al. 2009; Toll et al. 2017). Try your hand at visual arts activities, such as painting, drawing, or pottery, to facilitate the healing process (Stuckey et al. 2010). Give it a try and see how you feel. Also, refer to the American Art Therapy Association website www.arttherapy.org for more guidance.

Go ahead and draw in the book below (unless it's a library book or your friend's copy!) (Figure 15-2). Draw your favorite cartoon character, a stick figure, or even a few circles. Just get a pencil or pen and allow yourself to be creative.

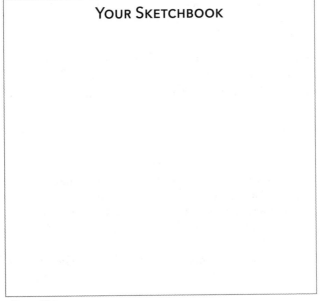

Figure 15-2

Another approach is to observe some art and photographs to help soothe your mind and body. A study shows that nurses can use photographic imagery, such as a sunset over a lake, a rock-covered river, or an autumn waterfall, as a restorative intervention in a hospital setting (Hanson et al. 2013). Consider the following websites to bring relaxing art and photography into your world:

- Leanne Venier, leannevenier.com
- Mangelsen Images of Nature Gallery, mangelsen.com
- National Gallery of Art, nga.gov
- Peter Lik Fine Art Photography, lik.com
- The Ansel Adams Gallery, anseladams.com
- The John Muir Exhibit, vault.sierraclub.org/john_muir_exhibit
- Thomas Kinkade Company, thomaskinkade.com

HEAL WITH HONEY

Products of the honeybee include bee venom, honey, pollen, royal jelly, propolis, and beeswax. According to the American Apitherapy Society, apitherapy (from the Latin *apis*, which means "bee") is the medicinal use of products made by honeybees.

Honey can benefit wound healing (Weissenstein et al. 2014), reduce post tonsillectomy pain (Mohebbi et al. 2014), and has antioxidant and anti-inflammatory properties (Alvarez-Suarez et al. 2013) when used under the supervision of a medical practitioner.

A study by Paul et al. (2007) also indicates that buckwheat [a type of honey from buckwheat flowers] "honey may be a preferable treatment for the cough and sleep difficulty associated with childhood upper respiratory tract infection." Another study by Watanabe et al. (2014) indicates that "honey, in general, and particularly manuka honey [a type of honey from New Zealand made by bees that pollinate the manuka bush], has potent inhibitory activity against the influenza virus."

Check with your healthcare provider before using honey for any medical conditions since honey can negatively interact with certain medications, increase blood sugar, and cause allergic reactions in some people who are prone.

HEAL WITH WATER

Many cultures, such as the traditional Romans and Greeks, have long used the healing effects of water for recovery and recuperation (Bates et al. 1996; Brody et al. 2009; Vargas 2004; Wilk et al. 2014). Consider the following forms of healing in water:

- Ai Chi, clinicalaichi.org
- Aquatic therapy (may also be called hydrotherapy), atri.org and aquaticpt .org and wcpt.org/apti
- Bad Ragaz Ring Method, badragazringmethod.org/en

- Balneotherapy (medical use of baths), balneology.org
- Halliwick Aquatic Therapy, halliwick.org
- Hot tubs and spas, apsp.org
- Watsu, watsu.com

Other generic forms of healing from water may be found in these basic activities:

- Fishing
- Listening to waterfalls (outdoors or in the home)
- Sailing
- Scuba diving
- Swimming

CONSIDER HIPPOTHERAPY
(A FORM OF EQUESTRIAN THERAPY)

According to the Equestrian Therapy website (www.equestriantherapy.com), the four types of equine therapy include equine facilitated psychotherapy (EFP), equine facilitated learning (EFL), hippotherapy, and therapeutic riding. The authors of an article (Koca et al. 2015) state that "Hippotherapy is a form of physical, occupational and speech therapy in which a therapist uses the characteristic movements of a horse to provide carefully graded motor and sensory input." They further state that "Unlike therapeutic horseback riding (where specific riding skills are taught), the movement of the horse is a means to a treatment goal when utilizing hippotherapy as a treatment strategy." Finally, the authors indicate that hippotherapy may be used to treat individuals with neurological or other disabilities, such as multiple sclerosis (Vermöhlen et al. 2017), arthritis, autism, cerebral palsy, stroke, head injury, spinal cord injury, and also psychiatric and behavioral disorders.

HEAL WITH KNITTING, SEWING, AND CROCHET

Perhaps the old saying, "Busy hands are happy hands" is true. I believe there is nothing like being creative with your hands for the mind and body connection. Knitting, sewing, and crocheting are active forms of meditation. An article by Riley et al. (2013) finds that knitting can contribute to well-being. Give it a try.

CONSIDER BIOFEEDBACK TRAINING

Biofeedback is a type of training program using monitoring devices to help develop control over the nervous system by learning to control heart rate, blood pressure, skin temperature, brain waves, or to relax certain muscles (Venes 2017). Ask your physician if you may use biofeedback to help you reduce pain, muscle tension, and anxiety. For example, biofeedback using an app (see below for BrightHearts) may help children to relax and manage pain while in the hospital (Morrow et al. 2017) and other types of biofeedback may help individuals with facial palsy heal at home (Vol et al. 2014) and reduce stress (Dillon et al. 2016) (see below for the Pip). For additional information on biofeedback, refer to the following:

- Association for Applied Psychophysiology and Biofeedback, Inc, aapb.org
- Bio-Medical Instruments (for consumers), bio-medical.com
- BrightHearts (for consumers), brightheartsapp.com
- NeuroSky, neurosky.com
- Noraxon (for clinicians), noraxon.com
- Pip, thepip.com

WEAR COMPRESSION GARMENTS

Ask your healthcare provider about compression garments and clothing to see if it may help you with recovery after aerobic and resistance exercise (Armstrong et al. 2015; Goto et al. 2014; Kraemer et al. 2010), managing lymphedema, and reducing the incidence of deep vein thrombosis (DVT) with anti-embolism stockings. For additional information on compression garments, refer to the following:

- Bauerfeind, bauerfeind.com
- Compressport, compressport.com
- JOBST, jobst-usa.com
- Lymphedema Products, lymphedemaproducts.com
- LympheDIVAs, lymphedivas.com
- Under Armour, underarmour.com
- Zensah, zensah.com

INFLAMMATION AND LIFESTYLE

Inflammation is defined as "An immunological defense against injury, infection, or allergy, marked by increases in regional blood flow, immigration of white blood cells, and release of chemical toxins. Inflammation is one way the body uses to protect itself from invasion by foreign organisms and to repair wounds to tissue. Clinical hallmarks of inflammation are redness, heat, swelling, pain, and loss of function of a body part" (Venes 2017).

Systemic inflammation (affecting the entire body) may produce joint and muscle pains, fever, organ dysfunction, and malaise (feeling of physical discomfort or uneasiness). Acute inflammation is the early response to tissue injury and most of the response takes place in the first 12 to 24 hours. Chronic inflammation is inflammation that goes on for weeks to months after tissue damage (Venes 2017). The following are some diseases associated with inflammation (Escott-Stump 2015): alcoholic liver disease, asthma, atherosclerotic cardiovascular disease, celiac disease, chronic obstructive pulmonary disease (COPD), Crohn's disease, cystic fibrosis, depression, diabetes mellitus, diverticular disease, fibromyalgia, food allergy, hypertension, irritable bowel syndrome (IBS), obesity, osteoarthritis, rheumatoid arthritis (RA), and ulcerative colitis.

The nutrition book *Nutrition and Diagnosis-Related Care* (Escott-Stump 2015) outlines the basic principles of the Mediterranean or an anti-inflammatory diet:

- Focus on a plant-based diet
- Focus on foods rich in antioxidants and phytochemicals
- Eat fresh and minimize processed foods
- Eat "super-foods" such as salmon, blueberries, bananas, broccoli, avocado, or dark chocolate (at least 70% cocoa)
- Drink green or oolong tea
- Use spices and herbs such as oregano, cinnamon, dill, turmeric, curcumin, ginger, or garlic

The nutrition book *Krause's Food & the Nutrition Care Process* (Mahan et al. 2017) states that after athletes are injured, the inflammatory stage of healing is affected by foods. The authors indicate that a "diet high in trans fats, saturated fats and some omega-6 vegetable oils has been shown to promote inflammation, whereas a diet high in monosaturated fat [such as olive and avocado] and essential omega-3 fats has been shown to be anti-inflammatory. The authors also state that "It is believed that nightshade plants aggravate the inflammation that causes pain, swelling, and stiffness in the joints of some patients with arthritis." Finally, the authors outline the following principles of the anti-inflammatory diet:

- Consume colorful vegetables and fruits, and also include anti-inflammatory spices and herbs such as turmeric, garlic, ginger, rosemary, oregano, cocoa, ginger, clove, coriander, cinnamon, nutmeg, black pepper, parsley, sage, dill, and basil.
- Eat a low glycemic diet.
- Eat nuts and seeds.
- Adjust the quality and quantity of fats to include olive oil, coconut oil, and avocados and decrease excess animal protein and omega-6 fatty acids (such as soybean, corn, safflower, and sunflower oils). Also, avoid hydrogenated fats and trans fats.
- Get adequate sources of probiotics from sources such as fermented and cultured foods.

- Be aware of any food allergies and food sensitivities and minimize or avoid these foods. Common food allergens include eggs, milk, fish, shellfish, wheat, tree nuts, peanuts, and soybeans.
- Avoid chemical and pesticides which can irritate your immune system. Use BPA-Free (Bisphenol A) cans. For more information, see the Environmental Working Group website www.ewg.org.
- Drink alcohol in moderation.
- Get enough sleep.
- Keep stress levels under control.

If you wish, you can review additional studies which in general discuss inflammation and diets (Cavicchia et al. 2009; Minihane et al. 2015; Olendzki et al. 2014) by going to the website www.PubMed.gov (US National Library of Medicine) and searching for the title of the article found in the References section. See the Dietary Inflammatory Index (Table 15-7). You may also want to get the free Dietary Inflammation Index (DII Screener) app at the Apple Store and additional information about the app at Connecting Health Innovations (http://chi-llc.net). Finally, go to the Arthritis Foundation website www.arthritis.org and search for "anti-inflammatory foods."

TABLE 15-7: DIETARY INFLAMMATORY INDEX

The following nutrients are arranged from the highest to lowest level of anti-inflammatory effects.

- Magnesium
- Turmeric
- Beta carotene
- Genistein
- Vitamin A
- Tea
- Quercetin
- Wine (red)
- Luteolin
- Vitamin E

Adapted from Cavicchia et al. (2009) and Shivappa et al. (2014).

In the end, I think we can all do ourselves a favor by reducing all potentially inflammatory things in our lifestyle (such a poor diet, chronic stress, lack of sleep, lack of exercise, or improper exercise) to keep our bodies healthy.

HABITS AND LIFESTYLE

Table 15-8 outlines various habit changes that may influence your overall health and well-being.

TABLE 15-8: LIFESTYLE HABITS FOR HEALTH AND HEALING

REASONS TO STOP SMOKING	REASONS TO AVOID SOFT DRINKS	REASONS TO LIMIT ALCOHOL	REASONS TO LIMIT CAFFEINE
Help reduce risk of cancer (Gullett et al. 2010; Rostron et al. 2014)	**Help reduce risk of cancer** (Mueller et al. 2010)	**Help reduce risk of cancer** (Cao et al. 2015; Mahan et al. 2012)	
Help protect your bones (Scolaro et al. 2014)	**Help protect your bones** (Høstmark et al. 2011; Tucker et al. 2006)	**Help protect your bones** (Tarantino et al. 2017)	**Help protect your bones** (Hallstrom et al. 2006, 2013)
Help protect your spine (Akmal et al. 2004; Behrend et al. 2012; Feldman et al. 1999; Goldberg et al. 2000; Lee et al. 2015; Sanden et al. 2011)	**Help reduce risk of asthma** (Shi et al. 2012)	**Help improve your immune system** (Bode et al. 2003)	
Help protect your vision (Cheng et al. 2000; Coleman et al. 2010; Delcourt et al. 1998; Myers et al. 2014)		**Help protect your vision** (Adams et al. 2012; Chong et al. 2008)	
Help lower your blood pressure (Virdis et al. 2010)	**Help lower your blood pressure** (Chen et al. 2010)	**Help lower your blood pressure** (Appel et al. 2003)	
Help protect your hearing (Cruickshanks et al. 1998; Dawes et al. 2014; Nakanishi et al. 2000; Sumit et al. 2015)	**Help reduce risk of diabetes** (Hu et al. 2010; Odegaard et al. 2010)	**Help prevent problems with reaction time** (Ogden et al. 2004; Welford 1980)	
Help protect your teeth (Kerdvongbundit et al. 2000; Machuca et al. 2000)	**Help protect your teeth** (Cheng 2009; Lee et al. 2010; Sohn et al. 2006)		

Help maintain your muscles (Rom et al. 2012)		**Help maintain your muscles** (Preedy et al. 2001)	
Help reduce risk of an abdominal aneurysm (Forsdahl et al. 2009)	**Help reduce risk of obesity** (Cohen et al. 2010; Fowler et al. 2015; Funtikova et al. 2015)	**Help reduce risk of obesity** (Wang et al. 2010)	
Help reduce mental health problems (Gurillo et al. 2015)	**Help reduce mental health problems** (Shi et al. 2010)	**Help yourself sleep better** (Jefferson et al. 2005; Kryger et al. 2016; Morita et al. 2012; Van Reen et al. 2011)	**Help yourself sleep better** (Ancoli-Israel 1996; Attarian 2010)
Help yourself live longer (Jha 2009; Jha et al. 2013; Office on Smoking and Health 2013)		**Help yourself heal faster** (Jung et al. 2011)	
Help yourself think better (Hagger-Johnson et al. 2013)		**Help yourself think better** (Hagger-Johnson et al. 2013; Kabai 2014; Sabia et al. 2014)	
Help reduce risk of depression (Clyde et al. 2013)		**Help reduce risk of depression** (Gilman et al. 2001; Schuckit et al. 2013)	
Help yourself breathe better (Lou et al. 2013; Orozco-Levi et al. 2012)			
Look better (Ernster et al. 1995; Kadunce et al. 1991; Kvaavik et al. 2010; Mosley et al. 1996; Trueb 2003)			

Did You Know?

- The nervous system, not including the brain and spine, can regrow about 1mm per day (Aminoff et al. 2013; Castro et al. 2002; Sunderland 1991).
- The majority of fractures, not counting surgical wounds, heal in 4 to 8 weeks (McKinnis 2014).
- A fully mature fibrous scar requires 12 to 18 months [for healing] and is about 20% to 30% weaker than normal skin" (Goodman et al. 2015).
- It is safe to adopt a 'wait-and-watch' policy for cases of massive disc herniation if there are any early signs of clinical improvement. Initial follow-up at an average of 23.2 months revealed that 83% had a complete and sustained recovery at the initial follow-up. A massive disc herniation can pursue a favorable clinical course. If early progress is shown, the long-term prognosis is very good and even a massive disc herniation can be treated conservatively (Benson et al. 2010).
- "Joint effusion increases intraarticular pressure and afferent activity, which contributes to muscle inhibition. In fact, even small increases in fluid in a joint (as little as 10 mL) can produce a 50% to 60% decrease in maximal voluntary contractions of the quadriceps" (Andrews et al. 2012, p. 43). In other words, knee swelling may cause your knee to give out while walking.

Some additional factors that influence healing include the following: age; coexisting conditions such as diabetes, presence of infection, types of tissue involved (muscle, tendon, ligament, bone, or skin), types of trauma, medications, and hormones. Keep in mind that almost any activity can become therapeutic if it has meaning to a person.

Finally, let's remember the wise words of Norman Cousins, an American journalist: "In the healing equation, therefore, the physician brings the best that medical science has to offer, and the patient brings the best that millions of years of evolution have to offer" (Carlson et al. 1989).

Box 14: Holistic Healing

Balance between Yin and Yang

One alternative medical system is Traditional Chinese medicine (TCM). The TCM system "is based on the theory that disease results from improper flow of life force [called qi]. The movement of qi is restored by balancing the opposing forces of yin and yang, which manifest in the body as heat and cold, external and internal, and deficiency and excess." The TCM uses various practices such as massage, acupuncture, diet, herbs, and meditative exercise (qigong) to restore qi and health (Porter et al. 2011). Yin-yang is an ancient Chinese philosophical concept of complementary opposites. In TCM the goal is to have proper balance between Chinese *yin* (such as the moon, dark, passive) and Chinese *yang* (such as the sun, bright, active) (Venes 2017).

YIN	YANG
• Moon	• Sun
• Dark	• Light
• Feminine	• Masculine
• Water	• Fire
• Cold	• Heat
• Passive	• Active

ADDITIONAL RESOURCES

- All Things Healing, allthingshealing.com
- American Art Therapy Association, arttherapy.org
- American College of Lifestyle Medicine, lifestylemedicine.org
- American Journal of Lifestyle Medicine, journals.sagepub.com/home/ajl
- American Music Therapy Association, musictherapy.org
- Animal Planet, animalplanet.com
- Blue Zones, bluezones.com
- Color Matters, colormatters.com
- Healing Guide Retreats and Escapes, healingguide.org
- Healing Lifestyles & Spas, healinglifestyles.com
- Institute of Lifestyle Medicine, instituteoflifestylemedicine.org
- Music Heals, music-heals.com
- Spine Surgery Recovery, spine-surgery-recovery.com
- Vitamin D Council, vitamindcouncil.org
- Wound Healing Society, woundheal.org
- Refer to the book by Romy Rawlings *Healing Gardens* (1998).
- Refer to the book by Clare Cooper-Marcus and Marni Barnes *Healing Gardens: Therapeutic Benefits and Design Recommendations* (1999).
- Refer to the book by Suren Shrestha *How to Heal with Singing Bowls: Traditional Tibetan Healing Methods* (2013).
- Refer to the book by Clare Cooper-Marcus and Naomi Sachs *Therapeutic Landscapes: An Evidence-Based Approach to Designing Healing Gardens and Restorative Outdoor Spaces* (2014).
- Refer to the book by Carol Davis *Integrative Therapies in Rehabilitation: Evidence for Efficacy in Therapy, Prevention and Wellness* (2017).
- Refer to the Meir Schneider, PhD, LMT School for Self-Healing website (and books) self-healing.org for inspiration and one person's life-long quest for self-healing knowledge.
- Refer to the products by *Energy Muse: Inspirational Jewelry* (jewelry, crystals, stones), energymuse.com
- Refer to the products by *Sunreed Instruments* (for sources of healings sounds), sunreed.com

REFERENCES

Abe Y, Kashiwagi K, Ishida S, et al. (2018). Risk factors for delayed healing at the free anterolateral thigh flap donor site. *Archives of Plastic Surgery* 45 (1): 51-57.

Abtahi AM, Granger EK, Tashjian RZ. (2015). Factors affecting healing after arthroscopic rotator cuff repair. *World Journal of Orthopedics* 6 (2): 211–220.

Academy of Geriatric Physical Therapy. (2018). Balance and falls special interest group. Madison, WI: Academy of Geriatric Physical Therapy. Retrieved on January 25, 2018 from https://geriatricspt.org/special-interest-groups/balance-falls/

Aleksiev AR. (2014). Ten-year follow-up of strengthening versus flexibility exercises with or without abdominal bracing in recurrent low back pain. *Spine (Phila Pa 1976)* 39 (13): 997–1003.

Al-Sharman A, Siengsukon CF. (2013). Sleep enhances learning of a functional motor task in young adults. *Physical Therapy* 93 (12): 1625–1635.

Altemus M, Rao B, Dhabhar FS, et al. (2001). Stress-induced changes in skin barrier function in healthy women. *Journal of Investigative Dermatology* 117 (2): 309–317.

Altug Z. (2011). Energy Conservation Guide for Older Adults. *GeriNotes* (Section on Geriatrics, American Physical Therapy Association) 18 (1): 8.

Altug Z. (2010). Joint protection guide for older adults. *GeriNotes* (Section on Geriatrics, American Physical Therapy Association) 17 (5): 11.

Aminoff MJ, Boller F, Swaab DF. (Eds.). (2013). *Peripheral Nerve Disorders* (Volume 115, 3rd Series). New York, NY: Elsevier.

Andrews JR, Harrelson GL, Wilk KE. (2012). *Physical Rehabilitation of the Injured Athlete*, 4th ed. Philadelphia, PA: Elsevier Saunders.

Armstrong SA, Till ES, Maloney SR, et al. (2015). Compression socks and functional recovery following marathon running: A randomized controlled trial. *Journal of Strength and Conditioning Research* 29 (2): 528–533.

Avishai E, Yeghiazaryan K, Golubnitschaja O. (2017). Impaired wound healing: Facts and hypotheses for multi-professional considerations in predictive, preventive and personalised medicine. *EPMA Journal,* 8 (1): 23–33.

Azeemi ST, Raza SM. (2005). A critical analysis of chromotherapy and its scientific evolution. *Evidence-based Complementary and Alternative* 2 (4): 481–488.

Barton J, Pretty J. (2010). What is the best dose of nature and green exercise for improving mental health? A multi-study analysis. *Environmental Science & Technology* 44 (10): 3947–3955.

Bates A, Hanson N. (1996). *Aquatic Exercise Therapy.* Philadelphia, PA: WB Saunders Company.

Beauchemin KM, Hays P. (1996). Sunny hospital rooms expedite recovery from severe and refractory depressions. *Journal of Affective Disorders* 40 (1–2): 49–51.

Beauchemin KM, Hays P. (1998). Dying in the dark: Sunshine, gender and outcomes in myocardial infarction. *Journal of the Royal Society of Medicine* 91 (7): 352–354.

Benson RT, Tavares SP, Robertson SC, et al. (2010). Conservatively treated massive prolapsed discs: A 7-year follow-up. *Annals of the Royal College of the Surgeons of England* 92 (2): 147–153.

Berman D, Oren JH, Bendo J, et al. (2017). The effect of smoking on spinal fusion. *International Journal of Spine Surgery* 11: 29.

Bitensky L, Hart JP, Catterall A, et al. (1988). Circulating vitamin K levels in patients with fractures. *Journal of Bone and Joint Surgery. British Volume* 70 (4): 663–664.

Bogunovic L, Kim AD, Beamer BS, et al. (2010). Hypovitaminosis D in patients scheduled to undergo orthopaedic surgery: A single-center analysis. *Journal of Bone and Joint Surgery. American Volume* 92 (13): 2300–2304.

Bozcuk H, Ozcan K, Erdogan C, et al. (2017). A comparative study of art therapy in cancer patients receiving chemotherapy and improvement in quality of life by watercolor painting. *Complementary Therapies in Medicine* 30: 67-72.

Bradt J, Dileo C, Shim M. (2013). Music interventions for preoperative anxiety. *Cochrane Database of Systematic Reviews* 6, Cd006908.

Broadbent E, Kahokehr A, Booth RJ, et al. (2012). A brief relaxation intervention reduces stress and improves surgical wound healing response: A randomised trial. *Brain, Behavior and Immunity* 26 (2): 212–217.

Brody LT, Geigle PR. (2009). *Aquatic Exercise for Rehabilitation and Training*. Champaign, IL: Human Kinetics.

Brown RP, Gerbarg PL. (2009). Yoga breathing, meditation, and longevity. *Annals of the New York Academy of Sciences* 1172: 54–62.

Buckle J. (2003). *Clinical Aromatherapy: Essential Oils in Practice*, 2nd ed. Louis, MO: Elsevier Churchill Livingstone.

Burke DT, Al-Adawi S, Lee YT, et al. (2007). Martial arts as sport and therapy. *Journal of Sports Medicine and Physical Fitness* 47 (1): 96–102.

Burton CM, King LA. (2004). The health benefits of writing about intensely positive experiences. *Journal of Research in Personality* 38 (2): 150–163.

Carlson R, Shield B. (1989). *Healers on Healing*. Los Angeles, CA: Jeremy P. Tarcher, Inc.

Carroll R. (2005). Finding the words to say it: The healing power of poetry. *Evidence-Based Complementary and Alternative Medicine* 2 (2): 161–172.

Castro AJ, Merchut MP, Neafsey EJ, et al. (2002). *Neuroscience: An Outline Approach*. St. Louis, MO: Mosby.

Cavicchia PP, Steck SE, Hurley TG, et al. (2009). A new dietary inflammatory index predicts interval changes in serum high-sensitivity C-reactive protein. *The Journal of Nutrition* 139 (12): 2365–2372.

Chiasson AM, Linda Baldwin A, McLaughlin C, et al. (2013). The effect of live spontaneous harp music on patients in the intensive care unit. *Evidence-based and Complementary and Alternative Medicine* 2013: 428731.

Coenen P, Parry S, Willenberg L, et al. (2017). Associations of prolonged standing with musculoskeletal symptoms-a systematic review of laboratory studies. *Gait & Posture 58*: 310-318.

Cooper-Marcus C, Barnes M. (Eds.). (1999). *Healing Gardens: Therapeutic Benefits and Design Recommendations*. New York, NY: John Wiley & Sons.

Cooper-Marcus C, Sachs NA. (2014). *Therapeutic Landscapes: An Evidence-Based Approach to Designing Healing Gardens and Restorative Outdoor Spaces*. Hoboken, NJ: John Wiley & Sons.

Crane JN. (2009). Religion and cancer: Examining the possible connections. *Journal of Psychosocial Oncology* 27 (4): 469–486.

Cupal DD, Brewer BW. (2001). Effects of relaxation and guided imagery on knee strength, reinjury anxiety, and pain following anterior cruciate ligament reconstruction. *Rehabilitation Psychology* 46 (1): 28–43.

Davis CM. (2017). *Integrative Therapies in Rehabilitation: Evidence for Efficacy in Therapy, Prevention and Wellness*, 4th ed. Thorofare, NJ: SLACK.

Delitto RS, Rose SJ. (1992). An electromyographic analysis of two techniques for squat lifting and lowering. *Physical Therapy* 72 (6): 438–448.

Dillon A, Kelly M, Robertson IH, et al. (2016). Smartphone applications utilizing biofeedback can aid stress reduction. *Frontiers in Psychology* 7: 832.

dos Santos Alves VL, Alves da Silva RJ, Avanzi O. (2014). Effect of a preoperative protocol of aerobic physical therapy on the quality of life of patients with adolescent idiopathic scoliosis: A randomized clinical study. *American Journal of Orthopedics (Belle Mead NJ)* 43 (6): E112–116.

Escott-Stump S. (2015). *Nutrition and Diagnosis-Related Care,* 8th ed. Philadelphia, PA: Wolters Kluwer.

Gerber L, Furst G, Shulman B, et. al. (1987). Patient education program to teach energy conservation behaviors to patients with rheumatoid arthritis: A pilot study. *Archives of Physical Medicine and Rehabilitation* 68 (7): 442–445.

Glaser R, Kiecolt-Glaser JK, Marucha PT, et al. (1999). Stress-related changes in proinflammatory cytokine production in wounds. *Archives of General Psychiatry* 56 (5): 450–456.

Goldman J. (2002). *Healing Sounds: The Power of Harmonics.* Rochester, VT: Healing Arts Press.

Goldman J, Goldman A. (2017). *The Humming Effect: Sound Healing for Health and Happiness.* Rochester, VT: Healing Arts Press.

Goldsby TL, Goldsby ME, McWalters M, et al. (2017). Effects of singing bowl sound meditation on mood, tension, and well-being: An observational study. *Journal of Evidence-Based Complementary & Alternative Medicine.* 22 (3): 401-406.

Goodman CC, Fuller KS. (2015). *Pathology: Implications for the Physical Therapist,* 4th ed. St. Louis, MO: Saunders Elsevier.

Goto K, Morishima T. (2014). Compression garment promotes muscular strength recovery after resistance exercise. *Medicine and Science in Sports and Exercise* 46 (12): 2265–2270.

Gouin JP, Kiecolt-Glaser JK, Malarkey WB, et al. (2008). The influence of anger expression on wound healing. *Brain Behavior and Immunity* 22 (5): 699–708.

Gyulai F, Raba K, Baranyai I, et al. (2015). BEMER therapy combined with physiotherapy in patients with musculoskeletal diseases: A randomised, controlled double blind follow-up pilot study. *Evidence-Based Complementary and Alternative Medicine* 245742.

Hanson H, Schroeter K, Hanson A, et al. (2013). Preferences for photographic art among hospitalized patients with cancer. *Oncology Nursing Forum* 40 (4): E337–345.

Hermann C. (2015). *Integral ecopsychological investigation of bonsai principles, meaning and healing.* (Unpublished doctoral thesis). University of Zululand, South Africa.

Hoogeboom TJ, Dronkers JJ, Hulzebos EH, et al. (2014). Merits of exercise therapy before and after major surgery. *Current Opinion in Anaesthesiology* 27 (2): 161–166.

Huddleston P. (2012). *Prepare for Surgery, Heal Faster: A Guide of Mind-Body Techniques,* 4th ed. Cambridge, MA: Angel River Press.

Humphrey R, Malone D. (2015). Effectiveness of preoperative physical therapy for elective cardiac surgery. *Physical Therapy* 95 (2): 160–166.

Hwang C, Ross V, Mahadevan U. (2012). Micronutrient deficiencies in inflammatory bowel disease: From A to zinc. *Inflammatory Bowel Diseases* 18 (10): 1961–1981.

Iversen MD, and Westby MD. (2014). Arthritis. In: O'Sullivan SB, Schmitz TJ, and Fulk GD. *Physical Rehabilitation,* 6th ed. Philadelphia, PA: FA Davis.

Jafarzadeh M, Arman S, Pour FF. (2013). Effect of aromatherapy with orange essential oil on salivary cortisol and pulse rate in children during dental treatment: A randomized controlled clinical trial. *Advanced Biomedical Research* 2: 10.

Jung MK, Callaci JJ, Lauing KL, et al. (2011). Alcohol exposure and mechanisms of tissue injury and repair. *Alcoholism, Clinical and Experimental Research* 35 (3): 392–399.

Kang J, Scholp A, Jiang JJ. (2017). A review of the physiological effects and mechanisms of singing. *Journal of Voice.* Electronic publication ahead of print.

Kassolik K, Andrzejewski W, Wilk I, et al. (2015). The effectiveness of massage based on the tensegrity principle compared with classical abdominal massage performed on patients with constipation. *Archives of Gerontology and Geriatrics* 61 (2): 202–211.

Kiecolt-Glaser K, Marucha PT, Malarkey WB, et al. (1995). Slowing of wound healing by psychological stress. *Lancet* 346 (8984): 1194–1196.

Kim MK, Kang SD. (2013). Effects of art therapy using color on purpose in life in patients with stroke and their caregivers. *Yonsei Medical Journal* 54 (1): 15–20.

Kligler B, Chaudhary S. (2007). Peppermint oil. *American Family Physician* 75 (7): 1027–1030.

Koca TT, Ataseven H. (2015). What is hippotherapy? The indications and effectiveness of hippotherapy. *Northern Clinics of Istanbul* 2 (3): 247–252.

Koschwanez HE, Kerse N, Darragh M, et al. (2013). Expressive writing and wound healing in older adults: A randomized controlled trial. *Psychosomatic Medicine* 75 (6): 581–590.

Kraemer WJ, Flanagan SD, Comstock BA, et al. (2010). Effects of a whole body compression garment on markers of recovery after a heavy resistance workout in men and women. *Journal of Strength and Conditioning Research.* 24 (3): 804–814.

Kratzing C. (2011). Preoperative nutrition and carbohydrate loading. *Proceedings of the Nutrition Society* 70 (3): 311–315.

Kross E, Bruehlman-Senecal E, Park J., et al. (2014). Self-talk as a regulatory mechanism: How you do it matters. *Journal of Personality and Social Psychology* 106 (2): 304–324.

Kumar S, Rampp T, Kessler C, et al. (2017). Effectiveness of ayurvedic massage (sahacharadi taila) in patients with chronic low back pain: A randomized controlled trial. *Journal of Alternative and Complementary Medicine* 23 (2): 109–115.

Lamplot JD, Angeline M, Angeles J, et al. (2014). Distinct effects of platelet-rich plasma and BMP13 on rotator cuff tendon injury healing in a rat model. *American Journal of Sports Medicine* 42 (12): 2877–2887.

Li Q, Kobayashi M, Kumeda S, et al. (2016). Effects of forest bathing on cardiovascular and metabolic parameters in middle-aged males. *Evidence-Based Complementary Alternative Medicine.* 2587381.

Lu FJH, Hsu Y. (2013). Injured athletes' rehabilitation beliefs and subjective well-being: The contribution of hope and social support. *Journal of Athletic Training* 48 (1): 92–98.

Lubetzky R, Mimouni FB, Dollberg S, et al. (2010). Effect of music by Mozart on energy expenditure in growing preterm infants. *Pediatrics.* 125 (1): e24–28.

Lyons LA. (2006). Why do cats purr? *Scientific American.* Retrieved on November 4, 2017 from www.scientificamerican.com/article/why-do-cats-purr/.

Maddison R, Prapavessis H, Clatworthy M, et al. (2012). Guided imagery to improve functional outcomes post-anterior cruciate ligament repair: Randomized-controlled pilot trial. *Scandinavian Journal of Medicine & Science in Sports* 22 (6): 816–821.

Mahan LK, Raymond JL. (2017). *Krause's Food & the Nutrition Care Process, 14*th *ed.* St. Louis, MO: Elsevier.

Mathiowetz VG, Finlayson ML, Matuska KM, et al. (2005). Randomized controlled trial of an energy conservation course for persons with multiple sclerosis. *Multiple Sclerosis* 11 (5): 592–601.

Matsumoto T, Asakura H, Hayashi T. (2013). Does lavender aromatherapy alleviate premenstrual emotional symptoms? A randomized crossover trial. *BioPsychoSocial Medicine* 7: 12.

Matsunaga M, Sato S, Isowa T, et al. (2009). Profiling of serum proteins influenced by warm partner contact in healthy couples. *Neuro Endocrinology Letters* 30 (2): 227–236.

McConnell AR, Brown CM, Shoda TM, et al. (2011). Friends with benefits: On the positive consequences of pet ownership. *Journal of Personality and Social Psychology* 101 (6): 1239–1252.

McCulloch JM, Kloth LC. (2010). *Wound Healing: Evidence-Based Management,* 4th ed. Philadelphia, PA: FA Davis.

McGill SM. (2016). *Low Back Disorders,* 3rd ed. Champaign IL: Human Kinetics.

McKinnis L. (2014). *Fundamental of Musculoskeletal Imaging,* 4th ed. Philadelphia, PA: FA Davis Company.

Meghani N, Tracy MF, Hadidi NN, et al. (2017). Part I: The effects of music for the symptom management of anxiety, pain, and insomnia in critically ill patients: An integrative review of current literature. *Dimensions of Critical Care Nursing* 36 (4): 234–243.

Minihane AM, Vinoy S, Russell WR, et al. (2015). Low-grade inflammation, diet composition and health: Current research evidence and its translation. *The British Journal of Nutrition* 114 (7): 999–1012.

Mitrione S. (2008). Therapeutic responses to natural environments: Using gardens to improve health care. *Minnesota Medicine* 91 (3): 31–34.

Moon S, Schmidt M, Smirnova IV, et al. (2017). Qigong exercise may reduce serum TNF-alpha levels and improve sleep in people with Parkinson's disease: A pilot study. *Medicines (Basel):* 4 (2).

Moriyama M, Moriyama H, Uda J, et al. (2016). Beneficial effects of the genus Aloe on wound healing, cell proliferation, and differentiation of epidermal keratinocytes. *PLoS One* 11 (10): e0164799.

Morrow AM, Burton KLO, Watanabe MM, et al. (2017). Developing Brighthearts: A pediatric biofeedback mediated relaxation app to manage procedural pain and anxiety. *Pain Practice.* Electronic publication ahead of print.

Ni CH, Hou WH, Kao CC, et al. (2013). The anxiolytic effect of aromatherapy on patients awaiting ambulatory surgery: A randomized controlled trial. *Evidence-based Complementary and Alternative Medicine* 927419.

Nilsson U. (2008). The anxiety- and pain-reducing effects of music interventions: A systematic review. *Association of Operating Room Nurses Journal* 87 (4): 780–807.

Nilsson U. (2009). Soothing music can increase oxytocin levels during bed rest after open-heart surgery: A randomised control trial. *Journal of Clinical Nursing* 18 (15): 2153–2161.

Olapour A, Behaeen K, Akhondzadeh R, et al. (2013). The effect of inhalation of aromatherapy blend containing lavender essential oil on cesarean postoperative pain. *Anesthesiology and Pain Medicine* 3 (1): 203–207.

Olendzki BC, Silverstein TD, Persuitte GM, et al. (2014). An anti-inflammatory diet as treatment for inflammatory bowel disease: A case series report. *Nutrition Journal* 13:5.

Oschman JL, Chevalier G, Brown R. (2015). The effects of grounding (earthing) on inflammation, the immune response, wound healing, and prevention and treatment of chronic inflammatory and autoimmune diseases. *Journal of Inflammation Research* 8: 83–96.

Patel M, Chipman J, Carlin BW, et al. (2008). Sleep in the intensive care unit setting. *Critical Care Nursing Quarterly* 31 (4): 309–318.

Paul IM, Beiler J, McMonagle A, et al. (2007). Effect of honey, dextromethorphan, and no treatment on nocturnal cough and sleep quality for coughing children and their parents. *Archives of Pediatric & Adolescent Medicine* 161 (12): 1140–1146.

Piatkowski J, Kern S, Ziemssen T. (2009). Effect of BEMER magnetic field therapy on the level of fatigue in patients with multiple sclerosis: A randomized, double-blind controlled trial. *Journal of Alternative and Complementary Medicine* 15 (5): 507–511.

Pludowski P, Holick MF, Pilz S, et al. (2013). Vitamin D effects on musculoskeletal health, immunity, autoimmunity, cardiovascular disease, cancer, fertility, pregnancy, dementia and mortality: A review of recent evidence. *Autoimmunity Reviews* 12 (10): 976–989.

Pongan E, Tillmann B, Leveque Y, et al. (2017). Can musical or painting interventions improve chronic pain, mood, quality of life, and cognition in patients with mild Alzheimer's disease? Evidence from a randomized controlled trial. *Journal of Alzheimers Disease* 60 (2): 663–677.

Raina P, Waltner-Toews D, Bonnett B, et al. (1999). Influence of companion animals on the physical and psychological health of older people: An analysis of a one-year longitudinal study. *Journal of the American Geriatrics Society* 47 (3): 323–329.

Rawlings R. (1998). *Healing Gardens.* Minocqua, WI: Willow Creek Press.

Reid D, Toole BJ, Knox S, et al. (2011). The relation between acute changes in the systemic inflammatory response and plasma 25-hydroxyvitamin D concentrations after elective knee arthroplasty. *American Journal of Clinical Nutrition* 93 (5): 1006–1011.

Rein G, Atkinson M, McCraty R. (1995). The physiological and psychological effects of compassion and anger. *Journal of Advancement in Medicine* 8 (2): 87–105.

Riley J, Corkhil B, Morris C. (2013). The benefits of knitting for personal and social wellbeing in adulthood: findings from an international survey. *British Journal of Occupational Therapy* 76 (2): 50–57.

Rollins JA. (2005). Tell me about it: drawing as a communication tool for children with cancer. *Journal of Pediatric Oncology Nursing* 22 (4): 203–221.

Roy B, Diez-Roux AV, Seeman T, et al. (2010). Association of optimism and pessimism with inflammation and hemostasis in the Multi-Ethnic Study of Atherosclerosis (MESA). *Psychosomatic Medicine* 72 (2): 134–140.

Sandén B, Försth P, Michaëlsson K. (2011). Smokers show less improvement than non-smokers 2 years after surgery for lumbar spinal stenosis: A study of 4555 patients from the Swedish spine register. *Spine (Philadelphia, Pa. 1976)* 36 (13): 1059–1064.

Sandrey MA. (2003). Acute and chronic tendon injuries: factors affecting the healing response and treatment. *Journal of Sports Rehabilitation* 12: 70–91.

Sasannejad P, Saeedi M, Shoeibi A, et al. (2012). Lavender essential oil in the treatment of migraine headache: A placebo-controlled clinical trial. *European Neurology* 67 (5): 288–291.

Schauss AG. (1979). Tranquilizing effect of color reduces aggressive behavior and potential violence. *Orthomolecular Psychiatry* 8 (4): 218–221.

Schauss AG. (1985). The physiological effect of color on the suppression of human aggression: Research on Baker-Miller pink. *International Journal for Biosocial Research* 7 (2): 55–64.

Shea MK, Booth SL, Massaro JM, et al. (2008). Vitamin K and vitamin D status: Associations with inflammatory markers in the Framingham Offspring Study. *American Journal of Epidemiology* 167 (3): 313–320.

Sheon RP. (1985). A joint protection guide for nonarticular rheumatic disorders. *Postgraduate Medicine* 77 (5): 329–338.

Sheon RP, and Orr PM. (1996). Appendix B: Joint protection guide for rheumatic disorders. In: Sheon RP, Moskowitz RW, and Goldberg VM. *Soft Tissue Rheumatic Pain: Recognition, Management and Prevention*, 3rd ed. Baltimore, MD: Williams & Wilkins.

Shivappa N, Steck SE, Hurley TG, et al. (2014). Designing and developing a literature-derived, population-based Dietary Inflammatory Index. *Public Health Nutrition* 17 (8): 1689–1696.

Shrestha S. (2013). *How to Heal With Singing Bowls: Traditional Tibetan Healing Methods*. Boulder CO: Sentient Publications.

Siengsukon CF, Al-Dughmi M, Stevens S. (2017). Sleep health promotion: Practical information for physical therapists. *Physical Therapy* 97 (8): 826–836.

Siengsukon CF, Boyd LA. (2009). Does sleep promote motor learning? Implications for physical rehabilitation. *Physical Therapy* 89 (4): 370–383.

Sinatra ST, Oschman JL, Chevalier G, et al. (2017). Electric nutrition: The surprising health and healing benefits of biological grounding (earthing). *Alternative Therapies in Health and Medicine* 23 (5): 8–16.

Sites DS, Johnson NT, Miller JA, et al. (2014). Controlled breathing with or without peppermint aromatherapy for postoperative nausea and/or vomiting symptom relief: A randomized controlled trial. *Journal of Perianesthesia Nursing* 29 (1): 12–19.

Soltani R, Soheilipour S, Hajhashemi V, et al. (2013). Evaluation of the effect of aromatherapy with lavender essential oil on post-tonsillectomy pain in pediatric patients: A randomized controlled trial. *International Journal of Pediatric Otorhinolaryngology* 77 (9): 1579–1581.

Stratos I, Li Z, Herlyn P, Rotter R, et al. (2013). Vitamin D increases cellular turnover and functionally restores the skeletal muscle after crush injury in rats. *American Journal Pathology* 182 (3): 895–904.

Stuckey HL, Nobel J. (2010). The connection between art, healing, and public health: A review of current literature. *American Journal of Public Health* 100 (2): 254–263.

Stults-Kolehmainen MA, Bartholomew JB, Sinha R. (2014). Chronic psychological stress impairs recovery of muscular function and somatic sensations over a 96-hour period. *Journal of Strength and Conditioning Research* 28 (7): 2007–2017.

Sunderland S. (1991). *Nerve Injuries and Their Repair: A Critical Appraisal.* London, England: WB Saunders Company.

Svensk AC, Oster I, Thyme KE, et al. (2009). Art therapy improves experienced quality of life among women undergoing treatment for breast cancer: A randomized controlled study. *European Journal of Cancer Care (Engl)* 18 (1): 69–77.

Tashjian RZ, Hollins AM, Kim H-K, et al. (2010). Factors affecting healing rates after arthroscopic double-row rotator cuff repair. *American Journal of Sports Medicine* 38 (12): 2435–2442.

Taylor B, Cheema A, Soslowsky L. (2017). Tendon pathology in hypercholesterolemia and familial hypercholesterolemia. *Current Rheumatology Reports* 19 (12): 76.

Thorud JC, Mortensen S, Thorud JL, et al. (2017). Effect of obesity on bone healing after foot and ankle long bone fractures. *Journal of Foot and Ankle Surgery* 56 (2): 258–262.

Thosar SS, Bielko SL, Mather KJ, et al. (2015). Effect of prolonged sitting and breaks in sitting time on endothelial function. *Medicine and Science in Sports and Exercise* 47 (4): 843–849.

Tisserand R, Young R. (2014). *Essential Oil Safety: A Guide for Health Care Professionals,* 2nd ed. St. Louis, MO: Churchill Livingstone Elsevier.

Toll E, Melfi BS. (2017). The healing power of paint. *JAMA* 317 (11): 1100–1102.

Toyoda Y, Fu RH, Li L, et al. (2018). Smoking as an independent risk factor for postoperative complications in plastic surgical procedures: A propensity score-matched analysis of 36,454 patients from the nsqip database from 2005 to 2014. *Plastic and Reconstructive Surgery* 141 (1): 226–236.

Travell JG, Simons DG. (1992). *Travell & Simons' Myofascial Pain and Dysfunction: The Trigger Point Manual.* (Volume 2)—*The Lower Extremities.* Baltimore MD: Williams & Wilkins.

Vaajoki A, Pietilä AM, Kankkunen P, et al. (2012). Effects of listening to music on pain intensity and pain distress after surgery: An intervention. *Journal of Clinical Nursing* 21 (5–6): 708–17.

Vargas LG. (2004). *Aquatic Therapy: Interventions and Applications.* Enumclaw, WA: Idyll Arbor.

Venes D. (Ed.). (2017). *Taber's Cyclopedic Medical Dictionary,* 23rd ed. Philadelphia, PA: FA Davis.

Vera-Garcia FJ, Elvira JL, Brown SH, et al. (2007). Effects of abdominal stabilization maneuvers on the control of spine motion and stability against sudden trunk perturbations. *Journal of Electromyography and Kinesiology* 17 (5): 556–567.

Vermohlen V, Schiller P, Schickendantz S, et al. (2017). Hippotherapy for patients with multiple sclerosis: A multicenter randomized controlled trial (MS-HIPPO). *Multiple Sclerosis.* Electronic publication ahead of print.

Voigt J. (2010/2011). The six healing sounds: Chinese mantras for purifying the body, mind, and soul. *Qi: The Journal of Traditional Eastern Health & Fitness* 20 (4).

Volk GF, Finkensieper M, Guntinas-Lichius O. (2014). EMG biofeedback training at home for patient with chronic facial palsy and defective healing. *Laryngorhinootologie* 93 (1): 15–24. [article in German].

Wadey R, Evans L, Hanton S, et al. (2013). Effect of dispositional optimism before and after injury. *Medicine and Science in Sports and Exercise* 45 (2): 387–394.

Warber SL, Ingerman S, Moura VL, et al. (2011). Healing the heart: A randomized pilot study of a spiritual retreat for depression in acute coronary syndrome patients. *Explore (NY)* 7 (4): 222–233.

Watanabe K, Rahmasari R, Matsunaga A, et al. (2014). Anti-influenza viral effects of honey in vitro: Potent high activity of manuka honey. *Archives of Medical Research* 45 (5): 359–365.

Weissenstein A, Luchter E, Bittmann S. (2014). Medical honey and its role in paediatric patients. *British Journal of Nursing* 23 (6): S30, s32–34.

Wentz I. (2017). *Hashimoto's Protocol: A 90-Day Plan for Reversing Thyroid Symptoms and Getting Your Life Back.* New York, NY: HarperOne,

Wilk KE, Joyner DM. (2014). *The Use of Aquatics in Orthopedics and Sports Medicine Rehabilitation and Physical Conditioning.* Thorofare, NY: SLACK, Incorporated.

Yavari Kia P, Safajou F, Shahnazi M, et al. (2014). The effect of lemon inhalation aromatherapy on nausea and vomiting of pregnancy: A double-blinded, randomized, controlled clinical trial. *Iranian Red Crescent Medical Journal* 16 (3): e14360.

Young GR. (1991). Energy conservation, occupational therapy, and the treatment of post-polio sequelae. *Orthopedics* 14 (11): 1233–1239.

Xie L, Kang H, Xu Q, et al. (2013). Sleep drives metabolite clearance from the adult brain. *Science* 342.

Reasons to Stop Smoking

Akmal M, Kesani A, Anand B, et al. (2004). Effect of nicotine on spinal disc cells: A cellular mechanism for disc degeneration. *Spine (Phila Pa 1976)* 29 (5): 568–575.

Behrend C, Prasarn M, Coyne E, et al. (2012). Smoking cessation related to improved patient-reported pain scores following spinal care. *Journal of Bone and Joint Surgery. American Volume* 94 (23): 2161–2166.

Cheng AC, Pang CP, Leung AT, et al. (2000). The association between cigarette smoking and ocular diseases. *Hong Kong Medical Journal* 6 (2): 195–202.

Clyde M, Smith KJ, Gariepy G, et al. (2013). The association between smoking and depression in a Canadian community-based sample with type 2 diabetes. *Canadian Journal of Diabetes* 37(3): 150–155.

Coleman AL, Seitzman RL, Cummings SR, et al. (2010). The association of smoking and alcohol use with age-related macular degeneration in the oldest old: The study of osteoporotic fractures. *American Journal of Ophthalmology* 149 (1): 160–169.

Cruickshanks KJ, Klein R, Klein BE, et al. (1998). Cigarette smoking and hearing loss: The epidemiology of hearing loss study. *JAMA* 279: 1715–1719.

Dawes P, Cruickshanks KJ, Moore DR, et al. (2014). Cigarette smoking, passive smoking, alcohol consumption, and hearing loss. *Journal of the Association for Research in Otolaryngology* 15 (4): 663–674.

Delcourt C, Diaz JL, Ponton-Sanches A, et al. (1998). Smoking and age-related macular degeneration. The POLA Study. *Archives of Ophthalmology* 116 (8): 1031–1035.

Feldman DE, Rossignol M, Shrier I, et al. (1999). Smoking: A risk factor for development of low back pain in adolescents. *Spine (Phila Pa 1976)* 24 (23): 2492–2496.

Forsdahl SH, Singh K, Solberg S, et al. (2009). Risk factors for abdominal aortic aneurysms: A 7-year prospective study: The Tromso Study, 1994–2001. *Circulation* 119 (16): 2202–2208.

Goldberg MS, Scott SC, Mayo NE. (2000). A review of the association between cigarette smoking and the development of nonspecific back pain and related outcomes. *Spine* 25 (8): 995–1014.

Gullett NP, Amin ARMR, Bayraktar S, et al. (2010). Cancer prevention with natural compounds. Seminars in Oncology 37 (3): 258–281.

Gurillo, P, Jauhar, S, Murray, RM, et al. (2015). Does tobacco use cause psychosis? Systematic review and meta-analysis. Lancet Psychiatry. Advance online publication.

Hagger-Johnson G, Sabia S, Brunner EJ, et al. (2013). Combined impact of smoking and heavy alcohol use on cognitive decline in early old age: Whitehall II prospective cohort study. *British Journal of Psychiatry* 203 (2): 120–125.

Jha P. (2009). Avoidable global cancer deaths and total deaths from smoking. *Nature Reviews. Cancer* 9: 655–664.

Jha P, Ramasundarahettige C, Landsman V, et al. (2013). 21st-century hazards of smoking and benefits of cessation in the United States. *New England Journal of Medicine* 368 (4): 341–350.

Kadunce DP, Burr R, Gress R, et al. (1991). Cigarette smoking: Risk factor for premature facial wrinkling. *Annals of Internal Medicine* 114 (10): 840–844.

Kerdvongbundit V, Wikesjo UM. (2000). Effect of smoking on periodontal health in molar teeth. *Journal of Periodontology* 71 (3): 433–437.

Kvaavik E, Batty D, Ursin G, et al. (2010). Influence of individual and combined health behaviors on total and cause-specific mortality in men and women: The United Kingdom health and lifestyle survey. *Archives of Internal Medicine* 170 (8): 711–718.

Lee JC, Lee SH, Peters C, et al. (2015). Adjacent segment pathology requiring reoperation after anterior cervical arthrodesis: The influence of smoking, sex, and number of operated levels. *Spine (Phila Pa 1976)* 40 (10): E571–577.

Lou P, Zhu Y, Chen P, et al. (2013). Supporting smoking cessation in chronic obstructive pulmonary disease with behavioral intervention: A randomized controlled trial. *BMC Family Practice* 14: 91.

Machuca G, Rosales I, Lacalle JR, et al. (2000). Effect of cigarette smoking on periodontal status of healthy young adults. *Journal of Periodontology* 71 (1): 73–78.

Mosley JG, and Gibbs ACC. (1996). Premature gray hair and hair loss among smokers: A new opportunity for health education? *British Medical Journal* 313: 1616.

Myers CE, Klein BE, Gangnon, R, et al. (2014). Cigarette smoking and the natural history of age-related macular degeneration: The Beaver Dam Eye Study. *Ophthalmology* 121 (10): 1949–1955.

Nakanishi N, Okamoto M, Nakamura K, et al. (2000). Cigarette smoking and risk for hearing impairment: A longitudinal study in Japanese male office workers. *Journal of Occupational and Environmental Medicine* 42 (11): 1045–1049.

Office on Smoking and Health. (2013). *Tobacco-related mortality*. Atlanta, GA: Centers for Disease Control and Prevention.

Orozco-Levi, M, Coronell C, Ramirez-Sarmiento A, et al. (2012). Injury of peripheral muscles in smokers with chronic obstructive pulmonary disease. *Ultrastructural Pathology* 36 (4): 228–238.

Rom O, Kaisari S, Aizenbud D, et al. (2012). Sarcopenia and smoking: A possible cellular model of cigarette smoke effects on muscle protein breakdown. *Annals of the New York Academy of Sciences* 1259: 47–53.

Rostron BL, Chang CM, Pechacek TF. (2014). Estimation of cigarette smoking-attributable morbidity in the United States. *JAMA Internal Medicine* 174 (12): 1922–1928.

Sanden B, Forsth P, Michaelsson K. (2011). Smokers show less improvement than nonsmokers two years after surgery for lumbar spinal stenosis: A study of 4555 patients from the Swedish spine register. *Spine (Phila Pa 1976)* 36 (13): 1059–1064.

Scolaro JA, Schenker ML, Yannascoli S, et al. (2014). Cigarette smoking increases complications following fracture: A systematic review. *Journal of Bone and Joint Surgery American Study* 96 (8): 674–681.

Sumit AF, Das A, Sharmin Z, et al. (2015). Cigarette smoking causes hearing impairment among Bangladeshi population. *PLoS One* 10 (3): e0118960.

Trueb RM. (2003). Association between smoking and hair loss: Another opportunity for health education against smoking? *Dermatology* 206 (3): 189–191.

Virdis A, Giannarelli C, Neves MF, et al. (2010). Cigarette smoking and hypertension. *Current Pharmaceutical Design* 16 (23), 2518-2525.

Volkow ND, Baler RD, Compton WM, et al. (2014). Adverse health effects of marijuana use. *New England Journal of Medicine* 370 (23): 2219–2227.

Volpp KG, Galvin R. (2014). Reward-based incentives for smoking cessation: How a carrot became a stick. *JAMA* 311 (9): 909–910.

Reasons to Avoid Soft Drinks

Chen L, Caballero B, Mitchell DC, et al. (2010). Reducing consumption of sugar-sweetened beverages is associated with reduced blood pressure. A prospective study among United States adults. *Circulation* 121 (22): 2398–2406.

Cheng R, Yang H, Shao My, et al. (2009). Dental erosion and severe tooth decay related to soft drinks: A case report and literature review. *Journal of Zhejiang University. Science B* 10 (5): 395–399.

Cohen DA, Sturm R, Scott M, et al. (2010). Not enough fruit and vegetables or too many cookies, candies, salty snacks, and soft drinks? *Public Health Reports; Hyattsville* 125 (1): 88–95.

Fowler SP, Williams K, Hazuda HP. (2015). Diet soda intake is associated with long-term increases in waist circumference in a biethnic cohort of older adults: The San Antonio longitudinal study of aging. *Journal of the American Geriatrics Society* 63 (4): 708–715.

Funtikova AN, Subirana I, Gomez SF, et al. (2015). Soft drink consumption is positively associated with increased waist circumference and 10-year incidence of abdominal obesity in Spanish adults. *Journal of Nutrition.* 145 (2): 328–334

Hostmark AT, Sogaard AJ, Alvaer K, et al. (2011). The Oslo health study: A dietary index estimating frequent intake of soft drinks and rare intake of fruit and vegetables is negatively associated with bone mineral density. *Journal of Osteoporosis 2011*: 102686.

Hu FB, and Malik VS. (2010). Sugar-sweetened beverages and risk of obesity and type 2 diabetes: Epidemiologic evidence. *Physiology & Behavior* 100 (1): 47–54.

Lee JG, Messer LB. (2010). Intake of sweet drinks and sweet treats versus reported and observed caries experience. *European Archives of Paediatric Dentistry* 11 (1): 5–17.

Mueller NT, Odegaard A, Anderson K, et al. (2010). Soft drink and juice consumption and risk of pancreatic cancer: The Singapore Chinese Health Study. *Cancer Epidemiology Biomarkers & Prevention* 19 (2): 447–455.

Odegaard AO, Koh WP, Arakawa K, et al. (2010). Soft drink and juice consumption and risk of physician-diagnosed incident type 2 diabetes: The Singapore Chinese Health Study. *American Journal of Epidemiology* 171 (6): 701–708.

Shi Z, Dal Grande E, Taylor AW, et al. (2012). Association between soft drink consumption and asthma and chronic obstructive pulmonary disease among adults in Australia. *Respirology* 17 (2): 363–369.

Shi Z, Taylor AW, Wittert G, et al. (2010). Soft drink consumption and mental health problems among adults in Australia. *Public Health Nutrition* 13 (7): 1073–1079.

Singh GM, Micha R, Khatibzadeh S, et al. (2015). Estimated global, regional, and national disease burdens related to sugar-sweetened beverage consumption in 2010. *Circulation*. Advance online publication.

Sohn W, Burt BA, Sowers MR. (2006). Carbonated soft drinks and dental caries in the primary dentition. *Journal of Dental Research* 85 (3): 262–266.

Tucker KL, Morita K, Qiao N, et al. (2006). Colas, but not other carbonated beverages, are associated with low bone mineral density in older women: The Framingham Osteoporosis Study. *American Journal of Clinical Nutrition* 84 (4): 936–942.

Reasons to Limit Alcohol

Adams MK, Chong EW, Williamson E, et al. (2012). 20/20—alcohol and age-related macular degeneration: The Melbourne Collaborative Cohort Study. *American Journal of Epidemiology* 176 (4): 289–298.

Appel LJ, Champagne CM, Harsha DW, et al. (2003). Effects of comprehensive lifestyle modification on blood pressure control: Main results of the premier clinical trial. *JAMA* 289 (16): 2083–2093.

Bode C, Bode JC. (2003). Effect of alcohol consumption on the gut. *Best Practice & Research. Clinical Gastroenterology* 17 (4): 575–592.

Cao Y, Willett WC, Rimm EB, et al. (2015). Light to moderate intake of alcohol, drinking patterns, and risk of cancer: Results from two prospective US cohort studies. *BMJ*. 351: h4238.

Chaves AA, Joshi MS, Coyle CM, et al. (2009). Vasoprotective endothelial effects of a standardized grape product in humans. *Vascular Pharmacology* 50 (1–2): 20–26.

Chong EW, Kreis AJ, Wong TY, et al. (2008). Alcohol consumption and the risk of age-related macular degeneration: A systematic review and meta-analysis. *American Journal Ophthalmology* 145 (4): 707–715.

Droste DW, Iliescu C, Vaillant M, et al. (2013). A daily glass of red wine associated with lifestyle changes independently improves blood lipids in patients with carotid arteriosclerosis: Results from a randomized controlled trial. *Nutrition Journal* 12 (1): 147.

Gilman SE, Abraham HD. (2001). A longitudinal study of the order of onset of alcohol dependence and major depression. *Drug and Alcohol Dependence* 63 (3): 277–286.

Goodman CC, Snyder TE. (2013). *Differential Diagnosis for Physical Therapists: Screening for Referral,* 5th ed. St. Louis, MO: Elsevier. www.differentialdiagnosisforpt.com.

Hagger-Johnson G, Sabia S, Brunner EJ, et al. (2013). Combined impact of smoking and heavy alcohol use on cognitive decline in early old age: Whitehall II prospective cohort study. *British Journal of Psychiatry* 203 (2): 120–125.

Jefferson CD, Drake CL, Scofield HM, et al. (2005). Sleep hygiene practices in a population-based sample of insomniacs. *Sleep* 28 (5): 611–615.

Jensen T, Retterstol LJ, Sandset PM, et al. (2006). A daily glass of red wine induces a prolonged reduction in plasma viscosity: A randomized controlled trial. *Blood Coagulation & Fibrinolysis* 17 (6): 471–476.

Jung MK, Callaci JJ, Lauing KL, et al. (2011). Alcohol exposure and mechanisms of tissue injury and repair. *Alcoholism, Clinical and Experimental Research* 35 (3): 392–399.

Kabai P. (2014). Alcohol consumption and cognitive decline in early old age. *Neurology* 83 (5): 476.

Kryger MH, Roth T, Dement WC. (2016). *Principles and Practice of Sleep Medicine,* 6th ed. Philadelphia, PA: Elsevier Saunders.

Mahan LK, Escott-Stump S, Raymond JL. (2012). *Krause's Food and the Nutrition Care Process,* 13th ed. St. Louis, MO: Elsevier Sanders.

Mash HB, Fullerton CS, Ramsawh HJ, et al. (2014). Risk for suicidal behaviors associated with alcohol and energy drink use in the US Army. *Social Psychiatry and Psychiatric Epidemiology* 49 (9): 1379–1387.

Matesa J. (2014). *The Recovering Body: Physical and Spiritual Fitness for Living Clean and Sober.* Center City, MN: Hazelden.

Morita E, Miyazaki S, Okawa M. (2012). Pilot study on the effects of a 1-day sleep education program: Influence on sleep of stopping alcohol intake at bedtime. *Nagoya Journal of Medical Science* 74 (3–4): 359–365.

Ogden EJ, Moskowitz H. (2004). Effects of alcohol and other drugs on driver performance. *Traffic Injury Prevention* 5 (3): 185–198.

Pennay A, Lubman D, Miller P. (2011). Combining energy drinks and alcohol: A recipe for trouble? *Australian Family Physician* 40 (3): 104–107.

Pesta DH, Angadi SS, Burtscher M, et al. (2013). The effects of caffeine, nicotine, ethanol, and tetrahydrocannabinol on exercise performance. *Nutrition & Metabolism (Lond)* 10 (1): 71.

Preedy VR, Adachi J, Ueno Y, et al. (2001). Alcoholic skeletal muscle myopathy: Definitions, features, contribution of neuropathy, impact and diagnosis. *European Journal of Neurology* 8 (6): 677–687.

Rachdaoui N, Sarkar DK. (2013). Effects of alcohol on the endocrine system. *Endocrinology and Metabolism Clinics of North America* 42 (3): 593–615.

Sabia S, Elbaz A, Britton A, et al. (2014). Alcohol consumption and cognitive decline in early old age. *Neurology* 82 (4): 332–339.

Schuckit MA, Smith TL, Kalmijn J. (2013). Relationships among independent major depressions, alcohol use, and other substance use and related problems over 30 years in 397 families. *Journal of Studies on Alcohol and Drugs* 74 (2): 271–279.

Shrotriya S, Agarwal R, Sclafani RA. (2015). A perspective on chemoprevention by resveratrol in head and neck squamous cell carcinoma. *Advances in Experimental Medicine and Biology* 815: 333–348.

Tarantino U, Iolascon G, Cianferotti L, et al. (2017). Clinical guidelines for the prevention and treatment of osteoporosis: summary statements and recommendations from the Italian Society for Orthopaedics and Traumatology. *Journal of Orthopaedics and Traumatology : Official Journal of the Italian Society of Orthopaedics and Traumatology* 18 (Suppl 1): 3–36.

van der Gaag MS, Sierksma A, Schaafsma G, et al. (2000). Moderate alcohol consumption and changes in postprandial lipoproteins of premenopausal and postmenopausal women: A diet-controlled, randomized intervention study. *Journal of Women's Health and Gender-Based Medicine* 9 (6): 607–616.

Van Reen E, Tarokh L, Rupp TL, et al. (2011). Does timing of alcohol administration affect sleep? *Sleep* 34 (2): 195–205.

Vasiliou V, Zakhari S, Seitz HK, et al. (Eds.). (2015). *Biological Basic of Alcohol-Induced Cancer.* Cham, Switzerland: Springer International Publishing.

Wang L, Lee IM, Manson JE, et al. (2010). Alcohol consumption, weight gain, and risk of becoming overweight in middle-aged and older women. *Archives of Internal Medicine* 170 (5): 453–461.

Welford AT. (Ed.) (1980). *Reaction Times.* New York, NY: Academic Press.

Wightman JD, Heuberger RA. (2015). Effect of grape and other berries on cardiovascular health. *Journal of the Science of Food and Agriculture* 95 (8): 1584–1597.

Zakhari S, Vasiliou V, Guo QM (Eds.). (2011). *Alcohol and Cancer.* New York, NY: Springer.

Reasons to Limit Caffeine

Ancoli-Israel S. (1996). *All I Want Is a Good Night's Sleep.* St. Louis, MO: Mosby-Yearbook.

Attarian HP. (2010). *Sleep Disorders in Women: A Guide to Practical Management.* Totowa, New Jersey: Humana Press.

Goodman CC, Snyder TE. (2013). *Differential Diagnosis for Physical Therapists: Screening for Referral,* 5th ed. St. Louis, MO: Elsevier. www.differentialdiagnosisforpt.com.

Hallstrom H, Byberg L, Glynn A, et al. (2013). Long-term coffee consumption in relation to fracture risk and bone mineral density in women. *American Journal of Epidemiology* 178 (6): 898–909.

Hallstrom H, Wolk A, Glynn A, et al. (2006). Coffee, tea and caffeine consumption in relation to osteoporotic fracture risk in a cohort of Swedish women. *Osteoporos International* 17 (7): 1055–1064.

James JE, Kristjansson AL, Sigfusdottir ID. (2015). A gender-specific analysis of adolescent dietary caffeine, alcohol consumption, anger, and violent behavior. *Substance Use & Misuse* 50 (2): 257–267.

Vilarim MM, Rocha Araujo DM, Nardi AE. (2011). Caffeine challenge test and panic disorder: A systematic literature review. *Expert Review of Neurotherapeutics* 11 (8): 1185–1195.

Holistic Healing Boxes

Women's Health Highlights

American Congress of Obstetricians and Gynecologists (ACOG). (2011). *Exercise During Pregnancy*. Washington, DC: American Congress of Obstetricians and Gynecologists.

Baccetti S, Da Fre M, Becorpi A, et al. (2014). Acupuncture and traditional Chinese medicine for hot flushes in menopause: A randomized trial. *Journal of Alternative and Complementary Medicine* 20 (7): 550–557.

Bowles KA, Steele JR. (2013). Effects of strap cushions and strap orientation on comfort and sports bra performance. *Medicine and Science in Sports and Exercise* 45 (6): 1113–1119.

Brown N, White J, Brasher A, et al. (2014). An investigation into breast support and sports bra use in female runners of the 2012 London marathon. *Journal of Sports Sciences* 32 (9): 801–809.

Hoefs J, Jagroo D. (2014). *Your Best Pregnancy: The Ultimate Guide to Easing the Aches, Pains, and Uncomfortable Side Effects During Each Stage of Your Pregnancy*. New York, NY: Demos Medical Publishing.

Irion JM, Irion GL. (2010). *Women's Health in Physical Therapy*. Baltimore, MD: Wolters Kluwer Lippincott Williams & Wilkins.

Litos K. (2014). Progressive therapeutic exercise program for successful treatment of a postpartum woman with a severe diastasis recti abdominis. *Journal of Women's Health Physical Therapy* 38 (2): 58–73.

McGhee DE. (2009). *Sports bra design and bra fit: Minimizing exercise-induced breast discomfort*. Doctor of Philosophy thesis. School of Health Sciences, University of Wollongong. http://ro.uow.edu.au/theses/3854/.

McGhee DE, Steele JR. (2010). Optimising breast support in female patients through correct bra fit: A cross-sectional study. *Journal of Science and Medicine in Sport* 13 (6): 568–572.

McGhee DE, Steele JR, Munro BJ. (2010). Education improves bra knowledge and fit, and level of breast support in adolescent female athletes: A cluster-randomised trial. *Journal of Physiotherapy* 56 (1): 19–24.

Mika A, Oleksy L, Mika P, et al. (2012). The effect of walking in high- and low-heeled shoes on erector spinae activity and pelvis kinematics during gait. *American Journal of Physical Medicine and Rehabilitation* 91 (5): 425–434.

Milligan RA, Flenniken PM, Pugh LC. (1996). Positioning intervention to minimize fatigue in breastfeeding women. *Applied Nursing Research* 9 (2): 67–70.

Noble E. (2003). *Essential Exercises for the Childbearing Year*, 4th ed. Harwich, MA: New Life Images.

Perales M, Refoyo I, Coteron J., et al. (2015). Exercise during pregnancy attenuates prenatal depression: A randomized controlled trial. *Evaluation & the Health Professions* 38 (1): 59–72.

Venes D. (Ed.). (2017). *Taber's Cyclopedic Medical Dictionary*, 23rd ed. Philadelphia, PA: FA Davis.

Balance between Yin and Yang

Porter RS, Kaplan JL. (Eds.). (2011). *The Merck Manual of Diagnosis and Therapy*, 19th ed. Whitehouse Station, NJ: Merck Sharp & Dohme Corporation.

Venes D. (Ed.). (2017). *Taber's Cyclopedic Medical Dictionary*, 23rd ed. Philadelphia, PA: FA Davis.

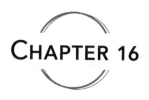

CHAPTER 16

IMPROVING YOUR BRAIN HEALTH

"Let food be thy medicine and medicine be thy food."

—Hippocrates

Cognition can be defined as thinking skills, language use, perception, calculation, awareness, memory, reasoning, judgment, learning, intellect, social skills, and imagination (Venes 2017). Cognitive function (or "executive function") impairments in individuals can lead to difficulties with activities of daily living such as dressing, eating, bathing, toileting, and walking. Additionally, a decline of cognitive function can result in reduced quality of life and problems with social engagement, driving skills, work-related tasks, money management, shopping, and operating communication devices (Jobe et al. 2001).

The following areas show promise in enhancing cognitive function, or slowing its decline, and also in maintaining mental stability:

AEROBIC TRAINING

Engaging in any aerobic exercise and physical activity, such as walking or jogging, elevates heart health but can also keep your brain healthy (Alves et al. 2014; Baker et al. 2010; Buck et al. 2008; Carvalho et al. 2014; Chapman et al. 2015; Chapman et al. 2013; Chang et al. 2015; Fabel et al. 2008; Hillman et al. 2003, 2009; Li et al. 2014; Nanda et al. 2013; Pontifex et al. 2009; ten Brinke 2015; Voss et al. 2010; Winter et al. 2007; Wu et al. 2011; Zhao et al. 2014; Zhu et al. 2014). Some studies have shown certain aspects of cognition in children can improve with exercise (Drollette et al. 2014; Fedewa et al. 2011; Kirkendall 1986; Lees et al. 2013; Tomporowski et al. 2008).

A study by Gauthier et al. (2015) indicates that "cognitive status in aging is linked to vascular health, and that preservation of vessel elasticity may be one of the key mechanisms by which physical exercise helps to alleviate cognitive aging." These findings are in line with other research, which studied older women (Brown et al. 2010). Moreover, a study by Guiney et al. (2015) shows that healthy young adults, ages 18 to 30, who engage in physical activity might improve their cognitive function. An article by Phillips et al. (2015) states that "In summary, the data presented here suggests that moderate physical activity—a target that is practical, well tolerated, and likely to optimize exercise adherence—can be used to improve cognitive function and reduce the slope of cognitive decline in people with dementia of the Alzheimer disease type."

So walk, bike, hike, swim, or do some other aerobic activity at least three to five times per week.

Dancing

Tango dancing and mindfulness meditation can be effective complementary additions for the treatment of depression as a part of stress-management programs (Pinniger et al. 2012). A different study shows that the Ngoma ceremony, a tradition that involves rhythms with drums and dance, may help with stress and healing (Vinesett et al. 2017).

Here are a few of my favorite songs I use to get clients at community centers up and moving before I begin class. I've been told these songs energize the mind and body, and also help relieve stress. So give the following tunes a listen when you try some of your new dance moves:

- Beatles, "Twist and Shout," YouTube: http://bit.ly/1r0lebL
- Chuck Berry, "Johnny B. Goode," YouTube: http://bit.ly/1jmTLw2
- Chubby Checker, "Let's Twist Again," YouTube: http://bit.ly/1hSav1Z

Diet and Medical Conditions

Be aware of your diet and how it can impact certain medical conditions. For example, a study by Lichtwark et al. (2014) indicates that in people with celiac disease, particularly in those who have just been diagnosed, "cognitive performance improves with adherence to the gluten-free diet in parallel to mucosal healing. Suboptimal levels of cognition in untreated coeliac [celiac] disease may affect the performance of everyday tasks." Celiac disease is an immunologic intolerance to dietary wheat products, especially gluten and gliadin (Venes 2017). See your physician and discuss any concerns you may have regarding your sensitivity to gluten or any other food.

EAT QUALITY FOODS

Quality foods can help enhance your brain function. The following are studies showing the link between food and cognitive function:

- Even following a short-term (10 days in this study) Mediterranean-style diet has the potential to enhance certain aspects of mood, cognition, and cardiovascular function in young healthy adults (Lee et al. 2015).
- Smyth et al. (2015) indicate that a "higher diet quality was associated with a reduced risk of cognitive decline. Improved diet quality represents an important potential target for reducing the global burden of cognitive decline."
- Valls-Pedret et al. (2015) indicate that "In an older population [average age in the study was 66.9 years], a Mediterranean diet supplemented with olive oil or nuts is associated with improved cognitive function."

FOLIC ACID

A study by Agnew-Blais et al. (2015) indicates that "folate intake below the Recommended Daily Allowance may increase risk for MCI [mild cognitive impairment]/probable dementia in later life."

FOOD FOR THOUGHT

An article by Rampersaud et al. (2005) indicates "that breakfast consumption may improve cognitive function related to memory, test grades, and school attendance" in children and adolescents. Also, a balanced diet with sufficient calories and nutrients is needed to prevent nutritional imbalances. The following foods and nutrients have been shown to positively affect cognitive function:

- *Blueberries*—Krikorian et al. (2010) indicate that "moderate-term blueberry supplementation can confer neurocognitive benefit."
- *Fish and omega-3 oils*—Barberger-Gateau et al. (2007) indicate that "frequent consumption of fruits and vegetables, fish, and omega-3 rich oils may decrease the risk of dementia and Alzheimer's disease."
- *Green leafy vegetables*—Kang et al. (2005) indicate that "women consuming the most green leafy vegetables also experienced slower [cognitive] decline than women consuming the least amount."
- *Plants/Extracts*—Plants and their extracts, such as saffron, ginseng, sage, lemon balm, and Ginkgo biloba, have produced some promising clinical data for individuals with dementia pathologies such as Alzheimer's disease (Howes et al. 2011).
- *Pomegranate juice*—Bookheimer et al. (2013) indicate that "results suggest a role for pomegranate juice in augmenting memory function through task-related increases in functional brain activity."

- *Turmeric*—Ng et al. (2006) indicate that "curcumin, from the curry spice turmeric, has been shown to possess potent antioxidant and anti-inflammatory properties and to reduce beta-amyloid and plaque burden in experimental studies" and also that "those who consumed curry 'occasionally' and 'often or very often' had significantly better MMSE [mini-mental state examination] scores than did subjects who 'never or rarely' consumed curry."
- *Water*—Water helps to prevent dehydration, which may impair mood and cognitive performance (Cheuvront et al. 2014; Masento et al. 2014).

GUT AND BRAIN HEALTH

More than likely, one of the next big areas that medicine will focus on is the interactions between the gastrointestinal system and the brain and how this can affect our sense of well-being. Therefore, exploring all options to improve health is a part of good medical practice and wellness.

The body's largest immune organ is the gastrointestinal tract. It has nearly 100 trillion bacteria, or about one kilogram of bacteria in the adult gut which are essential for health (Dinan et al. 2015; Foster et al. 2013; Severance et al. 2015). Microorganisms make up about one to three percent of our body mass (that's two to six pounds of bacteria in a 200-pound adult) (Human Microbiome Project 2015).

According to the Human Microbiome Project website (http://hmpdacc. org), microorganisms in the human body "produce some vitamins that we do not have the genes to make, break down our food to extract nutrients we need to survive, teach our immune systems how to recognize dangerous invaders and even produce helpful anti-inflammatory compounds that fight off other disease-causing microbes."

LET'S SEE WHAT RESEARCH SAYS . . .

- McKean et al. (2016) state that "probiotic consumption may have a positive effect on psychological symptoms of depression, anxiety, and perceived stress in healthy human volunteers."
- Huang et al. (2016) conclude that "probiotics were associated with a significant reduction in depression."
- Keightley et al. (2015) state that "Psychological treatments are known to improve functional gastrointestinal disorders, the next wave of research may involve preventative microbiological gut based treatments for primary psychological presentations, both to treat the presenting complaint and inoculate against later functional gastrointestinal disorders."

- Severance et al. (2015) state that "With accumulating evidence supporting newly discovered gut-brain physiological pathways, treatments to ameliorate brain symptoms of schizophrenia should be supplemented with therapies to correct gastrointestinal dysfunction."

IMPROVING GUT AND BRAIN FUNCTION

The following are some tips to help improve digestion and maintain a healthy gastrointestinal system:

- Follow medical treatment guidelines for conditions such as irritable bowel syndrome, celiac disease, and Crohn's disease.
- Get regular dental checkups. Also, brush and floss your teeth and massage your gums daily to keep your mouth healthy.
- Identify and control food allergens, intolerances, and sensitivities (Daulatzai 2015; Nemani et al. 2015) and malabsorption problems (such as lactose or fructose intolerance).
- Control your stress.
- Don't smoke (Fujiwara et al. 2011).
- Limit alcohol consumption (Swanson et al. 2010).
- Limit caffeine consumption (Heizer et al. 2009).
- Get enough sleep to help prevent stress and ensure full recovery (Chen et al. 2011).
- Exercise daily to help digestion and prevent constipation (Klare et al. 2015).
- Eat slowly not only to prevent overeating, but also to aid in proper digestion.
- Avoid large meals (Heizer et al. 2009).
- Practice mindfulness meditation.
- Eat a varied and balanced diet to avoid nutritional deficiencies.
- Wash your hands thoroughly before eating to prevent gastrointestinal illness (Aiello et al. 2008).
- Consider storing your floss, toothbrush, and gum massager outside of your bathroom to avoid cross contamination from your toilet (American Society for Microbiology 2015).
- Consider seeing a health care practitioner specializing in aromatherapy massage for relief of constipation, indigestion, nausea, or loss of appetite using essential oils.
- Consider seeing an acupuncturist for acupuncture and acupressure techniques for gastrointestinal health (Cross 2001).
- Include prebiotics and probiotics into your diet (Scott et al. 2015; Tillisch et al. 2013). For further information, refer to the following two tables (Table 16-1 and 16-2) and the International Scientific Association for Probiotics and Prebiotics website isappscience.org.

TABLE 16-1: PREBIOTIC FOODS

Prebiotics are nutrients that stimulate the growth or health of bacteria living in the large intestine (Venes 2017).

Prebiotics from foods can reduce the prevalence and duration of infectious and antibiotic-associated diarrhea, reduce the inflammation and symptoms of inflammatory bowel disease, protect against colon cancer, enhance the bioavailability and uptake of minerals (such as calcium, magnesium, and possibly iron), lower some risk for cardiovascular disease, and promote weight loss and prevent obesity (Slavin 2013).

Prebiotics occur naturally in foods such as (Gensler 2008; Hyde 2017):
· Fruits (such as apples or bananas)
· Vegetables (such as asparagus, bok choy, broccoli stems, potatoes, cauliflower stems, garlic, Jerusalem artichokes, leeks, or onions)
· Barley
· Flax
· Legumes
· Oats

TABLE 16-2: PROBIOTIC FOODS

Probiotics are defined as having a favorable or health-promoting effect on living cells and tissues (Venes 2017).

Probiotics from foods or supplements can prevent hypercholesterolemia (excessive amount of cholesterol in the blood), upper respiratory tract infections, bacterial vaginosis (vaginal infection), and antibiotic-associated diarrhea, help manage constipation, and reduce recurrent urinary tract infections and irritable bowel syndrome symptoms (Taibi et al. 2014).

Probiotics occur naturally in foods such as (Gensler 2008; Hyde 2017):
· Cultured or fermented vegetables (such as *sauerkraut or kimchi). For example, see the Healing Movement website* http://healingmovement.net
· Eggplant
· Kefir (fermented milk). For example, see the Lifeway website http://lifewaykefir. com and Redwood Hill Farm website www.redwoodhill.com
· Kombucha tea (fermented drink typically containing tea, sugar, bacteria, and yeast)
· Miso (mixture containing fermented soybeans)
· Roquefort cheese (French cheese) (Petyaev et al. 2013)
· Tempeh (fermented soybeans)
· Yogurt

DID YOU KNOW?

• "It takes about 3 to 4 weeks for a complete turnover of all gut cells throughout the digestive tract" (Goodman et al. 2015).

- "Because two-thirds of all immune system function and 90% of serotonin function take place in the gut, healing the gut can assist in bringing both of these functions back into balance. Serotonin is needed to produce melatonin, which is an essential component for good, restful sleep; the proper amount of circulating and functioning serotonin is also needed to stabilize mood" (Goodman et al. 2015).

MEDITATION

A study by Wells et al. (2013) indicates that "Mindfulness-Based Stress Reduction (MBSR) may have a positive impact on the regions of the brain most related to mild cognitive impairment and Alzheimer's disease." Another article indicates mindfulness meditation reduces anxiety (Zeidan et al. 2014).

MEMORY FITNESS PROGRAM

Look into enrolling in a memory fitness program at your local college, university, or community center. A study by Miller et al. (2012) indicates that "a 6-week healthy lifestyle program can improve both encoding and recalling of new verbal information, as well as self-perception of memory ability in older adults residing in continuing care retirement communities." Another study by Small et al. (2006) states that "a short-term healthy lifestyle program combining mental and physical exercise, stress reduction, and healthy diet was associated with significant effects on cognitive function and brain metabolism."

MINIMIZE POLLUTION

A study by Wilker et al. (2015) suggests that "Air pollution is associated with insidious effects on structural brain aging even in dementia and stroke-free persons."

NET-STEP EXERCISE

A study by Kitazawa et al. (2015) created a simple recreational stepping program using a Fumanet to maintain cognitive health and gait function. The name "Fumanet Exercise" originates from the words *fumanai* (which means "to avoid stepping on something" in Japanese) and "net exercise (stepping in and out of a grid-like apparatus on the floor)" (Sompo Japan Research Institute 2010). Also, view the video at links.lww.com/JGPT/A4 for the basics of how to perform the stepping program.

Night and Day

Get adequate rest, relaxation, and sleep. A study by Yoo et al. (2007) indicates that "results demonstrate that an absence of prior sleep substantially compromises the neural and behavioral capacity for committing new experiences to memory. It therefore appears that sleep before learning is critical in preparing the human brain for next-day memory formation—a worrying finding considering society's increasing erosion of sleep time." On the flip side, get enough natural bright light every day to increase the brain's serotonin levels needed to enhance mood and vitality (Brawley 2009).

No Smoking and Limited Alcohol

A study by Hagger-Johnson et al. (2013) indicates that "smokers who drank alcohol heavily had a 36% faster cognitive decline, equivalent to an age-effect of 2 extra years over 10-year follow-up, compared with individuals who were non-smoking moderate drinkers." Another study by Sabia et al. (2014) indicates that "excessive alcohol consumption in men was associated with faster cognitive decline compared with light to moderate alcohol consumption" (Kabai 2014).

Rocking Chair

A single session of rocking in a rocking chair for 30 minutes might increase blood flow to the brain (Pierce et al. 2009).

Soothing Music

Listening to music leads to positive changes in a person's emotional state and decreases the severity of behavioral disorders (Narme et al. 2013). Music also appears to reduce depression in elderly individuals (Chu et al. 2013). A study by Pongan et al. (2017) suggests that "singing and painting interventions may reduce pain and improve mood, quality of life, and cognition in patients with mild Alzheimer's disease, with differential effects of painting for depression and singing for memory performance."

Here are a few of my favorite songs I sometimes use to help relax my patients and clients as they perform the relaxation breathing techniques I prescribe. So give the following songs a try:

- Sarah Chang, Jules Massenet, Meditation From Thais, YouTube: bit. ly/2zT2tDv
- Pachelbel, Canon In D Major, YouTube: bit.ly/1f9m14H

STABLE BLOOD GLUCOSE LEVELS

Keep your blood sugar levels stable throughout your life. The following are studies showing the link between blood glucose and cognitive function:

- Weinstein et al. (2015) indicate that "hyperglycemia [high blood sugar levels] is associated with subtle brain injury and impaired attention and memory even in young adults, indicating that brain injury is an early manifestation of impaired glucose metabolism."
- Roberts et al. (2014) indicate that "Midlife onset of diabetes may affect late-life cognition through loss of brain volume."
- Young et al. (2014) indicate that "The ability to control the levels of blood glucose was related to mood and cognition."
- Crane et al. (2013) indicate that "higher glucose levels may be a risk factor for dementia, even among persons without diabetes."

STABLE BLOOD PRESSURE

Reducing your blood pressure can affect cognitive function in a positive way. One study (Roberts et al. 2014) indicates that elevated blood pressure levels among middle-aged individuals may bring about ischemia, or interrupted blood supply to vital tissues, which can negatively affect brain function. An article by Nagai et al. (2010) concludes that such damage "is associated with cognitive impairment. Accordingly, strict blood pressure control including during sleep may have a neuroprotective effect on the brain, and thereby prevent the incidence of dementia."

CEASE STEROID USE FOR MUSCLE BUILDING

Some studies have shown that androgenic-anabolic steroid use among regular gym users may impair memory (Heffernan et al. 2015).

STRENGTH TRAINING

Many studies show that engaging in strength training exercises (using resistance) has positive effects on cognitive function (Altug 2014; Brown et al. 2009; Cancela Carral et al. 2007; Cassilhas et al. 2007; Chang et al. 2009, 2012, 2014; Forte et al. 2013; Fragala et al. 2014; Kimura et al. 2010; Komulainen et al. 2010; Liu-Ambrose et al. 2008, 2010, 2012; Ozkaya et al. 2005; Perrig-Chiello et al. 1998; Tsutsumi et al. 1997).

- Gordon et al. (2017) conclude that "Resistance exercise training significantly improves anxiety symptoms among both healthy participants and participants with a physical or mental illness."
- Fiatarone et al. (2014) indicate that "resistance training significantly improved global cognitive function, with maintenance of executive and global benefits over 18 months" in men and women ages 55 or above with mild cognitive impairment. Basic executive function is typically thought of as working memory, flexible thinking, and self-control, while global cognition are abilities such as general knowledge, attention, language, and recall.
- Fragala et al. (2014) indicate that "resistance exercise training may be an effective means to preserve or improve spatial awareness and reaction with aging" in adults over 60 years old.
- Liu-Ambrose et al. (2010) indicate that "twelve months of once-weekly or twice-weekly resistance training benefited the executive cognitive function of selective attention and conflict resolution among senior women [ages 65 to 75]."

So why wait? Start doing some resistance training at least twice a week. Use equipment such as hand and ankle weights, or do exercises like push-ups that use the weight of your own body as resistance.

Stress Relief

Reduce daily stress levels (Lupien et al. 2005). A study indicates that controlling "anxiety symptoms may help delay memory decline in otherwise healthy older adults" (Pietrzak et al. 2014).

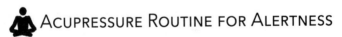 Acupressure Routine for Alertness

See an acupuncturist for detailed instructions. Try stimulating the following acupressure points (Table 16-3) for three minutes each to help increase your alertness before a test (Harris et al. 2005):

Table 16-3: Self-Acupressure for Alertness

Si Shen Chong point	Lightly tap the top of the head
LI 4 point	Massage the web space between the thumb and index finger

ST 36 POINT	Massage the point located about four finger widths down from the bottom of your knee cap, on the outer boundary of your shin bone
K 1 POINT	Massage the front portion of the bottom of your foot between the web space of the second and third toe
UB 10 POINT	Massage the depression at the outer border of the back of your neck within the hairline

TEST-TAKING STRATEGIES

Should you be physically active (such as walking, walking in place, or doing simple calisthenics) just before a major test or other mentally difficult task (such as a physician before surgery, a speaker before a lecture, or an airline pilot just before taking off or landing)? Even though some researchers suggest that the results of cognitive improvement with exercise should be interpreted cautiously based on current studies, it would be simple to get some exercise before a test or a mentally challenging task—and why wait for clarification when something like that could give you an advantage? How much would school and work performance improve if every student and worker was allowed multiple mini-exercise breaks throughout the day, especially before a mentally challenging task?

Perhaps the reason some people get good ideas during a shower or long walk is increased blood flow to the brain. Or is it due to the relaxation? Either way, engaging in low-key activities is good for you. Why not get up and move around or go for a 10- to 30-minute walk, and see what happens? Maybe even make your next meeting a "walking meeting" with your client or staff. You would be in good company since many great thinkers, like Aristotle, Ludwig van Beethoven, Charles Darwin, Charles Dickens, Albert Einstein, Steve Jobs, and Friedrich Nietzsche, used walking as a part of their thinking and creative process.

TEST-TAKING ROUTINE

As with any athletic program, there is a trial-and-error period to find the precise combination of what will work on test day. Try some or all of the following tips before your next test:

- The most important part is to study your materials well in advance of a test. No all-nighters!
- Ideally, you should handwrite your study materials for increased retention and learning (Mueller et al. 2014).
- Learn by using different strategies. First, hear it and see it (audio-visual), then practice what you learned (or discuss it in a group), and finally,

teach the technique or concept to someone else. In medical circles there is an adage which states: "See one, do one, teach one." It may be an old-school concept, but give it a try.

- Get enough sleep the previous night (and ideally, for the entire week leading up to the test).
- Identify the ideal pre-test meal several months in advance for optimal concentration. Determine what mixture of fat, carbohydrate, and protein you need for optimal performance.
- Eat a healthful breakfast before the test.
- Get some natural outdoor sunlight in the morning before the test.
- Perform light exercises, such as walking or calisthenics, for 10 to 30 minutes to invigorate your body and increase blood flow to your brain before the test.
- Use diaphragmatic breathing to relax before the test. Just before your test (or any intense mental task), close your eyes to relax, and breathe diaphragmatically 10 times in a slow and controlled manner.
- To reduce anxiety before the test, consider trying the Emotional Freedom Technique (Benor et al. 2009).
- Try smelling a little rosemary oil (Diego et al. 1998) or peppermint oil (Moss et al. 2008) before a test to help increase your alertness. Just remember, peppermint to "pep" you up.
- Finally, read the book *Skill* by physician Christopher Ahmad, MD. He is a high-performance orthopedic surgeon for the New York Yankees. Another great book to improve performance is *The Talent Code* by best-selling author Daniel Coyle. In both amazing books you will find many strategies to help you fine-tune your study and preparation habits.

VITAMIN D

The following studies are related to vitamin D and cognition, indicating that having your vitamin D level checked is another good reason to get annual medical checkups:

- Afzal et al. (2014) find that a vitamin D deficiency was associated with increased risk of Alzheimer's disease and dementia.
- Pettersen et al. (2014) indicate that "vitamin D3 insufficiency and seasonal declines ≥ [greater than or equal to] 15 nmol/L were associated with inferior working memory/executive functioning."
- Llewellyn et al. (2010) indicate that "low levels of vitamin D were associated with substantial cognitive decline in the elderly population studied over a six-year period."
- Seamans et al. (2010) indicate that "low vitamin D status was associated with a reduced capacity for SWM (spatial working memory), particularly in women" in several European countries.

Yoga or Tai Chi

Studies indicate that yoga may lead to improvements in cognitive function (Gothe et al. 2014; Hariprasad et al. 2013). Another study indicates that "mind-body exercise with integrated cognitive and motor coordination may help with the preservation of global ability in elders at risk of cognitive decline" (Lam et al. 2012).

Play Some Mind Games

A study by Miller (2013) indicates that "participating in a computerized brain exercise program over 6 months improves cognitive abilities in older adults." Try the following games to stimulate your brain cells:

- Bridge, bridgebase.com
- Cards, solitaire-cardgame.com
- Chess, chess.com
- Crossword puzzles, boatloadpuzzles.com
- Dakim BrainFitness, dakim.com
- Fit Brains, fitbrains.com
- Lumosity, lumosity.com
- Sudoku, 247sudoku.com

Stay Engaged in Life

Be socially interactive by joining clubs, volunteering, or teaching (Ybarra et al. 2008). Experience something beyond your normal activities. Go to a museum, opera, theater, or sporting event. Try something new and novel in your life, such as the following:

- Art—take drawing, painting, or sculpting classes
- Community involvement—volunteer, coach, or organize in your community
- Continued education—take a class at a community college (Hatch et al. 2007)
- Cooking—learn to cook and try new recipes
- Dance—take ballroom, hip-hop, or tango classes
- Language—take French or Chinese classes (Alladi et al. 2013; Craik et al. 2010)
- Math—do occasional simple arithmetic in your head
- Music—take lessons in flute, piano, or guitar
- Poetry—uncover hidden meanings or pen your own poems
- Reading—read newspapers, books, or magazines
- Writing—try journaling, writing prose, or work on your own novel!

BRAIN FITNESS COORDINATION EXERCISE ROUTINE

Simple coordination exercises improve cognitive function in men and women ages 66 to 90 (Kwok et al. 2011). Try the following modified movement circuit while sitting in a chair:

- Keep your eyes focused ahead while turning your head slowly to the right and left. Now keep your eyes focused ahead while moving your head slowly up and down.
- Touch your nose, alternating right and left index fingers. Now touch your ears, again alternating right and left index fingers.
- Turn the palms of both hands alternately to face up and down with elbows bent to 90 degrees.
- Touch your right or left shoulder, hip, or knee depending on the verbal commands of a training partner. Slowly increase the speed of the verbal commands. Try it with your eyes closed.
- Draw patterns (such as a circle, triangle, square, or rectangle) or letters of the alphabet in the air in front of your body with your right or left hand. Try this, too, with your eyes closed.
- Slide the heel of your right leg up along your left shin. Alternate legs. Again, try it with your closed eyes.

DID YOU KNOW?

- The metabolism of the brain accounts for about 15 percent of the total metabolism in the body under resting but awake conditions. The mass of the brain is only 2 percent of total body mass (Hall 2011).
- "Collectively, the brain, liver, heart, and kidneys account for approximately 60% to 70% of resting energy expenditure in adults, whereas their combined weight is less than 6% of total body weight. Skeletal muscle comprises 40% to 50% of total body weight and accounts for only 20% to 30% of resting energy expenditure" (Javed et al. 2010).

BOX 15: HOLISTIC HEALING

RANDOM ACTS OF KINDNESS

Help heal yourself and others around you by practicing some random acts of kindness:

- Smile more when interacting with individuals in daily life
- Speak gently with someone who is angry
- Drive respectfully
- Create a small scholarship fund for your local high school or college

- Send a handwritten note to thank someone for helping you
- Donate (blood, food, books, supplies to a local school, or magazines to a nursing home)
- Volunteer (hospital, school, animal shelter, nursing home, youth sports organization, or place of worship)
- Plant a tree
- Pick up trash
- Recycle
- Periodically offer free professional advice and services (pro bono)
- Help a neighbor

Jot down here your choices for random acts of kindness:

1. _____
2. _____
3. _____

ADDITIONAL RESOURCES

- American Gut Project, americangut.org
- American Psychiatric Association, psychiatry.org
- American Psychological Association, apa.org
- Association for Applied Sport Psychology, appliedsportpsych.org
- BrainHQ, brainhq.com
- Brain Injury Association of America, biausa.org
- Fit Brains, fitbrains.com

REFERENCES

Afzal S, Bojesen SE, Nordestgaard BG. (2014). Reduced 25-hydroxyvitamin D and risk of Alzheimer's disease and vascular dementia. *Alzheimer's & Dementia* 10 (3): 296–302.

Agnew-Blais JC, Wassertheil-Smoller S, Kang JH, et al. (2015). Folate, vitamin B-6, and vitamin B-12 intake and mild cognitive impairment and probable dementia in the Women's Health Initiative Memory Study. *Journal of the Academy of Nutrition and Dietetics* 115 (2): 231–241.

Aiello AE, Coulborn RM, Perez V, et al. (2008). Effect of hand hygiene on infectious disease risk in the community setting: A meta-analysis. *American Journal of Public Health* 98 (8): 1372–1381.

Alladi S, Bak TH, Duggirala V, et al. (2013). Bilingualism delays age at onset of dementia, independent of education and immigration status. *Neurology* 81 (22): 1938–1944.

Altug Z. (2014). Resistance exercise to improve cognitive function. *Strength and Conditioning Journal* 36 (6): 46–50.

Alves CR, Tessaro VH, Teixeira LA, et al. (2014). Influence of acute high-intensity aerobic interval exercise bout on selective attention and short-term memory tasks. *Perceptual and Motor Skills* 118 (1): 63–72.

American Society for Microbiology. (2015). *Toothbrush contamination in communal bathrooms.* American Society for Microbiology. Retrieved on November 4, 2017 from www.asm.org/index.php/press-releases/93536-toothbrush-contamination-in-communal-bathrooms

Baker LD, Frank LL, Foster-Schubert K, et al. (2010). Aerobic exercise improves cognition for older adults with glucose intolerance, a risk factor for Alzheimer's disease. *Journal of Alzheimer's Disease* 22 (2): 569–579.

Barberger-Gateau P, Raffaitin C, Letenneur L, et al. (2007). Dietary patterns and risk of dementia: The Three-City cohort study. *Neurology* 69 (20): 1921–1930.

Barral JP. (2007). *Visceral Manipulation II*, revised edition. Seattle, WA: Eastland Press.

Barral JP, Mercier P. (2005). *Visceral Manipulation*, revised edition. Seattle, WA: Eastland Press.

Benor DJ., Ledger K, Toussaint L, et al. (2009). Pilot study of emotional freedom techniques, wholistic hybrid derived from eye movement desensitization and reprocessing and emotional freedom technique, and cognitive behavioral therapy for treatment of test anxiety in university students. *Explore (NY)* 5 (6): 338–340.

Bookheimer SY, Renner BA, Ekstrom A, et al. (2013). Pomegranate juice augments memory and FMRI activity in middle-aged and older adults with mild memory complaints. *Evidence-Based Complementary and Alternative Medicine* 946298.

Brawley EC. (2009). Enriching light design. *NeuroRehabilitation* 25 (3): 189–199.

Bredesen DE. (2014). Reversal of cognitive decline: A novel therapeutic program. *Aging (Albany NY)* 6 (9): 707–717.

Brown AD, McMorris CA, Longman RS, et al. (2010). Effects of cardiorespiratory fitness and cerebral blood flow on cognitive outcomes in older women. *Neurobiology of Aging* 31 (12): 2047–2057.

Brown AK, Liu-Ambrose T, Tate R, et al. (2009). The effect of group-based exercise on cognitive performance and mood in seniors residing in intermediate care and self-care retirement facilities: A randomised controlled trial. *British Journal of Sports Medicine* 43 (8): 608–614.

Buck SM, Hillman CH, Castelli DM. (2008). The relation of aerobic fitness to Stroop task performance in preadolescent children. *Medicine and Science in Sports and Exercise* 40 (1): 166–172.

Cancela Carral JM, Ayan Perez C. (2007). Effects of high-intensity combined training on women over 65. *Gerontology* 53 (6): 340–346.

Carpenter S. (2012). That gut feeling. *Monitor on Psychology* 43 (8): 50.

Carvalho A, Rea IM, Parimon T, et al. (2014). Physical activity and cognitive function in individuals over 60 years of age: A systematic review. *Clinical Interventions in Aging* 9: 661–682.

Cassilhas RC, Viana VA, Grassmann V, et al. (2007). The impact of resistance exercise on the cognitive function of the elderly. *Medicine and Science in Sports and Exercise* 39 (8): 1401–1407.

Chang YK, Chu CH Wang CC et al. (2015). Dose–response relation between exercise duration and cognition. *Medicine & Science in Sports & Exercise* 47 (1): 159–165.

Chang YK, Etnier JL. (2009). Effects of an acute bout of localized resistance exercise on cognitive performance in middle-aged adults: A randomized controlled trial study. *Psychology of Sport and Exercise* 10 (1): 19–24.

Chang YK, Ku PW, Tomporowski PD, et al. (2012). Effects of acute resistance exercise on late-middle-age adults' goal planning. *Medicine and Science in Sports and Exercise* 44 (9): 1773–1779.

Chang YK, Tsai CL, Huang CC, et al. (2014). Effects of acute resistance exercise on cognition in late middle-aged adults: General or specific cognitive improvement? *Journal of Science and Medicine in Sport* 17 (1): 51–55.

Chen CL, Liu TT, Yi CH, et al. (2011). Evidence for altered anorectal function in irritable bowel syndrome patients with sleep disturbance. *Digestion* 84 (3): 247–251.

Chapman SB, Aslan S, Spence JS, et al. (2013). Shorter term aerobic exercise improves brain, cognition, and cardiovascular fitness in aging. *Frontiers in Aging Neuroscience* 5: 75.

Chapman SB, Aslan S, Spence JS, et al. (2015). Neural mechanisms of brain plasticity with complex cognitive training in healthy seniors. *Cerebral Cortex* 25 (2): 396–405.

Cheuvront SN, Kenefick RW. (2014). Dehydration: Physiology, assessment, and performance effects. *Comprehensive Physiology* 4 (1): 257–285.

Chodzko-Zajko O, Kramer A, Poon L. (2009). *Enhancing Cognitive Functioning and Brain Plasticity* (Volume 3). Champaign, IL: Human Kinetics.

Chu H, Yang CY, Lin Y, et al. (2013). The Impact of group music therapy on depression and cognition in elderly persons with dementia: A randomized controlled study. *Biological Research for Nursing* 16 (2): 209–217.

Craik FI, Bialystok E, Freedman M. (2010). Delaying the onset of Alzheimer disease: Bilingualism as a form of cognitive reserve. *Neurology* 75 (19): 1726–1729.

Crane PK, Walker R, Hubbard RA, et al. (2013). Glucose levels and risk of dementia. *New England Journal of Medicine* 369 (6): 540–548.

Cross JR. (2001). *Acupressure & Reflextherapy in the Treatment of Medical Conditions*. London, England: Butterworth-Heinemann.

Daulatzai MA. (2015). Non-celiac gluten sensitivity triggers gut dysbiosis, neuroinflammation, gut-brain axis dysfunction, and vulnerability for dementia. *CNS & Neurological Disorders Drug Targets* 14 (1): 110–131.

Diego MA, Jones NA, Field T, et al. (1998). Aromatherapy positively affects mood, EEG patterns of alertness and math computations. *International Journal of Neuroscience* 96 (3-4): 217–224.

Di Lazzaro V, Capone F, Cammarota G, et al. (2014). Dramatic improvement of Parkinsonian symptoms after gluten-free diet introduction in a patient with silent celiac disease. *Journal of Neurology* 261 (2): 443–445.

Dinan TG, Stilling RM, Stanton C, et al. (2015). Collective unconscious: How gut microbes shape human behavior. *Journal of Psychiatric Research* 63: 1–9.

Drollette ES, Scudder MR, Raine LB, et al. (2014). Acute exercise facilitates brain function and cognition in children who need it most: An ERP study of individual differences in inhibitory control capacity. *Developmental Cognitive Neuroscience* 7: 53–64.

Fabel K, Kempermann G. (2008). Physical activity and the regulation of neurogenesis in the adult and aging brain. *NeuroMolecular Medicine* 10 (2): 59–66.

Fedewa AL, Ahn S. (2011). The effects of physical activity and physical fitness on children's achievement and cognitive outcomes: A meta-analysis. *Research Quarterly for Exercise and Sport* 82 (3): 521–535.

Fernandez A, Goldberg E, Michelon P. (2013). *The SharpBrains Guide to Brain Fitness*. San Francisco, CA: SharpBrain Inc. http://sharpbrains.com.

Fiatarone Singh MA, Gates N, Saigal N, et al. (2014). The study of mental and resistance training (SMART) study-resistance training and/or cognitive training in mild cognitive impairment: A randomized, double-blind, double-sham controlled trial. *Journal of the American Medical Directors Association* 15 (12): 873–880.

Forte R, Boreham CA, Leite JC, et al. (2013). Enhancing cognitive functioning in the elderly: Multicomponent vs resistance training. *Clinical Interventions in Aging* 8: 19–27.

Foster JA, and McVey Neufeld KA. (2013). Gut-brain axis: How the microbiome influences anxiety and depression. *Trends in Neurosciences* 36 (5): 305–312.

Fragala MS, Beyer KS, Jajtner AR, et al. (2014). Resistance exercise may improve spatial awareness and visual reaction in older adults. *Journal of Strength and Conditioning Research* 28 (8): 2079–2087.

Fujiwara Y, Kubo M, Kohata Y. (2011). Cigarette smoking and its association with overlapping gastroesophageal reflux disease, functional dyspepsia, or irritable bowel syndrome. *Internal Medicine (Tokyo, Japan)* 50 (21): 2443–2447.

Gauthier CJ, Lefort M, Mekary S, et al. (2015). Hearts and minds: Linking vascular rigidity and aerobic fitness with cognitive aging. *Neurobiology of Aging* 36 (1): 304–314.

Gensler TO. (2008). *Probiotic and Prebiotic Recipes for Health: 100 Recipes That Battle Colitis, Candidiasis, Food Allergies, and Other Digestive Disorders.* Beverly, MA: Fair Wind Press.

Goodman CC, Fuller KS. (2015). *Pathology: Implications for the Physical Therapist,* 4rd ed. St. Louis, MO: Elsevier Saunders.

Gordon BR, McDowell CP, Lyons M, et al. (2017). The effects of resistance exercise training on anxiety: A meta-analysis and meta-regression analysis of randomized controlled trials. *Sports Medicine* 47 (12):2521-2532.

Gothe NP, Kramer AF, McAuley E. (2014). The effects of an 8-week hatha yoga intervention on executive function in older adults. *Journals of Gerontology. Series A, Biological Sciences and Medical Sciences* 69 (9): 1109–1116.

Guiney H, Lucas SJ, Cotter JD, et al. (2015). Evidence cerebral blood-flow regulation mediates exercise-cognition links in healthy young adults. *Neuropsychology* 29 (1): 1–9.

Hagger-Johnson G, Sabia S, Brunner EJ, et al. (2013). Combined impact of smoking and heavy alcohol use on cognitive decline in early old age: Whitehall II prospective cohort study. *British Journal of Psychiatry* 203 (2): 120–125.

Hall JE. (2011). *Guyton and Hall Textbook of Medical Physiology,* 12th ed. Philadelphia, PA: Saunders Elsevier.

Hariprasad VR, Koparde V, Sivakumar PT, et al. (2013). Randomized clinical trial of yoga-based intervention in residents from elderly homes: Effects on cognitive function. *Indian Journal Psychiatry* 55 (Supplement 3): S357–363.

Harris RE, Jeter J, Chan P, et al. (2005). Using acupressure to modify alertness in the classroom: A single-blinded, randomized, cross-over trial. *Journal of Alternative and Complementary Medicine* 11 (4): 673–679.

Hatch SL, Feinstein L, Link BG, et al. (2007). The continuing benefits of education: Adult education and midlife cognitive ability in the British 1946 birth cohort. *Journals of Gerontology. Series B, Psychological Sciences and Social Sciences* 62 (6): S404–414.

Heffernan TM, Battersby L, Bishop P, et al. (2015). Everyday memory deficits associated with anabolic-androgenic steroid use in regular gymnasium users. *The Open Psychiatry Journal* 9: 1–6.

Heizer WD, Southern S, McGovern, S. (2009). The role of diet in symptoms of irritable bowel syndrome in adults: A narrative review. *Journal of the American Dietetic Association* 109 (7): 1204–1214.

Hillman CH, Pontifex MB, Raine LB, et al. (2009). The effect of acute treadmill walking on cognitive control and academic achievement in preadolescent children. *Neuroscience* 159 (3): 1044–1054.

Hillman CH, Snook EM, Jerome GJ. (2003). Acute cardiovascular exercise and executive control function. *International Journal of Psychophysiology* 48 (3): 307–314.

Howes MJ, and Perry E. (2011). The role of phytochemicals in the treatment and prevention of dementia. *Drugs & Aging* 28 (6): 439–468.

Huang R, Wang, K, Hu J. (2016). Effect of probiotics on depression: A systematic review and meta-analysis of randomized controlled trials. *Nutrients* 8 (8).

Hulsken S, Martin A, Mohajeri MH, et al. (2013). Food-derived serotonergic modulators: Effects on mood and cognition. *Nutrition Research Reviews* 26 (2): 223–234.

Human Microbiome Project. (2015). *About the Human Microbiome Project.* Bethesda, MD: National Institutes of Health. Retrieved on November 4, 2017 from http://hmpdacc.org

Hyde J. (2017). *The Gut Makeover.* New York, NY: Bloomsbury.

Javed F, He Q, Davidson LE, et al. (2010). Brain and high metabolic rate organ mass: Contributions to resting energy expenditure beyond fat-free mass. *American Journal of Clinical Nutrition* 91 (4): 907–912.

Jobe JB, Smith DM, Ball K, et al. (2001). ACTIVE: a cognitive intervention trial to promote independence in older adults. *Controlled Clinical Trials* 22 (4): 453–479.

Kabai P. (2014). Alcohol consumption and cognitive decline in early old age. *Neurology* 83 (5): 476.

Kang JH, Ascherio A, Grodstein F. (2005). Fruit and vegetable consumption and cognitive decline in aging women. *Annals of Neurology* 57 (5): 713–720.

Keightley PC, Koloski NA, Talley NJ. (2015). Pathways in gut-brain communication: Evidence for distinct gut-to-brain and brain-to-gut syndromes. *Australian and New Zealand Journal of Psychiatry* 49 (3): 207–214.

Kimura K, Obuchi S, Arai T, et al. (2010). The influence of short-term strength training on health-related quality of life and executive cognitive function. *Journal of Physiological Anthropology* 29 (3): 95–101.

Kirkendall DR. (1986). Effects of physical activity on intellectual development and academic performance. In: Lee M, Eckert HM, and Stull GA. (Eds.). *Effects of Physical Activity on Children: A Special Tribute to Mabel Lee.* Champaign, IL: Human Kinetics.

Kitazawa K, Showa S, Hiraoka A, et al. (2015). Effect of a dual-task net-step exercise on cognitive and gait function in older adults. *Journal of Geriatric Physical Therapy* 38 (3): 133–140.

Klare P, Nigg J, Nold J, et al. (2015). The impact of a ten-week physical exercise program on health-related quality of life in patients with inflammatory bowel disease: A prospective randomized controlled trial. *Digestion* 91 (3): 239–247.

Komulainen P, Kivipelto M, Lakka TA, et al. (2010). Exercise, fitness and cognition—A randomised controlled trial in older individuals: The DR's EXTRA study. *European Geriatric Medicine* 1 (5): 266–272.

Krikorian R, Shidler MD, Nash TA, et al. (2010). Blueberry supplementation improves memory in older adults. *Journal of Agricultural and Food Chemistry* 58 (7): 3996–4000.

Kwok TC, Lam KC, Wong PS, et al. (2011). Effectiveness of coordination exercise in improving cognitive function in older adults: A prospective study. *Clinical Interventions in Aging* 6: 261–267.

Lam LC, Chau RC, Wong BM, et al. (2012). A 1-year randomized controlled trial comparing mind body exercise (Tai Chi) with stretching and toning exercise on cognitive function in older Chinese adults at risk of cognitive decline. *Journal of the American Medical Directors Association* 13 (6): 568.e15–20.

Lee J, Pase M, Pipingas A, et al. (2015). Switching to a 10-day Mediterranean-style diet improves mood and cardiovascular function in a controlled crossover study. *Nutrition* 31 (5): 647–652.

Lees C, Hopkins J. (2013). Effect of aerobic exercise on cognition, academic achievement, and psychosocial function in children: A systematic review of randomized control trials. *Preventing Chronic Disease* 10: E174.

Li L, Men WW, Chang YK, et al. (2014). Acute aerobic exercise increases cortical activity during working memory: A functional MRI study in female college students. *PLoS One* 9 (6): e99222.

Lichtwark IT, Newnham ED, Robinson SR, et al. (2014). Cognitive impairment in coeliac disease improves on a gluten-free diet and correlates with histological and serological indices of disease severity. *Alimentary Pharmacology & Therapeutics* 40 (2): 160–170.

Liu-Ambrose T, Donaldson MG, Ahamed Y, et al. (2008). Otago home-based strength and balance retraining improves executive functioning in older fallers: A randomized controlled trial. *Journal of the American Geriatrics Society* 56 (10): 1821–1830.

Liu-Ambrose T, Nagamatsu LS, Graf P, et al. (2010). Resistance training and executive functions: A 12-month randomized controlled trial. *Archives of Internal Medicine* 170 (2): 170–178.

Liu-Ambrose T, Nagamatsu LS, Voss MW, et al. (2012). Resistance training and functional plasticity of the aging brain: A 12-month randomized controlled trial. *Neurobiology of Aging* 33 (8): 1690–1698.

Llewellyn DJ, Lang IA, Langa KM, et al. (2010). Vitamin D and risk of cognitive decline in elderly persons. *Archives of Internal Medicine* 170 (13): 1135–1141.

Lounsbury H. (2014). *Fix Your Mood With Food: The "Live Natural, Live Well" Approach to Whole Body Health.* Guilford, CT: Globe Pequot Press.

Lupien SJ, Fiocco A, Wan N, et al. (2005). Stress hormones and human memory function across the lifespan. *Psychoneuroendocrinology* 30 (3): 225–242.

Masento NA, Golightly M, Field DT, et al. (2014). Effects of hydration status on cognitive performance and mood. *British Journal of Nutrition* 111 (10): 1841–1852.

Mayer EA, Knight R, Mazmanian SK, et al. (2014). Gut microbes and the brain: Paradigm shift in neuroscience. *Journal of Neuroscience* 34 (46): 15490–15496.

McKean J, Naug H, Nikbakht E, et al. (2017). Probiotics and subclinical psychological symptoms in healthy participants: A systematic review and meta-analysis. *Journal of Alternative and Complementary Medicine* 23 (4): 249–258.

Miller KJ, Dye RV, Kim J, et al. (2013). Effect of a computerized brain exercise program on cognitive performance in older adults. *American Journal of Geriatric Psychiatry* 21 (7): 655–663.

Miller KJ, Siddarth P, Gaines JM, et al. (2012). The memory fitness program: Cognitive effects of a healthy aging intervention. *American Journal of Geriatric Psychiatry* 20 (6): 514–523.

Moss M, Hewitt S, Moss L, et al. (2008). Modulation of cognitive performance and mood by aromas of peppermint and ylang-ylang. *International Journal of Neuroscience* 118 (1): 59–77.

Mueller PA, Oppenheimer DM. (2014). The pen is mightier than the keyboard: Advantages of longhand over laptop note taking. *Psychological Science* 25 (6): 1159–1168.

Nagai M, Hoshide S, Kario K. (2010). Hypertension and dementia. *American Journal of Hypertension* 23 (2): 116–124.

Nanda B, Balde J, Manjunatha S. (2013). The acute effects of a single bout of moderate-intensity aerobic exercise on cognitive functions in healthy adult males. *Journal of Clinical and Diagnostic Research* 7 (9): 1883–1885.

Narme P, Clément S, Ehrlé N, et al. (2013). Efficacy of musical interventions in dementia: Evidence from a randomized controlled trial. *Journal of Alzheimer's Disease* 38 (2): 359–369.

Nemani K, Hosseini Ghomi R, McCormick B, et al. (2015). Schizophrenia and the gut-brain axis. *Prognosis in Neuropsychopharmacol & Biological Psychiatry* 56: 155–160.

Ng TP, Chiam PC, Lee T, et al. (2006). Curry consumption and cognitive function in the elderly. *American Journal of Epidemiology* 164 (9): 898–906

Ozkaya GY, Aydin H, Toraman FN, et al. (2005). Effect of strength and endurance training on cognition in older people. *Journal of Sports Science and Medicine* 4 (3): 300–313.

Perrig-Chiello P, Perrig WJ, Ehrsam R, et al. (1998). The effects of resistance training on well-being and memory in elderly volunteers. *Age and Ageing* 27 (4): 469–475.

Pettersen JA, Fontes S, Duke CL. (2014). The effects of vitamin D insufficiency and seasonal decrease on cognition. *Canadian Journal of Neurological Sciences* 41 (4): 459–465.

Petyaev IM, Zigangirova NA, Kobets NV, et al. (2013). Roquefort cheese proteins inhibit *Chlamydia pneumoniae* propagation and LPS-Induced leukocyte migration. *The Scientific World Journal* 140591.

Phillips C, Akif Baktir M, Das D, et al. (2015). The link between physical activity and cognitive dysfunction in Alzheimer disease. *Physical Therapy* 95 (7): 1046–1060.

Pierce C, Pecen J, McLeod KJ. (2009). Influence of seated rocking on blood pressure in the elderly: A pilot clinical study. *Biological Research for Nursing* 11 (2): 144–151.

Pietrzak RH, Scott JC, Neumeister A, et al. (2014). Anxiety symptoms, cerebral amyloid burden and memory decline in healthy older adults without dementia: 3-year prospective cohort study. *British Journal of Psychiatry* 204: 400–401.

Pinniger R, Brown RF, Thorsteinsson, et al. (2012). Argentine tango dance compared to mindfulness meditation and a waiting-list control: A randomised trial for treating depression. *Complementary Therapies in Medicine* 20 (6): 377–384.

Pongan E, Tillmann B, Leveque Y, et al. (2017). Can musical or painting interventions improve chronic pain, mood, quality of life, and cognition in patients with mild Alzheimer's disease? Evidence from a randomized controlled trial. *Journal of Alzheimer's Disease* 60 (2): 663–677.

Pontifex MB, Hillman CH, Fernhall B, et al. (2009). The effect of acute aerobic and resistance exercise on working memory. *Medicine and Science in Sports and Exercise* 41 (4): 927–934.

Poon L, Chodzko-Zajko W, Tomporowski P. (2006). *Active Living, Cognitive Functioning, and Aging* (Volume 1). Champaign IL: Human Kinetics.

Rampersaud GC, Pereira MA, Girard BL, et al. (2005). Breakfast habits, nutritional status, body weight, and academic performance in children and adolescents. *Journal of the American Dietetic Association* 105 (5): 743–760.

Roberts RO, Knopman DS, Przybelski SA, et al. (2014). Association of Type 2 diabetes with brain atrophy and cognitive impairment. *Neurology* 82 (13): 1132–1141.

Sabia S, Elbaz A, Britton A, et al. (2014). Alcohol consumption and cognitive decline in early old age. *Neurology* 82 (4): 332–339.

Seamans KM, Hill TR, Scully L, et al. (2010). Vitamin D status and measures of cognitive function in healthy older European adults. *European Journal of Clinical Nutrition* 64 (10): 1172–1178.

Scott KP, Antoine JM, Midtvedt T, et al. (2015). Manipulating the gut microbiota to maintain health and treat disease. *Microbial Ecology in Health and Disease* 26: 25877.

Severance EG, Prandovszky E, Castiglione J, et al. (2015). Gastroenterology issues in schizophrenia: Why the gut matters. *Current Psychiatry Reports* 17 (5): 574.

Sharon G, Garg N, Debelius J, et al. (2014). Specialized metabolites from the microbiome in health and disease. *Cell Metabolism* 20 (5): 719–730.

Slavin J. (2013). Fiber and prebiotics: Mechanisms and health benefits. *Nutrients* 5 (4): 1417–1435.

Small G, Vorgan G. (2004). *The Memory Prescription: Dr. Gary Small's 14-Day Plan to Keep Your Brain and Body Young*. New York, NY: Hyperion.

Small GW, Silverman DH, Siddarth P, et al. (2006). Effects of a 14-day healthy longevity lifestyle program on cognition and brain function. *American Journal of Geriatric Psychiatry* 14 (6): 538–545.

Smyth A, Dehghan, M, O'Donnell M, et al. (2015). Healthy eating and reduced risk of cognitive decline: A cohort from 40 countries. *Neurology* 84 (22): 2258–2265.

Somer E. (1999). *Food & Mood: The Complete Guide to Eating Well and Feeling Your Best*, 2nd ed. New York, NY: Henry Holt and Company.

Sompo Japan Research Institute. (2010). A non-profit organization, community health promotion support meeting "one to three" and its health promotion activities for the elderly using the FUMANET exercise. Disease Management Reporter in Japan 18: 1–8. www.sj-ri.co.jp/eng/disease/pdf/eng_dmr-18.pdf

Spirduso W, Poon L, Chodzko-Zajko W. (2008). *Exercise and Its Mediating Effects on Cognition* (Volume 2). Champaign IL: Human Kinetics.

Swanson GR, Sedghi S, Farhadi A, et al. (2010). Pattern of alcohol consumption and its effect on gastrointestinal symptoms in inflammatory bowel disease. *Alcohol* 44 (3): 223–228.

Taibi A, Comelli EM. (2014). Practical approaches to probiotics use. *Applied Physiology, Nutrition, and Metabolism* 39 (8): 980–986.

ten Brinke LF, Bolandzadeh N, Nagamatsu LS, et al. (2015). Aerobic exercise increases hippocampal volume in older women with probable mild cognitive impairment: A 6-month randomised controlled trial. *British Journal of Sports Medicine* 49 (4): 248–254.

Tillisch K, Labus J, Kilpatrick L, et al. (2013). Consumption of fermented milk product with probiotic modulates brain activity. *Gastroenterology* 144 (7): 1394–1401.

Tomporowski PD, Davis CL, Miller PH, et al. (2008). Exercise and children's intelligence, cognition, and academic achievement. *Educational Psychology Review* 20 (2): 111–131.

Tsutsumi T, Don BM, Zaichkowsky LD, et al. (1997). Physical fitness and psychological benefits of strength training in community dwelling older adults. *Applied Human Science* 16 (6): 257–266.

Valls-Pedret C., Sala-Vila A., Serra-Mir M, et al. (2015). Mediterranean diet and age-related cognitive decline: A randomized clinical trial. *JAMA Internal Medicine* 175 (7): 1094–1103.

Venes D. (Ed.). (2017). *Taber's Cyclopedic Medical Dictionary*, 23rd ed. Philadelphia, PA: FA Davis.

Vinesett AL, Whaley RR, Woods-Giscombe C, et al. (2017). Modified African Ngoma healing ceremony for stress reduction: A pilot study. *Journal of Alternative and Complementary Medicine 23* (10): 800-804.

Voss MW, Prakash RS, Erickson KI, et al. (2010). Plasticity of brain networks in a randomized intervention trial of exercise training in older adults. *Frontiers in Aging Neuroscience* 2: 32.

Weinstein G, Maillard P, Himali JJ, et al. (2015). Glucose indices are associated with cognitive and structural brain measures in young adults. *Neurology* 84 (23): 2329–2337.

Wells RE, Yeh GY, Kerr CE, et al. (2013). Meditation's impact on default mode network and hippocampus in mild cognitive impairment: A pilot study. *Neuroscience Letter* 556: 15–19.

White BA, Horwath CC, Conner TS. (2013). Many apples a day keep the blues away—Daily experiences of negative and positive affect and food consumption in young adults. *British Journal of Health Psychology* 18 (4): 782–798.

Wilker EH, Preis SR, Beiser AS, et al. (2015). Long-term exposure to fine particulate matter, residential proximity to major roads and measures of brain structure. *Stroke* 46 (5): 1161–1166.

Winter B, Breitenstein C, Mooren FC, et al. (2007). High impact running improves learning. *Neurobiology of Learning and Memory* 87 (4): 597–609.

Wu CT, Pontifex MB, Raine LB, et al. (2011). Aerobic fitness and response variability in preadolescent children performing a cognitive control task. *Neuropsychology* 25 (3): 333–341.

Ybarra O, Burnstein E, Winkielman P, et al. (2008). Mental exercising through simple socializing: Social interaction promotes general cognitive functioning. *Personality & Social Psychology Bulletin* 34 (2): 248–259.

Yoo SS, Hu PT, Gujar N, et al. (2007). A deficit in the ability to form new human memories without sleep. *Nature Neuroscience* 10 (3): 385–392.

Young H, Benton D. (2014). The nature of the control of blood glucose in those with poorer glucose tolerance influences mood and cognition. *Metabolic Brain Disease* 29 (3): 721–728.

Zeidan F, Martucci KT, Kraft RA, et al. (2014). Neural correlates of mindfulness meditation-related anxiety relief. *Social Cognitive and Affective Neuroscience* 9 (6): 751–759.

Zhao E, Tranovich MJ, Wright VJ. (2014). The role of mobility as a protective factor of cognitive functioning in aging adults: A review. *Sports Health* 6 (1): 63–69.

Zhou L, Foster JA. (2015). Psychobiotics and the gut-brain axis: In the pursuit of happiness. *Neuropsychiatric Disease and Treatment* 11: 715–723.

Zhu N, Jacobs DR, Schreiner PJ, et al. (2014). Cardiorespiratory fitness and cognitive function in middle age: The CARDIA study. *Neurology* 82 (15): 1339–1346.

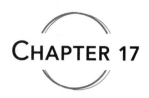

CHAPTER 17

SUSTAINABLE WEIGHT LOSS GUIDE

"The part can never be well unless the whole is well."

—Plato

Individuals wanting to lose weight have a goal of getting in shape and staying in shape. Most people want sustainable results. Controlling stress, getting adequate sleep, eating quality foods, engaging in some fun exercises, and also doing meditative movements, such as tai chi and qigong, may go a long way in helping many people attain their weight loss goal as compared to other unsustainable higher intensity workouts and gimmick diets. If you have a high-paced lifestyle, consider slowing down and giving the gentler and more mindful approach a try for your weight loss and weight maintenance goals. If you need some evidence, an article by Kushner et al. (2014) indicates that for a weight-loss program to be effective, a person needs to focus on comprehensive lifestyle changes, such as healthful eating, physical activity, and stress management. So, lifestyle changes win again.

Here is an interesting fact you can use. One pound of muscle (lean body mass) burns 14 calories per day, while one pound of fat burns only two calories per day (Heber 1999; Heber et al. 2001). As you increase lean body mass, you burn more calories during activity *and* while resting. Now I think that's pretty neat.

The following are some tips to help you with your weight-loss goals:

SEE YOUR PHYSICIAN

Your doctor can facilitate a weight-loss plan and guide you throughout the entire process. For example, an undiagnosed or untreated medical condition, such as a thyroid issue, might affect weight gain.

Brush Your Teeth after All Meals

Brushing your teeth provides a cue that mealtime is finished. In a study published in the *Journal of the Japan Society for the Study of Obesity*, Dr. Takashi Wada indicates that individuals who stay slim tend to brush their teeth after each meal (British Dental Journal News 2005).

Focus on Mindful Eating

A study by Dalen et al. (2010) indicates that "focused mindfulness-based intervention can result in significant changes in weight, eating behavior, and psychological distress in obese individuals."

Get Enough Sleep

- Inadequate or reduced sleep can lead to weight gain (Hasler et al. 2004; Nedeltcheva et al. 2010; Patel 2009; Patel et al. 2006).
- Sleeping less might lead to eating more (Brondel et al. 2010; Nedeltcheva et al. 2009).

Improve Your Diet

Don't let the overwhelming amount of information related to nutrition derail your weight-loss program. Any amount of improvement is better than none. Consider the following nutrition tips for losing weight:

- All diets should focus on being composed of healthful foods (such as fresh fruits and vegetables, seafood, yogurt, nuts, seeds, and grass-fed meat) rather than focusing on just calories or carbohydrate and fat content. Healthful foods are essential for healing, recovery, and maintaining physical and mental wellness.
- Find the best combination of foods for your system.
- Eliminate foods to which you have allergies or sensitivities.
- Eat a healthful breakfast.
- Johnston et al. (2014) conclude that any low-carbohydrate or low-fat diet leads to weight loss.
- Exercise alone is not enough to lose weight—a healthful diet is essential (Caudwell et al. 2009).
- Use smaller plates, bowls, spoons, and forks, and don't supersize your meals (Rolls 2003).
- Gilhooly et al. (2007) indicate that the "portion size of craved foods and frequency of giving into food cravings appear to be important areas for focus in lifestyle modification programs for long-term weight loss."
- Eat small bite sizes to avoid overeating (Zijlstra et al. 2009) and chew your food thoroughly.

- Reduce sugar intake by having fruit juices, jellies, jams, soft drinks, candies, cakes, cookies, and pies only in moderation.
- Reduce carbohydrate intake by limiting foods made from grains, such as breads, pastas, and cereals.
- Alcohol is a source of calories, and can contribute to weight gain and obesity. Consume only light to moderate amounts of alcohol (Wang et al. 2010), or avoid it altogether.
- Try a FODMAP (which stands for fermentable oligosaccharides, disaccharides, monosaccharides, and polyols) diet to determine if you have sensitivity to specific foods identified in the FODMAP list (Gibson et al. 2010). See the discussion about FODMAPS in chapter 4: Nutrition for Life. Also, see the FODMAP Friendly website fodmapfriendly.com and The Monash Low FODMAP Diet website and Appmonashfodmap.com for additional information about this strategy.

Try the following sample plans according to what you consider a reasonable change:

- Plan A—reduce unhealthful sugar and fat from your diet by 75 percent
- Plan B—reduce unhealthful sugar and fat from your diet by 50 percent
- Plan C—reduce unhealthful sugar and fat from your diet by 25 percent

Box 16: Holistic Healing

MANAGING OSTEOARTHRITIS

Osteoarthritis is a type of arthritis marked by progressive cartilage deterioration in synovial joints and vertebrae. Risk factors include aging, obesity, overuse or abuse of joints (repetitive motions, bending, lifting) as in sports or strenuous occupations, instability of joints, excessive mobility, immobilization, and trauma (Venes 2017).

Obesity has been linked with osteoarthritis (Coggon et al. 2001; Felson 1995). One preliminary study shows that weight loss and exercise (resistance training and walking) regimes lead to reductions in knee pain (Messier et al. 2000). Another study indicates that the combination of modest dietary weight loss combined with moderate exercise (resistance training and walking) provides reduction in pain and improvements in performance measures of mobility (walking and stair-climbing) in older overweight and obese adults with knee osteoarthritis (Messier et al. 2004).

Being overweight is an important modifiable risk factor in osteoarthritis of the knee and hips (Derman et al. 2014; Felson 1995, 1996; Vad et al. 2002). Overloading the hip and knee joints can lead to cartilage breakdown or failure of other structures, such as ligaments (Felson et al. 2000). Researchers (Felson et al. 2000) state that "for each one-pound increase in weight, the overall force across the knee in a single-leg stance increases two to three pounds. This load effect probably explains most of the increased risk for osteoarthritis of the knee and hip among overweight persons."

LET'S SEE WHAT OTHER RESEARCH SAYS . . .

- "Hand exercises were well tolerated and significantly improved activity performance, grip strength, pain, and fatigue in women with hand osteoarthritis" (Hennig et al. 2014).
- "Current evidence supports the use of acupuncture as an alternative for traditional analgesics in patients with osteoarthritis" (Manyanga et al. 2014).
- "Therapeutic aquatic exercise is effective in managing symptoms associated with lower limb osteoarthritis" (Waller et al. 2014).
- "Participants who have osteoarthritis of the knee benefit from self-massage intervention therapy" (Atkins et al. 2013).
- Consuming ginger may reduce muscle pain after exercise and in individuals with osteoarthritis (Black et al. 2010).
- Natural thermal mineral waters improve pain and function in individuals with knee osteoarthritis (Harzy et al. 2009).
- "Massage therapy seems to be efficacious in the treatment of osteoarthritis of the knee" (Perlman et al. 2006).

The following are some resources to consider for managing osteoarthritis:

- American Arthritis Society, americanarthritis.org
- Arthritis Foundation, arthritis.org
- Osteoarthritis Research Society International, oarsi.org
- The Arthritis Society, arthritis.ca

INCREASE YOUR PHYSICAL ACTIVITY

Consider the following exercise tips for losing weight:

- Inactivity can lead to weight gain (Leskinen et al. 2009).
- Exercise is needed to help sustain weight loss (Jakicic et al. 2008).
- In addition to aerobic exercise, add resistance training (Idoate et al. 2011; Strasser et al. 2011).

REDUCE STRESS

- Excess stress can lead to weight gain (Bose et al. 2009).
- Try relaxation, mindfulness meditation, yoga, qigong, or tai chi to reduce stress levels.

TRACK YOUR PROGRESS

The National Weight Control Registry (where you share your success story), www.nwcr.ws. Most registry members report keeping weight off by maintaining a low-calorie, low-fat diet and high levels of activity. Reported statistics of registry participants as of February 2018 include:

- 78 percent eat breakfast every day.
- 75 percent weigh themselves at least once a week.

- 62 percent watch less than 10 hours of television per week.
- 90 percent exercise, on average, about one hour per day.

Don't let limited time derail your weight-loss exercise program. Any amount of activity is better than none. Keep the following in mind as you do your personalized exercise program for weight loss:

- Not everyone loses body weight with a primarily aerobic exercise program (in which you train five days a week with aerobic exercises). Therefore, try increasing your strength training from one or two to two or three times per week to see if this ignites your weight loss or continues your weight-loss momentum.
- Try substituting swimming, hiking, bicycling, or sports like basketball or tennis into your aerobic days to see if it fits better into your lifestyle and provides more variety.
- Try substituting yoga, Pilates, tai chi, qigong, or dancing to see if mind and body exercises fit better into your strength-training days and provide more variety and relaxation.

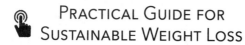 ## PRACTICAL GUIDE FOR SUSTAINABLE WEIGHT LOSS

Let's be honest here. There is not one easy way to lose weight and keep it off. If there was one way or <u>the</u> way, then we would all do it this way. This is only <u>a</u> way for you to try. At some point, you have to set aside all the research articles and books and learn to listen to your body. I outline here what has worked for my patients and clients. See if this strategy (or an adapted version) will work for you.

- **Step 1:** Make sure you are controlling your stress (refer to chapter 2) and getting enough sleep (refer to chapter 3) every night. Stress control and sleep are listed first as Step 1 because I feel it is essential to control these factors before you do anything else. This may be your missing link.
- **Step 2:** For the first two months, rather than focusing on counting calories and stressing over every bite, concentrate on consuming wholesome foods your great-grandmother would recognize. Don't obsess over eating organic and non-GMO foods (genetically modified organisms). Get rid of all junk foods and just eat real foods. Eating real foods will include a variety of proteins (vegetarian or non-vegetarian depending on your personal approach), plenty of vegetables, some fruits, some nuts and seeds (if you tolerate them), and healthy oils (like olive oil) in your diet. If you get good results with this approach, you may not need to count calories. Later, you can

consider choosing more organic and non-GMO foods which fit your budget and philosophy.

- **Step 3:** For at least the first two months, avoid alcohol, soft drinks (and hopefully you avoid this forever), and fruit juices (too high in sugar) and focus more on water and herbal tea (if you tolerate tea) as your beverages.
- **Step 4:** Chew each bite of food 20 times (Hyde 2017). Slow down and enjoy each bite.
- **Step 5:** Try consuming some probiotic foods to help improve your gut health (Hyde 2017). Refer to chapter 16 for a list of probiotic foods or take a probiotic supplement if you are unable to consume these foods.
- **Step 6:** Engage in some *fun* exercise or activity. Please don't punish yourself with exercise (Hyde 2017) or grueling workouts. You are aiming to find a sustainable activity and movement program you enjoy. This could be accomplished with walking, hiking, weight training, yoga, Pilates, tai chi, qigong, sports (like tennis), or a combination. See the Sample Exercise Plans for Weight Loss (Table 17-1) and Sample Exercise Programs for Weight Loss in this chapter.

Try this very simple 6-step approach for two months and see what kind of progress you make. Sometimes, all you need is simplicity and the basics for success. If you are happy with the results at the end of two months, then keep going until you reach your goals. Depending on how much weight you need to lose, it may take you three to twelve months or more to achieve your goals. But wait, what is considered success? You could say the success is in terms of lost pounds, or you are now wearing a smaller dress size or pants, you are satisfied that you improved your health, you are happier and enjoying life with more energy, or some combination. Remember, success is not just about your weight on the scale or the inches lost. And if you do determine you are successful on your own terms, then reward yourself with a nice gift, go shopping, go to a movie, or plan that special vacation.

If you are not making any progress in your health after two months, consult with your physician for another full checkup (in addition to your yearly checkup) to discuss your goals of wanting to lose weight. After you see your physician, consider seeing a physical therapist for a customized exercise program, and finally, see a dietitian for a personalized nutrition program.

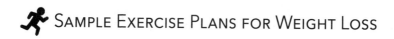

Sample Exercise Plans for Weight Loss

Table 17-1: Exercise Plans for Weight Loss

Plan A—when you have plenty of time
Plan B—when you have a moderate amount of time
Plan C—when you have a limited amount of time

MONDAY (STRENGTH)	Plan A—10 minutes of mobility exercises / 30 minutes of strength exercises / 5 minutes of stretching Plan B—10 minutes of mobility exercises / 15 minutes of strength exercises / 5 minutes of stretching Plan C—5 minutes of mobility exercises / 5 minutes of strength exercises / 5 minutes of stretching
TUESDAY (AEROBIC)	Plan A—walk 30 to 60 minutes in the morning, afternoon, or evening Plan B—walk 15 minutes in the afternoon / 15 minutes in the evening Plan C—walk 10 minutes in the morning / 10 minutes in the afternoon / 10 minutes the evening
WEDNESDAY (STRENGTH)	Plan A—10 minutes of mobility exercises / 30 minutes of strength exercises / 5 minutes of stretching Plan B—10 minutes of mobility exercises / 15 minutes of strength exercises / 5 minutes of stretching Plan C—5 minutes of mobility exercises / 5 minutes of strength exercises / 5 minutes of stretching
THURSDAY (AEROBIC)	Plan A—walk 30 to 60 minutes in the morning, afternoon, or evening Plan B—walk 15 minutes in the afternoon / 15 minutes in the evening Plan C—walk 10 minutes in the morning / 10 minutes in the afternoon / 10 minutes in the evening
FRIDAY (AEROBIC)	Plan A—walk 30 to 60 minutes in the morning, afternoon, or evening Plan B—walk 15 minutes in the afternoon / 15 minutes in the evening Plan C—walk 10 minutes in the morning / 10 minutes in the afternoon / 10 minutes in the evening
SATURDAY (STRENGTH)	Plan A—10 minutes of mobility exercises / 30 minutes of strength exercises / 5 minutes of stretching Plan B—10 minutes of mobility exercises / 15 minutes of strength exercises / 5 minutes of stretching Plan C—5 minutes of mobility exercises / 5 minutes of strength exercises / 5 minutes of stretching
SUNDAY	Day off

SAMPLE EXERCISE PROGRAMS FOR WEIGHT LOSS

PROGRAM 1: TRADITIONAL WEIGHT LOSS ROUTINE

The following routine is for beginner and intermediate level individuals. All of the exercises outlined in this section are explained in chapter 13.

Aerobic Routine (select one or combine)
- Outdoor Walking
- Hiking
- Aquatic Walking (if joints are painful)
- Stationary Bicycle (recumbent)

Dynamic Warm-Up Routine
- Tai Chi Steps
- Shoulder March

Strength Routine
- Shortstop Squats
- Elastic High Rows
- Elevated Push-Ups
- Bird Dog

Flexibility Routine
- Yawn Stretch
- Squat Stretch
- Calf Stretch

PROGRAM 2: INTEGRATIVE WEIGHT LOSS ROUTINE

The following routine is for beginner and intermediate level individuals.

Aerobic Routine (select one or combine)
- Refer to the Mindfulness Walking Program in chapter 1
- Refer to the Labyrinth Walking Program in chapter 1
- Refer to the Track, Park, or Neighborhood Circuit in chapter 12.

Mobility / Strength / Balance Routine (select one or combine)
- Tai Chi Training (choose a style such as Yang, Chen, Wu, Hao, or Sun)
- Qigong Training (choose a style such as Eight Strands of Brocade Qigong or Tai Chi Qigong)
- Yoga Training (choose a style such as Ashtanga, Bikram, Hatha, Iyengar, or Kundalini)

Healthy Teeth and Gums
for a Healthy Body

The mouth is the gateway into the body, and periodontal disease has been associated with systemic inflammatory conditions such as arthritis, obesity, kidney disease, and Alzheimer's disease (Tornwall et al. 2012). An article by Lee et al. (2013) indicates that regular dental checkups can help reduce the incidence of a stroke. So, make sure you brush, floss, and massage your gums.

Use a gum massager (with a rubber tip stimulator) as directed by your dentist and dental hygienist to keep your gums healthy (Kazmierczak et al. 1994). As an example, refer to the www.gumbrand.com website for a gum stimulator device. Your mouth will feel amazing after the gentle massage.

Also, consider storing your floss, toothbrush, and gum massager outside of your bathroom to avoid cross contamination from your toilet (American Society for Microbiology 2017). It may not be a bad idea to keep your shaver and cosmetics outside the bathroom as well.

The following websites can help you learn more about taking care of your teeth and gums:

- American Dental Association, ada.org
- American Dental Hygienists' Association, adha.org

Box 18: Holistic Healing

Tips to Manage Constipation

Constipation is a problem that might cause headaches and is associated with other issues, such as anxiety, depression, abdominal bloating, abdominal or hamstring cramps, fatigue, and lower-back pain (Altug 2016). However, further research is needed in these areas. If you have chronic constipation (or diarrhea, for that matter), see your physician. There might be a medical reason or medication side effect that needs to be addressed.

If you have constipation only periodically, try the following suggestions:

- Be careful of taking excess calcium supplements at one time or eating too much dairy, such as yogurt or cheese (Jackson et al. 2006; Prince et al. 2006).
- Do not hold your breath when you are having a bowel movement, especially when constipated. Individuals have suffered strokes or heart attacks from prolonged breath-holding and bearing down during bowel movements (Kollef et al. 1991; Sikirov 1990). A proper breathing technique during a bowel movement is to use a "huffing" type of breathing—breathing out with small breaths (Harrington et al. 2006; Storrie 1997). Breathing out in this manner activates

abdominal muscles and assists with the propulsion of stools, while minimizing stress to the heart and small blood vessels in the brain. A Valsalva maneuver (trying to breathe out forcibly with the air passages in the mouth and nose closed) has been shown to create excessive pressure on blood vessels in the heart and brain, possibly leading to rupture (Vlak et al. 2011).

- The natural bowel movement posture for a human is the squatting position (Bajwa et al. 2009; Sikirov 1989, 2003). A change in your posture and position might help with a normal bowel movement. Here are three methods you can try:
  - » Lean forward at the trunk with your forearms on top of your thighs.
  - » Modify your current toilet posture by placing a small footstool or box, approximately six inches in height, in front of your toilet (Storrie 1997). Put your feet on the stool, and lean your trunk forward approximately 45 degrees. Rest your forearms on your upper thighs for support and relaxation. This seated position on a Western toilet comes closest to the natural squat style for emptying the bowels. Refer to the Squatty Potty website (squattypotty.com) for more information about modifying your position on the toilet.
  - » Look for a toilet seat that has a slight dip or downward curve in the back of the seat to help position the body properly for bowel movement.
- The following simple exercises while lying supine (faceup) in bed may help increase gastrointestinal mobility (McMillan 1921):
  - » Repeated alternate single knee-to-chest movements (for example, do 1 set of 10 repetitions).
  - » Repeated double knee-to-chest movements (for example, do 1 set of 10 repetitions).
  - » Small single leg circle movements (for example, do 1 set of 5 repetitions).
  - » As an alternate technique, try the Squat Stretch in chapter 13.

ADDITIONAL RESOURCES

- American Diabetes Association, diabetes.org
- Obesity Society, obesity.org (see the Resources section for *Your Weight Matters Magazine*)
- Pro-Change Behavior Systems—Transtheoretical Model, prochange.com

REFERENCES

Bose M, Oliván B, Laferrère B. (2009). Stress and obesity: The role of the hypothalamic-pituitary-adrenal axis in metabolic disease. *Current Opinion in Endocrinology, Diabetes, and Obesity* 16 (5): 340–346.

British Dental Journal News. (2005). Brushing teeth for all around health. *British Dental Journal* 198: 257.

Brondel L, Romer MA, Nougues PM, et al. (2010). Acute partial sleep deprivation increases food intake in healthy men. *American Journal of Clinical Nutrition* 91 (6): 1550–1559.

Caudwell P, Hopkins M, King NA, et al. (2009). Exercise alone is not enough: Weight loss also needs a healthy (Mediterranean) diet? *Public Health Nutrition* 12 (9A): 1663–1666.

Dalen J, Smith BW, Shelley BM, et al. (2010). Pilot study: Mindful eating and living (MEAL): Weight, eating behavior, and psychological outcomes associated with a mindfulness-based intervention for people with obesity. *Complementary Therapies in Medicine* 18 (6): 260–264.

Gibson PR, Shepherd SJ. (2010). Evidence-based dietary management of functional gastrointestinal symptoms: The FODMAP approach. *Journal of Gastroenterology and Hepatology* 25 (2): 252–258.

Gilhooly CH, Das SK, Golden JK, et al. (2007). Food cravings and energy regulation: The characteristics of craved foods and their relationship with eating behaviors and weight change during 6 months of dietary energy restriction. *International Journal of Obesity* 31 (12): 1849–1858.

Hasler G, Buysse DJ, Klaghofer R, et al. (2004). The association between short sleep duration and obesity in young adults: A 13-year prospective study. *Sleep* 27 (4): 661–666.

Heber D. (1999). *The Resolution Diet: Keeping the Promise of Permanent Weight Loss.* Garden City Park, NY: Avery Publishing Group.

Heber D, Bowerman S. (2001). *What Color is Your Diet? The 7 Colors of Health.* New York, NY: HarperCollins.

Hyde J. (2017). *The Gut Makeover.* New York, NY: Bloomsbury.

Idoate F, Ibañez J, Gorostiaga EM, et al. (2011). Weight-loss diet alone or combined with resistance training induces different regional visceral fat changes in obese women. *International Journal of Obesity* 35 (5): 700–713.

Jakicic JM, Marcus BH, Lang W, et al. (2008). Effect of exercise on 24-month weight loss maintenance in overweight women. *Archives of Internal Medicine* 168 (14): 1550–1559.

Johnston BC, Kanters S, Bandayrel K, et al. (2014). Comparison of weight loss among named diet programs in overweight and obese adults: A meta-analysis. *JAMA* 312 (9): 923–933.

Kushner RF, and Ryan DH. (2014). Assessment and lifestyle management of patients with obesity: Clinical recommendations from systematic reviews. *JAMA* 312 (9): 943–952.

Leskinen T, Sipilä S, Alen M, et al. (2009). Leisure-time physical activity and high-risk fat: A longitudinal population-based twin study. *International Journal of Obesity* 33 (11): 1211–1218.

Malhotra A, Noakes T, Phinney S. (2015). It is time to bust the myth of physical inactivity and obesity: You cannot outrun a bad diet. *British Journal of Sports Medicine.* Advance online publication.

Nedeltcheva AV, Kilkus JM, Imperial J, et al. (2009). Sleep curtailment is accompanied by increased intake of calories from snacks. *American Journal of Clinical Nutrition* 89 (1): 126–133.

Nedeltcheva AV, Kilkus JM, Imperial J, et al. (2010). Insufficient sleep undermines dietary efforts to reduce adiposity. *Annals of Internal Medicine* 153 (7): 435–441.

Patel SR. (2009). Reduced sleep as an obesity risk factor. *Obesity Review* 10 (Supplement 2): 61–68.

Patel SR, Malhotra A, White DP, et al. (2006). Association between reduced sleep and weight gain in women. *American Journal of Epidemiology* 164 (10): 947–954.

Rolls BJ. (2003). The supersizing of America: Portion size and the obesity epidemic. *Nutrition Today* 38 (2): 42–53.

Strasser B, Schobersberger W. (2011). Evidence for resistance training as a treatment therapy in obesity. *Journal of Obesity* pii: 482564.

Venes D. (Ed.). (2017). *Taber's Cyclopedic Medical Dictionary*, 23rd ed. Philadelphia, PA: FA Davis.

Wang L, Lee IM, Manson JE, et al. (2010). Alcohol consumption, weight gain, and risk of becoming overweight in middle-aged and older women. *Archives of Internal Medicine* 170 (5): 453–461.

Zijlstra N, de Wijk RA, Mars M, et al. (2009). Effect of bite size and oral processing time of a semisolid food on satiation. *American Journal of Clinical Nutrition* 90 (2): 269–275.

HOLISTIC HEALING BOXES

Managing Osteoarthritis

Atkins DV, Eichler DA. (2013). The effects of self-massage on osteoarthritis of the knee: A randomized, controlled trial. *International Journal of Therapeutic Massage & Bodywork* 6 (1): 4–14.

Black CD, Herring MP, Hurley DJ, et al. (2010). Ginger (Zingiber officinale) reduces muscle pain caused by eccentric exercise. *Journal of Pain* 11 (9): 894–903.

Buckwalter JA. (2003). Sports, joint injury, and posttraumatic osteoarthritis. *Journal of Orthopaedic & Sports Physical Therapy* 33 (10): 578–588.

Coggon D, Reading I, Croft P, et al. (2001). Knee osteoarthritis and obesity. *International Journal of Obesity* 25 (5): 622–627.

Derman PB, Fabricant PD, David G. (2014). The role of overweight and obesity in relation to the more rapid growth of total knee arthroplasty volume compared with total hip arthroplasty volume. *Journal of Bone and Joint Surgery* 96 (11): 922–928.

Felson DT. (1995). Weight and osteoarthritis. *Journal of Rheumatology* 43 (22): 7–9.

Felson DT. (1996). Weight and osteoarthritis. *American Journal of Clinical Nutrition* 63: 430S–432S.

Felson DT, Lawrence RC, Dieppe PA, et al. (2000). Osteoarthritis: New insights. Part 1: The disease and its risk factors. *Annals of Internal Medicine* 133 (8): 635–646.

Felson DT, Lawrence RC, Hochberg MC, et al. (2000). Osteoarthritis: New insights. Part 2: Treatment approaches. *Annals of Internal Medicine* 133 (9): 726–737.

Harzy T, Ghani N, Akasbi N, et al. (2009). Short- and long-term therapeutic effects of thermal mineral waters in knee osteoarthritis: A systematic review of randomized controlled trials. *Clinical Rheumatology* 28 (5): 501–507.

Hennig T, Haehre L, Hornburg VT, et al. (2015). Effect of home-based hand exercises in women with hand osteoarthritis: A randomised controlled trial. *Annals of the Rheumatic Diseases* 74 (8): 1501–1508.

Manyanga T, Froese M, Zarychanski R, et al. (2014). Pain management with acupuncture in osteoarthritis: A systematic review and meta-analysis. *BMC Complementary and Alternative Medicine* 14: 312.

Messier SP, Loeser RF, Miller GD, et al. (2004). Exercise and dietary weight loss in overweight and obese older adults with knee osteoarthritis: The Arthritis, Diet, and Activity Promotion Trial. *Arthritis and Rheumatism* 50 (5):1501–1510.

Messier SP, Loeser RF, Mitchell MN, et al. (2000). Exercise and weight loss in obese older adults with knee osteoarthritis: A preliminary study. *Journal of the American Geriatrics Society* 48 (9): 1062–1072.

Panahi Y, Rahimnia AR, Sharafi M, et al. (2014). Curcuminoid treatment for knee osteoarthritis: A randomized double-blind placebo-controlled trial. *Phytotherapy Research* 28 (11): 1625–1631.

Perlman AI, Sabina A, Williams AL, et al. (2006). Massage therapy for osteoarthritis of the knee: A randomized controlled trial. *Archives of Internal Medicine* 166 (22): 2533–2538.

Vad V, Hong HM, Zazzali M, et al. (2002). Exercise recommendations in athletes with early osteoarthritis of the knee. *Sports Medicine* 32 (11): 729–739.

Waller B, Ogonowska-Slodownik A, Vitor M, et al. (2014). Effect of therapeutic aquatic exercise on symptoms and function associated with lower limb osteoarthritis: Systematic review with meta-analysis. *Physical Therapy* 94 (10): 1383–1395.

Healthy Teeth and Gums for a Healthy Body

American Society for Microbiology. (2017). *Toothbrush contamination in communal bathrooms.* American Society for Microbiology. Retrieved on November 4, 2017 from www.asm.org/ index.php/press-releases/93536-toothbrush-contamination-in-communal-bathrooms.

Kazmierczak M, Mather M, Anderson TM, et al. (1994). An alternative to dental floss in a personal dental hygiene program. *Journal of Clinical Dentistry* 5 (1): 5–7.

Lee YL, Hu HY, Huang N, et al. (2013). Dental prophylaxis and periodontal treatment are protective factors to ischemic stroke. *Stroke* 44 (4): 1026–1030.

Tornwall RF, Chow AK. (2012).The association between periodontal disease and the systemic inflammatory conditions of obesity, arthritis, Alzheimer's and renal diseases. *Canadian Journal of Dental Hygiene* 46 (2): 115–123.

Tips to Manage Constipation

Altug Z. (2016). Constipation and low back pain in an athlete: A case report. *Orthopaedic Physical Therapy Practice.* 28 (3): 188–192.

Bajwa A, Emmanuel A. (2009). The physiology of continence and evacuation. *Best Practice & Research Clinical Gastroenterology* 23 (4): 477–485.

Harrington KL, Haskvitz EM. (2006). Managing a patient's constipation with physical therapy. *Physical Therapy* 86 (11): 1511–1519.

Jackson RD, LaCroix AZ, Gass M, et al. (2006). Calcium plus vitamin D supplementation and the risk of fractures. *New England Journal of Medicine* 354 (7): 669–683.

Kollef MH, Neelon-Kollef RA. (1991). Pulmonary embolism associated with the act of defecation. *Heart and Lung* 20: 451–454.

McMillan M. (1921). *Massage and Therapeutic Exercise.* Philadelphia, PA: WB Saunders.

Prince RL, Devine A, Dhaliwal SS, et al. (2006). Effects of calcium supplementation on clinical fracture and bone structure: Results of a 5-year, double-blind, placebo-controlled trial in elderly women. *Archives of Internal Medicine* 166 (8): 869–875.

Sikirov BA. (1989). Primary constipation: An underlying mechanism. *Medical Hypotheses* 28 (2): 71–73.

Sikirov BA. (1990). Cardio-vascular events at defecation: Are they unavoidable? *Medical Hypothesis* 32 (3): 231–233.

Sikirov D. (2003). Comparison of straining during defecation in three positions. *Digestive Diseases and Sciences* 48 (7): 1201–1205.

Storrie JB. (1997). Biofeedback: A first-line treatment for idiopathic constipation. *British Journal of Nursing* 6 (3): 152–158.

Vlak MH, Rinkel GJ, Greebe P, et al. (2011). Trigger factors and their attributable risk for rupture of intracranial aneurysms: A case-crossover study. *Stroke* 42 (7): 1878–1882.

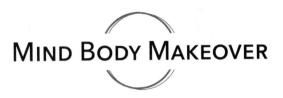

MIND BODY MAKEOVER

MESSAGE FROM THE AUTHOR

Thank you for allowing me to be a part of your journey in discovering your optimal mind body connections. Hopefully this book has armed you with the latest information about strategies you can use to explore ways to heal yourself and take charge of your life. What works for one person may not work for you. Take time to explore different strategies.

In summary, here are the following things you should consider for your personal Mind Body Makeover:

- Find a lifestyle which agrees with your mind and body.
  - » For example: Are you in the right job? Are you in the right relationship?
- Consume foods which agree with your body.
  - » For example: Do the foods you eat leave you feeling energized and refreshed or do they make you feel congested, bloated, painful, or lethargic?
- Be active, move, and exercise with sports and hobbies you find enjoyable.
  - » For example, are the movements and exercises you are doing improving your ability to function in daily life and make your mind and body feel better or do they leave you in pain, stiff, and totally drained?
- Sleep long enough to awaken feeling refreshed.
  - » For example, do you awaken naturally every morning or does it take two alarms and several cups of coffee before you are ready to tackle the day?
- Learn about your stress triggers and find ways to control them.
  - » For example, does the slightest word from someone or a change in traffic patterns get you to a point where you are worked up all day or are you able to roll along on a smooth path?
- Incorporate variety into your life.
  - » For example, try to vary the fruits, vegetables, fish, and meats you are eating. Also, try to vary the brands of products you are using

such as water and olive oil. Finally, vary your weekly exercises with movements such as qigong, tai chi, yoga, and walking.

- Challenge yourself with new skills.
    - » For example, try gardening or learn to cook. Both strategies may help reduce stress and also provide you with the healing powers of food.

This book plants the seeds, but it's up to you to water the seeds and nurture their growth. It is my sincere hope that you enjoy your journey in life with good mental and physical health and have the ability to pursue your dreams in life. Drop me a line to say hello and let me know how you are doing. You can also obtain free bonus information by staying in touch through social media. I wish you and your family good health and happiness.

Respectfully,

Z Altug, PT, DPT, MS, CSCS

Los Angeles
zaltug13@gmail.com
www.zmindbody.com

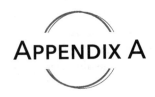

APPENDIX A

MEDICAL AND WELLNESS ASSOCIATIONS

Here is a list of associations you can use to obtain further quality information about medical conditions, wellness, fitness, and nutrition.

- Academic Consortium for Integrative Medicine & Health, imconsortium.org
- Academy of Integrative Health & Medicine, aihm.org
- Academy of Nutrition and Dietetics, eatright.org
- American Academy of Medical Acupuncture, medicalacupuncture.org
- American Art Therapy Association, arttherapy.org
- American Association for Marriage and Family Therapy, aamft.org
- American Association of Naturopathic Physicians, naturopathic.org
- American Chiropractic Association, acatoday.org
- American College of Lifestyle Medicine, lifestylemedicine.org
- American College of Preventive Medicine, acpm.org
- American College of Sports Medicine, acsm.org
- American Counseling Association, counseling.org
- American Institute of Homeopathy, homeopathyusa.org
- American Massage Therapy Association, amtamassage.org
- American Medical Association, ama-assn.org
- American Music Therapy Association, musictherapy.org
- American Naturopathic Medical Association, anma.org
- American Nurses Association, nursingworld.org
- American Occupational Therapy Association, aota.org
- American Orthopaedic Society for Sports Medicine, sportsmed.org
- American Osteopathic Association, osteopathic.org
- American Pharmacists Association, pharmacist.com
- American Physical Therapy Association, apta.org
- American Podiatric Medical Association, apma.org
- American Psychiatric Association, psychiatry.org
- American Psychological Association, apa.org
- American Speech-Language-Hearing Association, asha.org

- American Therapeutic Recreation Association, atra-online.com
- Australian Acupuncture & Chinese Medicine Association, acupuncture.org.au
- European Traditional Chinese Medicine Association, etcma.org
- Institute for Functional Medicine, ifm.org
- International Society for Japanese Kampo Medicine, isjkm.com
- National Center for Complementary and Integrative Health, nccih.nih.gov
- National Center for Homeopathy, homeopathycenter.org
- National Guild of Acupuncture & Oriental Medicine, ngaom.org
- National Osteoporosis Foundation, nof.org
- National Scoliosis Foundation, scoliosis.org
- National Strength and Conditioning Association, nsca.com
- North American Society of Homeopaths, homeopathy.org
- Scoliosis Research Society, srs.org
- The Accreditation Commission for Acupuncture and Oriental Medicine, acaom.org
- The Ayurvedic Institute, ayurveda.com
- The Institute of Lifestyle Medicine, instituteoflifestylemedicine.org
- The Society for Acupuncture Research, acupunctureresearch.org
- Traditional Chinese Medicine Association & Alumni, tcmaa.org
- Traditional Chinese Medicine World Foundation, tcmworld.org

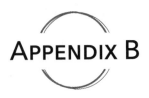

APPENDIX B

RESEARCH RESOURCE TO MANAGE HEALTH

The following are resources to help clinicians and other readers find clinically relevant research topics and articles. I bolded the top three sites I use most often.

- **American Physical Therapy Association, apta.org**
- Centre for Evidence-Based Medicine (University of Oxford), cebm.net
- ClinicalTrials, clinicaltrials.gov
- Cochrane Library, cochrane.org
- Cumulative Index of Nursing and Allied Health Literature, cinahl.com
- Google Scholar, scholar.google.com
- Library of Congress, loc.gov
- National Center for Biotechnology Information, ncbi.nlm.nih.gov
- National Guideline Clearinghouse, guideline.gov
- Orthopaedic Scores, orthopaedicscore.com
- OTseeker, otseeker.com
- Physiotherapy Evidence Database, pedro.org.au
- PICO (Patient, Intervention, Comparison, Outcome), pubmedhh.nlm.nih.gov
- **PTNow (APTA), ptnow.org**
- Public Library of Science, plos.org
- **PubMed, pubmed.gov**
- RAND Corporation, rand.org
- Rehabilitation Measures Database, rehabmeasures.org

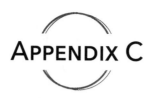

APPENDIX C

PRODUCTS FOR HOLISTIC LIVING

Disclaimer: Please note that I have not received any funding from the following products that are mentioned in this section. I simply list these as products I have used and provide them for your consideration for enhancing your holistic living options. Also, check out the health-related resources guide from Dr. Izabella Wentz, PharmD, FASCP at https://thyroidpharmacist.com/resources for additional books, supplements, personal care products, and cookware.

FOODS

CANNED FISH

- Sardines (BPA-free or bisphenol A liner)—Season Brand, seasonproducts .com
- Sardines (BPA-free liner)—WildPlanet, wildplanetfoods.com

CANNED FOODS (BPA-FREE LINER)

- Organic Butternut Squash, Organic Sweet Potato, Organic Pumpkin, farmersmarketfoods.com

PROBIOTIC FOODS

- Coconut Water Kefir—Tonix, mytonix.com
- Lifeway—lifewaykefir.com
- Non-dairy Super Probiotic Coconut Yogurt—New Earth Superfoods, newearthsuperfoods.com
- Raw Cultured Vegetables—Healing Movement, healingmovement.net
- Redwood Hill Farm—redwoodhill.com

PRODUCTS FOR MIXING FOODS AND SPICES

- Blender—Kitchen Aid, kitchenaid.com
- Mortar and pestle
  (I personally like the White Marble Mortars & Pestle, 2½" x 4½" which can fit into my hand for grinding herbs and spices, williams-sonoma.com, surlatable.com)

Supplements

- Magnesium—Natural CALM, naturalvitality.com
  (This is one of my secrets for staying calm and relaxed mentally and physically)
- Probiotics—Garden of Life, gardenoflife.com
- Probiotics—Renew Life, renewlife.com
- Pure Encapsulations, pureencapsulations.com

Water

- Evian, evian.com
- Fiji, fijiwater.com (bottle indicates BPA free)
- Icelandic Glacial, icelandicglacial.com (bottle indicates BPA free)

PERSONAL CARE PRODUCTS

Car Comfort

- Sacral and Lower Thoracic Support—YogaBack Company, yogaback.com

Cleaning Solutions

- Dishwashing Liquid—Meyer's Clean Day, mrsmeyers.com
- Hand Soap—Meyer's Clean Day, mrsmeyers.com
- Hand Soap—Williams Sonoma, williams-sonoma.com
- Hand Wipes—Seventh Generation Disinfecting Wipes, seventhgeneration

Cosmetic Safety

- Environmental Working Group, ewg.org
- Safe Cosmetics, Safecosmetics.org

Dental Care

- Floss—CocoFloss, cocofloss.com
- Gum Stimulator—GUM, gumbrand.com
- Toothbrush—Oral-B, oralb.com
- Toothpaste—Tom's Fluoride-Free Toothpaste, tomsofmaine.com

Deodorant

- Arm & Hammer Baking Soda, armandhammer.com
- Dr. Hauschka, dr.hauschka.com
- Weleda, weleda.com

Ergonomics

- Ergoweb, ergoweb.com
- Herman Miller, store.hermanmiller.com
- LEVO, levostore.com
- UCLA Ergonomics, ergonomics.ucla.edu
- VARIDESK, varidesk.com

Essential Oils–Aromatherapy

- Aura Cacia, auracacia.com
- Mountain Rose Herb, mountainroseherbs.com
- Vitality Works, vitalityworks.com
- Young Living, youngliving.com

Foot Care

- Massage—Acuball Mini, Acuball.com
- Massage—RAD Roller, radroller.com
- Pumi Bar, mrpumice.com
- Pumice Stone, earththerapeutics.com
- Shoes—New Balance, newbalance.com
- Shoes—On, on-running.com (for running)
- Shoes—Saucony, saucony.com (for running)
- Socks—Balega, balega.com
- Socks—CVS Non-binding Dress Socks, cvs.com
- Socks—Feetures, feeturesrunning.com
- Insoles—Spenco Rx—comfort insoles, spenco.com
- Insoles—Superfeet, superfeet.com/en-us
- Insoles—Surefoot, surefoot.com

Laundry

- Arm & Hammer Laundry Detergent, armandhammer.com
- Borox, 20muleteamlaudry.com

Shampoo

- California Baby, californiababy.com
- Lily of the Desert, lilyofthedesert.com

Shaving Gel

- Lily of the Desert, lilyofthedesert.com
- Weleda, weleda.com

Shower Filters

- Pelican Water System, pelicanwater.com
- Sprite, spritewater.com
- Water Chef Shower Filtration System, waterchef.com

Skin Moisturizer

- Gabriel Organics, gabrielcosmetics.com
- Lily of the Desert, lilyofthedesert.com

Sun Protection

- Goldcoast Sunwear, gcsunwear.com
- Solumbra, sunprecautions.com

INDEX

239, 243, 245, 252–53, 258–59, 265, 267–69, 272, 276, 282–84, 287, 293

soothing music 24, 35, 46, 252, 268

strength exercises ix, 171, 173, 179, 204, 289

stress ii, 1–2, 4, 7–12, 16–17, 21, 24–26, 28, 30, 33–38, 41, 48, 50, 61, 73, 78, 80, 86, 88–91, 98, 102–4, 113, 115, 118, 121, 123–24, 130–31, 133–35, 144, 179, 187, 200–204, 213–14, 221, 224–27, 230, 232, 236, 241, 243, 249, 250, 254, 262, 264–67, 270, 282–83, 286–87, 292, 296–97

stretching exercises 207–8

T

tai chi vii–viii, x, xii, 3, 5, 16, 25, 28, 34–35, 44, 49, 78–80, 83, 101–5, 109–14, 120, 153–58, 162, 170–73, 176–77, 187, 195, 216, 228, 235, 273, 279, 283, 286–90, 297, 307

test-taking strategies 271

trigger foods 9, 35, 56

V

vitamin D 34, 49, 59, 65, 170, 226, 253, 272, 280, 295

W

warm-up exercises viii, 171–74

weight loss vii, 54, 60–61, 67–69, 77, 82, 165, 213, 220, 266, 283–90, 293–94

Y

yoga vii, x, xii, 3–5, 16, 25, 28, 34–38, 40, 44, 46, 49, 78–80, 83–90, 94, 97–100, 103, 110, 155, 158, 160, 168, 170–72, 187, 195, 209, 215–16, 228, 249, 273, 278, 286–88, 290, 297, 307

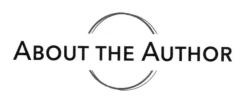

Z Altug, PT, DPT, MS, CSCS, is a licensed physical therapist and performance specialist with more than 28 years of experience in his field. He currently works at a private physical therapy clinic in Los Angeles. He graduated from the University of Pittsburgh with a Bachelor of Science degree in physical therapy and obtained his Master of Science degree in sport and exercise studies and a Bachelor of Science degree in physical education from West Virginia University. Z also completed a transitional Doctor of Physical Therapy (DPT) degree from the College of St. Scholastica in Duluth, Minnesota, and is a long-standing member of the American Physical Therapy Association, California Physical Therapy Association, and National Strength and Conditioning Association.

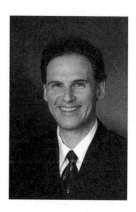

Z is certified by the National Strength and Conditioning Association (NSCA) as a certified strength and conditioning specialist (CSCS) and personal trainer (NSCA-CPT). Additionally, he was twice certified by USA Track & Field as a level 1 coach and twice by USA Weightlifting as a level 1 sport performance coach. Z also has completed workshops and classes in yoga, Tai Chi, Qigong, the Pilates method, the Feldenkrais Method, and the Alexander Technique to further expand his knowledge of body movement.

Beyond sharing his knowledge and experience with personal clients, Z extends his reach through writing. Z coauthored *2012 Healthy Lifestyle Wall and Engagement Calendars* (TF Publishing, 2011), *The Anti-Aging Fitness Prescription* (Hatherleigh Press, 2006), and the *Manual of Clinical Exercise Testing, Prescription and Rehabilitation* (Appleton & Lange, 1993).

Z enjoys participating in a variety of sports, learning about astronomy, and discussing new projects with his two rowdy cats at his home in Los Angeles.

For further information about Z Altug, please see the following social media sites:

- Website: zmindbody.com
- LinkedIn: linkedin.com/in/zaltug

- Facebook: facebook.com/zaltugfitness
- Twitter: twitter.com/zzenzone
- Instagram: instagram.com/zmindbody
- Goodreads (Blog): goodreads.com/author/show/15343007.Z_Altug

Scan to visit

www.zmindbody.com

ALSO LOOK FOR

YOGA FORMA:
A VISUAL RESOURCE GUIDE
FOR THE SPINE AND
LOWER BACK

BY ROMY PHILLIPS
WITH Z ALTUG

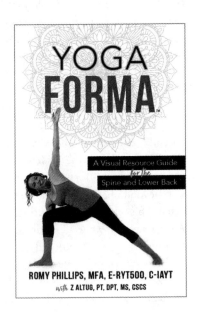